The Cognitive Basis of Polysemy

METALINGUISTICA

Edited by/herausgegeben von András Kertész

Volume/Band 19

PETER LANG
Frankfurt am Main · Berlin · Bern · Bruxelles · New York · Oxford · Wien

Marina Rakova/Gergely Pethő/Csilla Rákosi
(eds.)

The Cognitive Basis of Polysemy

New Sources of Evidence for Theories of Word Meaning

PETER LANG
Internationaler Verlag der Wissenschaften

Bibliographic Information published by the Deutsche Nationalbibliothek
The Deutsche Nationalbibliothek lists this publication in the Deutsche Nationalbibliografie; detailed bibliographic data is available in the internet at <http://www.d-nb.de>.

ISSN 0946-4174
ISBN 978-3-631-54094-7
US-ISBN 0-8204-7740-0

www.peterlang.de

METALINGUISTICA

Die Reihe ist ein Forum für Untersuchungen, die theoretische, methodologische und philosophische Probleme der linguistischen Forschung thematisieren.

The series is a forum for studies focusing on theoretical, methodological and philosophical problems of linguistic research.

Herausgeber/Editor

András Kertész
Universität Debrecen/University of Debrecen
Lehrstuhl für germanistische Linguistik/Department of German Linguistics
H-4010 Debrecen, Pf. 47.
Ungarn/Hungary

Herausgeberbeirat/Advisory Editorial Board

Contents

Introduction: Polysemy Matters

Polysemy is traditionally defined as the multiplicity of meaning, where the focus is on the meanings of individual words which are perceived as interrelated. However, this definition is fraught with unexpected pitfalls: what is it exactly for a word to have several distinct but related meanings? If by 'meaning' we understand a link between a word and a portion of the conceptual space, then presumably distinct meanings are expressed by the verb *open* in *John opened the door* and *John opened his eyes.* But if the meanings expressed are different, where should one locate the commonality that possibly exists between them? On the other hand, if we construe 'meaning' as that which is univocally expressed by a word type regardless of context (e.g. saying that *keep* always means 'keep'), we lose the intuitive perception of differences that sets apart the action of *keeping money in a wallet* and that of *keeping a crowd happy*. Either way, polysemy seems to evaporate.

This elusiveness of meaning also plays a curious role in setting up the recent intellectual climate for thinking about polysemy, and language in general. Although several monographs and volumes of collected papers emphasising the psychological intricacies and theoretical significance of the problem of polysemy have been published over the last decade, it continues to be associated in many minds with the narrowly specialised fields of computational linguistics or lexicography. Somewhat surprisingly, the renewed interest in the issues of human communication (a good deal of which depends on language production and understanding) left the problem of polysemy untouched. Thus, for example, in lexical pragmatics one finds countless discussions of how context modifies the "encoded" meaning of a word like *open*, while the more basic question of what exactly is semantically encoded hardly ever gets addressed. But even more surprising is perhaps the fact that such a landmark linguistics publication as Jackendoff's *Foundations of Language* allots polysemy some meagre four pages, pronouncing that most cases of a single word type having multiple interpretations are a matter of contingent similarity with nothing to explain it.

Here is not the place to go into the details of such views, and we believe that the reader is probably aware of the state of research on these issues. We feel that this denigration of polysemy is undeserved and hope that the articles presented in this volume support our view convincingly. There are many questions about the psychological representation of meanings, the types of relations existing between them or the interaction between meaning and grammar that remain unanswered, and *The Cognitive Basis of Polysemy* continues their exploration.

1. On What's in the Head

Linguists investigating polysemy generally accept as their working hypothesis the view that polysemous words must have more complex "entries" in the mental lexicon than single-meaning or merely ambiguous (homonymous) words. In developing this view they have mostly concentrated on logical polysemy or those words that multiply their meaning along some clearly definable parameters, e.g.: container – containee (*book, glass*) or producer – product (*chicken, mink*). From a purely theoretical standpoint, words like these can be grouped into a particular category because the meaning shifts they exhibit possess a certain degree of systematicity and can thus be explained through the application of transformational-generative rules. But do these rules and the representations on which they supposedly operate possess any psychological reality? The answer to this question should be sought from psycholinguists and cognitive psychologists.

Thus the first section of this volume is devoted to the cognitive reality of models of polysemy. It opens with an article by Ekaterini Klepousniotou which introduces the reader to the details of experimental work in psycholinguistics, providing important background on models of lexical access (whether the lexicon is autonomous or whether access to word meanings is modulated by context). Klepousniotou shows that psycholinguists were not always careful to distinguish between polysemy (one word with different related meanings) and homonymy (two different words with identical word forms) as well as between metonymically motivated (logical) and metaphorically motivated polysemy. She then reports on her own psycholinguistic and neurolinguistic research, where such distinctions were carefully drawn, and concludes that there is a continuum of representation ranging from homonyms to logical polysemes (whose senses are created on-line from complex core entries). Unlike them, metaphorically motivated polysemes (in her study, instances of nominal polysemy like *fox* or *star*), characterised by greater word and subject variability, must be distributed between these two end points, which suggests that a word may be at different stages of representation.

As becomes clear from this article, the nature of meaning representation is far from being well understood, and experimental results may be difficult to interpret because of a lack of consistency in the selection of materials. The next two articles deepen the reader's awareness of the complexities of psycholinguistic research and offer new challenges to both theoretical and experimental linguists.

Thus Gregory Murphy shows that theoretical and psychological perspectives may not fit each other very well. After analysing the space of logical possibilities for meaning representation and reviewing experimental evidence, Murphy concludes that what is parsimonious from the point of view of semantic theory is not necessarily such when one addresses the question of how meanings are represented in the minds of language users. Why should it be more cognitively economical to store in the mental lexicon complex entries and sense extension rules rather than represent all meanings of a word individually? Nothing in the mind/brain comes for free: the reduction in the number of entries stored inevitably increases the cognitive processing load. Besides, there seems to be little cognitive parsimony in having to infer those meanings of words that are all too familiar to us, but this processing model is implied by some theoretical accounts. Arguing for the consistency of meaning representation theories with what is known elsewhere in cognitive science and supporting his thesis with data from recent research on memory, Murphy convincingly defends the unfashionable view that all meanings of a polysemous word (logical polysemes being no exception) are represented in the lexicon explicitly.

On the other hand, inquiring into the nature of metaphorically polysemous words, Raymond Gibbs and Julia Lonergan come to reject the reality of the lexicon as that store of knowledge which contains whatever is necessary to generate the meanings of words across contexts. Contrasting data from lexicography, cognitive linguistics (conceptual metaphor theory) and psycholinguistics, they list difficulties facing the researcher set on delineating the meanings of a word: Do words have metaphoric meanings (e.g. *bulldozer*)? Can one univocally establish the core meaning of a word (e.g. *stand*)? Can one say what exactly its other meanings are? Cognitive linguistics tries to capture the intuition that words in context may have innumerable meanings without postulating a process that abstracts them and stores them in the lexicon. Noting the lack of agreement between both researchers and language speakers on what constitutes literal and metaphoric meanings, and referring to divergent evidence on the processing of abstract word meanings, Gibbs and Lonergan conclude that psychologically it makes little sense to separate meaning and use in context. Despite the appearance reinforced by dictionaries, human meaning representation is situational, imagistic, and driven by embodied information.

2. The Nature of Polysemy

The previous section may create the impression, especially in a reader new to the problem of polysemy, that the role of theoretical linguistics can be reduced to the elaboration of models which serve as points of departure for experimental researchers who either refute or improve them. However, as contributors to the previous section also note, the relationship between these two approaches is by no means linear because at later stages of linguistic theory formation, the theoretical approach may again become instrumental or even indispensable. For example, from the point of view of language processing, it may be impossible to establish the exact number of the possible meanings or senses of a word, but theoretical investigations of this issue may produce new testable evidence on what constitutes word meaning. Moreover, the elucidation of lexical and grammatical peculiarities associated with distinct meanings of a word may throw light on the psychological aspects of language processing, since the selection of lexical items and their composition into phrases is an observable manifestation of one's linguistic competence. Such painstakingly detailed analysis has always been the domain of theoretical linguists, who are concerned with formulating criteria along which distinctions must be drawn and creating the correct typology of different ways in which word meanings can relate to one another.

This section of the volume opens with an article by Anna Zalizniak, which gives a stimulating overview of the many kinds of ambiguity present in natural language. Numerous examples make the reader realise that the multiplicity of meaning is not confined to linguists' favoured cases but penetrates every corner of language, even if sometimes it goes unnoticed. Having thus set the mood for reflection on polysemy, Zalizniak isolates four types of non-zeugmatic meaning superposition and describes six approaches to the theoretical representation of polysemous words. While recognising the success of cognitive semantics, she argues that the meaning of many polysemes (especially abstract words) can be more effectively represented in terms of their conceptual schemata. A word's conceptual schema is a formula that has concrete content, but does not specify the values of the parameters that distinguish between its realisations in distinct meanings. She employs this approach to analyse some Russian words, and concludes that research into polysemy should combine dictionary-style descriptions of discrete meanings with the formulation of hypotheses about the way such systems of meanings may be represented in the minds of language speakers.

In his article Gergely Pethő emphasises the need to take into consideration a set of data that have been largely overlooked in polysemy research thus far: words showing non-systematic types of meaning variation. He takes issue with those approaches that draw a sharp distinction between metonymically motivated polysemy, which is seen as systematic and therefore describable by rules, and metaphorically motivated polysemy, which is perceived as unconstrained. Concentrating on nominal polysemy and distinguishing between several types within these two large groups, he shows that only in the case of regular polysemes related via focussing rules (e.g. *book*) can one detect nearly perfect systematicity. However, he argues, this systematicity is due to conceptual rather than linguistic factors. In all the other cases of metonymically motivated polysemy linguistic data do not confirm the existence of invariably reproducible productive patterns. This clear lack of "quantitative systematicity" also characterises metaphorically motivated polysemy: numerous examples (including those used in support of the conceptual metaphor theory) show that it is not thoroughly unsystematic or ungrounded. Pethő concludes that productivity cannot be reduced to quantitative systematicity and the neglect of metaphorically motivated polysemy is therefore unwarranted. He also notes that new types of evidence, in particular diachronic studies, might be required to gain a deeper understanding of how polysemy types exhibiting different degrees of systematicity come into being or disappear.

Finally, this section includes a translation of a seminal article by Georges Kleiber where he first developed the idea of meronomic integration. In this article Kleiber deals with examples of the kind *I'm parked in the square*. The explanation of such examples through a metonymically motivated change of the referent (which says that *I* no longer refers to the speaker, but to the speaker's car) is contradicted by anaphoric considerations. But, according to Kleiber, their explanation in terms of predicate change (as proposed by Nunberg) fares no better. The rules of predicate interpretation postulated by Nunberg cannot be rid of context dependence despite the constraint of noteworthiness. Besides, in many instances it is so evident to the hearer that by using words in their 'literal' sense the speaker intends to refer to something else that their assimilation under the notion of predicate change would be erroneous. Kleiber concludes that the problem must receive a pragmatic rather than semantic solution, and argues that it can be found in the principle of meronomisation or the pragmatic construal of part-whole relationships in discourse. He closes the article with providing an argument for the cognitive basis of referential phenomena and showing how the principle of meronomisation can be applied to a broader class of examples.

3. From Words to Constructions

Although many linguists believe that polysemy specifically affects the meaning of individual words, it has been noticed by several authors that the meanings of words often change when these words appear in different syntactic structures. Recent research in what may be called "constructional linguistics" has made it clear that more or less systematic semantic variations that are connected to consistent syntactic patterns are numerous and non-trivial, and also pose a significant challenge to the generative models of syntax. Some of the best known examples of this phenomenon are the resultative construction (e.g. *Phil hammered the metal flat*), where the presence of a secondary predicate in syntax forces a perfective interpretation for the verb, and the *way* construction, in which a 'change of location' reading is forced even with verbs that do not normally refer to movement (e.g. *Dora drank her way down the street*). In our view, the exploration of the relationship between syntactic constructions and polysemy is one of the most promising areas for future research. Besides, as linguists are becoming more and more willing to accept constructions as building blocks of linguistic structure (as lexical items, in a sense), we feel that it is reasonable to extend the term 'polysemy' from individual word meanings to grammatical constructions. Both sides of the coin, which are best examined in parallel, are dealt with in the articles included in this section.

Mária Ladányi's article is a very thorough analysis of the most pervasive patterns of systematic polysemy among Hungarian verbs. She emphasises that a verb's semantic variation is inseparable from those syntactic constructions that the verb appears in; in particular, she concentrates on different valency frames that verbs can occur with (i.e. what arguments a verb has and what nominal cases they carry). She also stresses that it is not just the more abstract syntactic description of these structures that correlates with the semantic alternation of a verb (i.e. its polysemy), but also the semantic content of the nouns that can appear as its arguments. In addition to her detailed empirical study, which could serve as a model for similar catalogues of verbal polysemy in other languages, Ladányi carefully explains and justifies the theoretical and methodological principles behind it, including a number of important remarks on the relationship between polysemy and morphology (more specifically, word formation), and the delimitation of different verb meanings.

In their turn, Ronnie Cann and Patricia Mabugu investigate semantic variation which is connected to a single structure, the applicative construction in the Bantu language ChiShona. The addition of a singularly productive applicative affix *-ir* to a large number of verbal stems increases their valency, and the applied object can be interpreted in several ways: as a beneficiary, maleficiary, goal, location, motive or source. Previous researchers concentrated on the syntax of the construction, believing the affix to be homonymous. In contrast to them, Cann and Mabugu argue that one can detect important similarities of meaning behind all the heterogeneity. They show that the correct interpretation of the applied object in context may be derived from a basic underspecified representation (which they identify as the goal relation) together with linguistic (a verb's lexical meaning) and non-linguistic (world knowledge) cues. Although they stress the descriptive nature of their enterprise, the way their approach allows for the integration of syntactic, semantic and pragmatic factors affecting the use of the applicative construction bears much promise of fruitful future developments.

The volume's final paper, written by Balázs Szilárd, addresses the issue of Hungarian verb formation by prefixation, concentrating specifically on semantic effects obtained through the addition of goal and of source particles to a verb as prefixes. The most important issue in the semantics of these verbal prefixes is how their perfectivising function should be accounted for (both goal and source particles, when added as a prefix, change a lexically imperfective base verb to a perfective one). Szilárd argues that those authors who believe that source particles, just like goal particles, express termination, and who thus derive the element of perfectivity from the notion of termination, are mistaken. He goes on to describe the spatial relations expressed by goal and source particles using a topological system of representation. He concludes that the element of perfectivity can be explained through the adoption of such a system of representation, without having to accept the implausible assumption that source particles express termination.

***

The recognition that polysemy matters and that a range of new types of evidence must be consulted for it to receive a psychologically viable explanation unites the contributors to this volume, who, from differing standpoints, urge one to take the problem of polysemy seriously. They also make it clear that there are many subtle matters involved in the understanding of the problem that require closer scrutiny and greater investigative effort. In conclusion we would like to thank the authors for their well-argued thought-provoking and most insightful articles. We also thank Ronnie Cann, Judit Gervain, Rachel Giora, Denis Gladkov, James R. Hurford, Éva Kardos, Ingrid Kaufmann, György Rákosi and Dan Wedgwood for their help at different stages of the editing process. We are deeply indebted to the editor of the series MetaLinguistica, András Kertész, for having suggested the idea of publishing this volume, and for his constant support of this project. Both the publication of the volume as a whole and of the individual papers in it were supported by the Research Group for Theoretical Linguistics of the Hungarian Academy of Sciences at the Universities of Debrecen, Pécs and Szeged.

Marina Rakova, Gergely Pethő, and Csilla Rákosi

Part I

On What's in the Head

Reconciling Linguistics and Psycholinguistics: On the Psychological Reality of Linguistic Polysemy*

Ekaterini Klepousniotou

Centre for Research on Language, Mind, and Brain, McGill University
1266 Pine Ave. West, Montreal, Qc H3G 1A8, Canada
E-mail: ekaterini.klepousniotou@mail.mcgill.ca

1. Introduction

For over thirty years, researchers from the fields of theoretical linguistics, computational linguistics, and psycholinguistics have conducted research on lexical ambiguity. Several terms have been used in an attempt to capture and describe the alternations of word meanings, and several assumptions have been made about how words with multiple meanings are stored and accessed from the mental lexicon.

Most work in psycholinguistics has concentrated on homonymy, while polysemous words have often been used interchangeably with homographs, homophones, or homonyms[1] to test models and theories of lexical access and lexical ambiguity processing (Schreuder & Flores d'Arcais 1989). However, it should be noted that "homographs", "homophones" and "homonyms" refer to three subtypes of ambiguous words that have distinct, unrelated meanings, while "polysemy" refers to ambiguous words with related senses. In other words, although psycholinguistic research has often dealt with lexical ambiguity, it has generally overlooked the semantics and the different types of it.

---

* Publication of the present paper was supported by the Research Group for Theoretical Linguistics of the Hungarian Academy of Sciences at the Universities of Debrecen, Pécs and Szeged. The studies discussed in this chapter were conducted while the author was a PhD student at McGill University. The neurolinguistic studies are part of the author's doctoral dissertation submitted to the School of Communication Sciences and Disorders at McGill University. Support was provided by McGill Majors Scholarships, Faculty of Medicine Internal Studentships and a CRLMB Postdoctoral Fellowship. A special thank you goes to Dr. Shari R. Baum for helpful comments on an earlier draft of this chapter.

1 Homography is the case where two words have the same written form, but different pronunciation and meaning, such as *wound*$_1$ which is the past tense of the verb *to wind*, and *wound*$_2$ which means 'a sore/cut'. Homophony is the case where two words are pronounced the same, but they have different written forms, as for example, *red* which refers to 'a colour', and *read* which is the past tense form of the verb *to read.* Finally, homonymy is the case where both the pronunciation and written form of two words are the same, but they have distinct and unrelated meanings, as for example, *bank*$_1$ which means 'a financial institution' and *bank*$_2$ which means 'the side of a river'.

On the other hand, theoretical, as well as computational, linguistics has focused mostly on the semantics of lexical ambiguity, making a distinction between two types. The first type is homonymy, in which a word form carries two (or more) distinct and unrelated meanings, such as pen_1 which means 'a writing device' and pen_2 which means 'an enclosure'. The other type of lexical ambiguity is polysemy, in which a single lexical item has several different but related senses, such as *rabbit*, which means 'the animal' and 'the meat of that animal' (Cruse 1986; Lyons 1977).

Thus, it seems that theories of psycholinguistics and theories of theoretical and computational linguistics have dealt with distinct but complementary aspects of lexical ambiguity. In particular, psycholinguistics has dealt with the issues of lexical ambiguity processing and storage in the mental lexicon. Theoretical and computational linguistics, on the other hand, have dealt with the issues of what lexical ambiguity really is, what types of lexical ambiguity exist in language and how word meanings are related.

Although dealing with the same subject, very often the theories in the two domains (i.e., psycholinguistics and theoretical and computational linguistics) have developed independently, without taking into consideration advances made in the other field. This situation may have led to misinterpretations about the nature of lexical ambiguity and as a consequence, misinterpretations about the storage and processing of lexical ambiguity. It is time to integrate the advances in understanding lexical ambiguity made in both domains in an attempt to further clarify this most interesting aspect of language and lexical processing.

Overall, in the present chapter, the most influential theories of individuation of word meaning from both theoretical and computational linguistics are briefly reviewed, and then the psycholinguistic, as well as neurolinguistic, theories on lexical ambiguity are briefly presented. Finally, the linguistic and psycholinguistic theories are brought together in an attempt to reconcile these two fields and find a common domain of analysis. A distinction is made between words with multiple, unrelated meanings (i.e., homonymy) and words with multiple, related senses (i.e., polysemy). Psycholinguistic (as well as neurolinguistic) evidence in favour of this theoretical distinction is discussed, and the implications for the nature of the mental representations and the access system that may exist for the two types of ambiguous words are presented.

2. Linguistic Theories on Lexical Ambiguity

2.1. Different Types of Lexical Ambiguity: Homonymy and Polysemy

The distinction between homonymy and polysemy was made early on in linguistic theory. Weinreich (1964) observed linguistic differences among ambiguous lexical items and distinguished between two types of lexical ambiguity. He called the first type of lexical ambiguity contrastive ambiguity. This is seen where a lexical item *accidentally* carries two distinct and unrelated meanings. For example, in the sentences *John lay down on the bank of the river* and *The Royal Bank is the largest bank in Montreal*, the word *bank* has the meanings 'river side' and 'financial institution'. Contrastive ambiguity is what traditionally has been called homonymy. Weinreich (1964) concluded that contrastive senses are contradictory in nature (i.e., only one sense is available at any given time), and the context and the discourse setting help in their disambiguation. In other words, the context selects the appropriate sense each time (Weinreich 1964).

The other type of ambiguity Weinreich (1964) referred to involves lexical senses which are manifestations of the same basic meaning of the word as it occurs in different contexts. For example, in the sentences *Mary painted the door* and *Mary walked through the door*, the word *door* in the first sentence refers to the 'physical object', whereas in the second sentence it refers to the 'aperture'. However, the basic meaning of the word is the same in both sentences. These sense distinctions are referred to as complementary polysemies (i.e., polysemy). Unlike senses in contrastive ambiguity, senses in complementary polysemy are not contradictory in nature. Rather, one sense seems more appropriate or "focused" for the interpretation of the word in the particular context.

Thus, traditionally, homonymy (or contrastive ambiguity) is the case where a lexical item "accidentally" carries two (or more) distinct and unrelated meanings, for example *bank*$_1$ which means 'a financial institution' and *bank*$_2$ which means 'the side of a river', whereas in polysemy a single lexical item has several different but related senses, for example *mouth*, meaning 'organ of body' and 'entrance of cave' (Cruse 1986; Lyons 1977).

The question, then, arises of how to distinguish between homonymy and polysemy. Lyons (1977) proposed two criteria for this distinction. The first criterion involves the etymological derivation of words, while the second criterion has to do with the "relatedness/unrelatedness of meaning". In fact, the distinction between homonymy and polysemy seems to correlate with the native speaker's feeling that certain meanings are connected and that others are not. Unrelatedness in meaning points to homonymy (Lyons 1977). However, it seems that "relatedness of meaning" is not an all or nothing relation, but rather a matter of degree. Apart from the clear-cut cases like *bank*, in a large number of instances there does not seem to be an agreement among native speakers as to whether the meanings of the words are related or not. For example, some native speakers claim that there is a connection between the meanings 'organ of hearing' and 'part of such cereal plants as wheat and barley' of the word *ear*, whereas others do not see any connection at all (Lyons 1977).

So it seems that the distinction between homonymy and polysemy is problematic, as there is no clear-cut dichotomy between the two. Rather, there seems to be a continuum from "pure" homonymy to "pure" polysemy. Two ways of circumventing, rather than solving, the problem of having a clear dichotomy between homonymy and polysemy are either to maximize homonymy or to maximize polysemy. Depending on the "solution" that is chosen, there are different implications about the representations of the ambiguous lexical items in the mental lexicon. In particular, if homonymy is maximized (e.g. Kempson 1977), every distinct meaning of an ambiguous word will be associated with a different word-form in the lexicon. As a result, there would be a highly expanded lexicon which would store separately every meaning a word has. On the other hand, maximization of polysemy (e.g. Lyons 1977) would result in a much reduced lexicon since the different meanings of a word would be associated with a single representation in the lexicon.

2.2. Different Types of Polysemy: Metonymic and Metaphorical

Even though the problem of distinguishing between homonymy and polysemy has not been resolved, at least for some cases, research on lexical ambiguity has continued. Most discussion in theoretical and computational linguistics has concentrated on polysemy. Polysemy is further divided into two types, which are basically motivated by two distinct figures of speech, namely metaphor and metonymy (Apresjan 1974). In metaphorical polysemy, a relation of analogy is assumed to hold between the senses of the word. The basic sense of metaphorical polysemy is literal, whereas the secondary sense was originally figurative when this use of the word emerged. For example, the ambiguous word *eye* has the literal basic sense 'organ of the body', and the secondary sense 'hole in a needle'. Metaphorically motivated polysemy seems to be quite unconstrained. There are cases where the primary and the derivative meanings keep a sufficiently large part of meaning in common, but there are also cases where the relatedness in meaning is not so obvious (Apresjan 1974).

The other type of polysemy is motivated by metonymy. In metonymic polysemy, the relation that is assumed to hold between the senses of the word is that of contiguity or connectedness. Apresjan (1974) claims that metonymically motivated polysemy respects the usual notion of lexical polysemy, which is the ability of a word to have several distinct but related meanings. Nunberg (1979), continuing the work of Apresjan (1974), also observed that the changes of meaning in metonymic polysemy are not accidental, as in the case of homonymy, but systematic or "regular", as Apresjan (1974) called them. In metonymic polysemy, both the basic and the secondary senses are quite literal (i.e., the secondary sense is not felt to be any more figurative than the basic sense). For example, the ambiguous word *rabbit* has the literal basic sense 'the animal', and the literal secondary sense 'the meat of that animal'. Drawing on the observation that homonymy and polysemy are relative concepts, it seems that some types of metaphorically motivated polysemy are closer to homonymy. On the other hand, metonymically motivated polysemy is a step further away from homonymy and possibly represents "pure" polysemy (Apresjan 1974).

Several types of metonymic changes of meaning (or shifts of meaning) have been identified, such as count/mass alternations (e.g. *lamb*: *I have two lambs* vs. *Would you like some more lamb?*), container/containee alternations (e.g. *bottle*: *He broke the bottle* vs. *He drank the whole bottle*), producer/product alternations (e.g. *Picasso*: *My grandfather had met Picasso* vs. *My grandfather owns a Picasso*), product/institution alternations (e.g. *newspaper*: *John read the newspaper* vs. *The newspaper fired the reporter*), and place/people alternations (e.g. *Washington*: *Washington is the capital of the United States* vs. *Washington voted for Bill Clinton*), to name just a few (Copestake & Briscoe 1995; Nunberg 1995; Pustejovsky 1995). These shifts of meaning, which seem to hold cross-linguistically to a great extent, are systematic in nature and, thus, in a way, predictable and productive.

2.3. The Mental Representation and Processing Implications of Homonymy and Polysemy

Having identified the different types of lexical ambiguity and the relations that hold among the multiple meanings/senses of ambiguous words, the question arises as to how these meanings/senses are stored. The linguistic distinctions between homonymous and polysemous words lead to the assumption that there must be different mental representations for the two types of ambiguous words in the lexicon. Although theoretical linguists have never explicitly tested their assumptions about the mental representations of ambiguous words, they have assumed that the linguistic distinctions must reflect differences in their representations. Thus, two broad classes of theoretical descriptions of the mental representation of lexically ambiguous items have emerged, as presented below.

In traditional computational models of the lexicon, words are assumed to be understood by selecting their intended sense from a short exhaustive list of potential senses which are stored in the mental lexicon (Clark & Gerrig 1983; Pustejovsky 1995). These models of lexical design and storage, which are often called Sense Enumeration Lexicons (SEL), make two main assumptions: a) all possible meanings for each word are listed in the mental lexicon, and b) the right meaning is selected among these enumerable meanings. So, under such accounts, homonymy and polysemy must be represented in the same way. Each meaning of a given ambiguous lexical item (irrespective of whether it is homonymous or polysemous) is stored separately in the mental lexicon. Within its specification, information about the syntactic category of the item as well as its broader meaning category can be found along with orthographic/ phonological information.

Nevertheless, Sense Enumeration Lexicons are faced with several limitations. In addition to the issue of parsimony (i.e., listing every nuance of meaning would result in a very uneconomical lexicon), the fact that the senses of polysemous words are logically related (unlike the distinct and unrelated meanings of homonymous words) is not captured in their representations. In addition, it seems that SELs cannot account for the creative use of language. Since they posit that all meanings/senses have to be listed in order to be selected, such lexicons cannot account for the fact that words are used creatively and assume new senses in novel contexts all the time.

More recently, in order to account for the inadequacies of SELs, lexicons have been proposed where the multiple senses of words are not listed, but rather generated from one central sense (Copestake & Briscoe 1995; Pustejovsky 1995). These lexicons, which have been developed within computational linguistics, draw on observations made earlier by Nunberg (1979), Apresjan (1974) and Cruse (1986) on the "extended reference" of words. Under this view, the lexicon is seen not as a static set of word senses where everything is stored, but rather as an active "generator" of new senses. According to such models, there is a core set of word senses, with greater internal structure than is assumed in traditional theories, which is used to generate a larger set of word senses when individual lexical items are combined together (Pustejovsky 1995).

In addition, some researchers (e.g. Copestake & Briscoe 1995; but cf. Pustejovsky 1995) assume a set of rules (known as sense extension rules) stored in the lexicon which can operate on a basic sense of a lexical item, which is also stored in the lexicon, in order to derive an extended sense of that item. Sense extension rules can apply to both metonymic and metaphorical transfers, as well as account for novel senses of words. For example, a common novel sense extension is when we use the physical object to refer to the human as in sentences like *The ham sandwich in table 3 asked for the bill*, where *the ham sandwich* refers to 'the person who ate it' (Nunberg 1995). These more recent lexicons, therefore, draw a distinction between homonymous and polysemous words. In the case of homonymy, the distinct meanings are stored separately, whereas in the case of polysemy, only the basic/core sense of the word is stored in the lexicon while the extended senses are created, when required, possibly by means of lexical rules.

Although theoretical linguists have not tested their implicit storage assumptions of ambiguous words, it is expected that there might be a distinction in processing depending on whether all the meanings/senses of ambiguous words are assumed to be stored in the lexicon, or whether there is only a basic/core meaning representation stored in the lexicon. Crucially, the two broad classes of theoretical accounts of lexical storage discussed above make different predictions about the processing of ambiguous words. In particular, accounts which hold that the meanings of ambiguous words are listed separately in the mental lexicon, irrespective of whether the ambiguous word is homonymous or polysemous, would predict that all ambiguous words are processed in a similar way, given the fact that they are assumed to have similar representations. On the other hand, accounts that support that the meanings of homonymous words are listed separately in the mental lexicon, whereas the senses of polysemous words are derived from a basic/core sense, which is stored in the lexicon, would predict that there is differential processing depending on the type of ambiguity.

3. Psycholinguistic Models of Lexical Ambiguity

3.1. Models of Lexical Ambiguity Processing

In the psycholinguistic literature, the processing of ambiguous words, focusing on homonymy, has received a great deal of attention. The main concern of these studies has been whether or not lexical access is an autonomous process (i.e., whether lexical access is interactive or modular[2]). So, if it is shown that only the contextually appropriate meaning is activated, then this would be evidence that lexical access is not autonomous and the interactive view would be supported. If, on the other hand, it is shown that all meanings of an ambiguous word are activated despite any contextual biases, then this would be evidence for the autonomy of lexical access and the notion of modularity in language processing.

---

2 It should be noted here that the interactive and the modular views are two different conceptions about the organisation of cognitive functions in general, while the different access models (e.g. the context-dependent/selective model and the exhaustive/multiple access model) discussed below specifically deal with the question of how lexical information is accessed.

According to the interactive view (McClelland 1987), higher level information (i.e., sentence level information which includes syntactic and semantic specifications) can be used to constrain the processing of other types of information (e.g. word recognition) as soon as it is useful (Swinney 1991). The context-dependent or selective access model, which in its strongest form holds that only the meaning of the ambiguous word that is compatible with the context is activated (Simpson 1984; 1994), has been influenced by the lexical storage and access assumptions of the interactive activation point of view (McClelland 1987). The main assumption of this model is that if sentence context is found to constrain processing only to the meaning that is appropriate in that context, then this is taken as evidence that lexical processing is influenced by semantic activity that occurs at a higher level. Several studies exploring the nature and the effects of context on the activation of meaning have found evidence in favour of the selective access model, thus supporting the interactive view of the lexicon (e.g. Glucksberg, Kreuz & Rho 1986; Simpson 1981; Tabossi 1988; Van Petten & Kutas 1987).

On the other hand, according to the modularity view (Fodor 1983), the lexicon is an independent module that is not affected by higher level semantic representations such as those arising from the processing of a sentence (Simpson 1994). Thus, if the multiple meanings of ambiguous words are all activated regardless of context, then this is taken as evidence in favour of the modular view (Simpson & Kang 1994). The processes that take place in the lexicon are autonomous, in that they are not affected by information from other sources. Only after the completion of the internal operations of an autonomous module are the results of these processes available for use by other processes (Swinney 1991). The exhaustive or multiple access model, which in its strongest form holds that all the meanings of an ambiguous word are activated upon its presentation (Simpson 1984; 1994), has been influenced by the modularity point of view (Fodor 1983). This model also has found support from a variety of studies which have shown that all the meanings of an ambiguous word are initially activated regardless of context (Conrad 1974; Kintsch & Mross 1985; Lucas 1987; Oden & Spira 1983; Onifer & Swinney 1981; Seidenberg, Tanenhaus, Leiman & Bienkowski 1982; Swinney 1979; Tanenhaus, Leiman & Seidenberg 1979).

Thus, there is still no consensus as to whether access is selective or exhaustive. However, a more careful examination of the psycholinguistic studies mentioned above may point toward a solution to this problem. In particular, looking at the results obtained in the studies of the proponents of the selective access model, we observe that there are instances where they find evidence that all the meanings of the ambiguous word have been accessed (e.g. Simpson 1981; Tabossi 1988; Tabossi, Colombo & Job 1987; Tabossi & Zardon 1993; Van Petten & Kutas 1987). Similarly, looking at the studies of the proponents of the exhaustive or multiple access model, we observe that there is evidence in favour of the selective access model (e.g. Oden & Spira 1983; Onifer & Swinney 1981; Seidenberg et al. 1982; Swinney 1979; Tanenhaus et al. 1979). Thus, looking more closely at the results of studies on lexical ambiguity processing collectively, we can sketch a model that seems to lie somewhere between the strong versions of both the selective access and the multiple access models. According to this "middle ground" model, there seems to be activation of all meanings initially. However, within 200 ms there seems to be selection of the appropriate meaning. The studies also seem to suggest that a highly constraining context may lead to selective access of the appropriate meaning only. Simpson (1984, 1994) suggests that the results of the studies on lexical ambiguity processing could be explained better by having a "hybrid" model where all meanings are activated, but the degree of activation would be sensitive to the relative frequency of the meanings, and the context in which the ambiguous word occurs.

This kind of "middle ground" hybrid model has, in fact, found empirical support from studies using a variety of methods, such as ambiguity detection (Neill, Hilliard & Cooper 1988) and eye movements (Duffy, Morris & Rayner 1988; Pacht & Rayner 1993; Rayner, Binder & Duffy 1999; Rayner & Duffy 1986; Rayner & Frazier 1989; Rayner, Pacht & Duffy 1994). In particular, based on these studies, Rayner and his colleagues argued that pure exhaustive access and pure selective access models cannot actually capture the processes involved in the activation of ambiguous words (Rayner & Morris 1991). Instead, they suggested that a revised version of the exhaustive access model, namely the "reordered access" model, can account for the observed results (Duffy et al. 1988). According to this "hybrid" model, the meanings of an ambiguous word are always exhaustively accessed, but prior context affects the access process by increasing the availability of the contextually appropriate meaning without affecting the alternative meaning (Rayner & Morris 1991). This can lead to a re-ordering of the times that the dominant and the subordinate meanings of an ambiguous word become available to post-access processes (i.e., all meanings are activated simultaneously but the degree of activation depends on frequency and type of context).

3.2. Processing Multiple Meanings versus Multiple Senses

As discussed above, examining, overall, the results of the studies on lexical ambiguity processing (in particular homonymy), a model has been described that seems to lie somewhere between the strong versions of both the selective access and the multiple access models. In short, according to this hybrid model, activation of all meanings seems to occur initially (although in different degrees), followed, within 200 ms, by selection of the appropriate meaning.

As far as the representation of ambiguous words is concerned, based on homonymy, some studies of context effects on lexical ambiguity processing have proposed that ambiguous words have a single phonological/orthographic representation linked to multiple semantic and syntactic representations (e.g. Seidenberg et al. 1982). Seidenberg et al. (1982), in particular, argued that meanings from a single syntactic category, such as noun-noun ambiguous words, share a representation, whereas meanings from different syntactic categories, such as noun-verb ambiguous words, have separate representations.

In addition, most research that has compared the processing of ambiguous and unambiguous words in isolation has proposed that ambiguous words have a separate entry for each of their meanings (e.g. Forster & Bednall 1976; Jastrzembski 1981; Millis & Button 1989; Rubenstein, Lewis & Rubenstein 1971). These studies report that ambiguous words are accessed faster than unambiguous words and that ambiguous words with many meanings are accessed faster than ambiguous words with fewer meanings (while all types of words are matched for frequency). It was argued that ambiguous words are recognised faster than unambiguous words because they have more than one entry in the mental lexicon, which makes it likely that some of their entries will be in the set of candidates for activation sooner than an entry for a non-ambiguous word (Rubenstein, Garfield & Millikan 1970). Further support for the hypothesis that homonymous words have multiple entries in the mental lexicon comes from priming studies that found that the facilitation effects observed for repeated words do not emerge for ambiguous words when different meanings are primed on separate trials (e.g. *runner-race* followed later by *ethnic-race*) (Masson & Freedman 1990). This result, which is contrary to the strong repetition priming effects that are usually seen in lexical decision tasks, suggests that separate entries of the ambiguous word are processed on the two trials (Kellas, Ferraro & Simpson 1988).

However, conclusions about the storage and processing of lexical ambiguity as a whole should not be drawn based on the evidence we have for homonymy only. As discussed in the first part of the chapter, a theoretical distinction exists between two types of lexical ambiguity, namely homonymy and polysemy. It should, therefore, be investigated whether this theoretical distinction reflects real differences in representation and processing patterns. In the next section, psycholinguistic and neurolinguistic studies of lexical ambiguity addressing processing and representation issues are discussed.

4. Bridging Linguistic and Psycholinguistic Theories: Experimental Evidence for the Theoretical Distinction between Homonymy and Polysemy

Although psycholinguistic studies focusing on the semantics of ambiguous words are rare, there are a few studies that either treat this issue directly or provide indirect evidence for the differences in processing between homonymy and polysemy (e.g. Azuma & Van Orden 1997; Frazier & Rayner 1990; Frisson & Pickering 1999; Rodd, Gaskell & Marslen-Wilson 2002; Williams 1992; but cf. Klein & Murphy 2001, 2002 who report no differences between homonymy and polysemy).

In the sections that follow, a series of studies will be discussed that were designed to investigate whether the different meanings/senses of the three types of ambiguous words, namely homonymous words, words exhibiting metaphorically motivated polysemy and words exhibiting metonymically motivated polysemy[3], are accessed differentially and whether they are stored differently in the mental lexicon. More specifically, this series of studies were designed to investigate the source of the processing advantage found in previous lexical decision studies for words with multiple meanings (i.e., the "ambiguity advantage" effect; e.g. Jastrzembski 1981; Rubenstein et al. 1970) and to address the following questions:

---

3 It should be noted here that the terms "metaphor" and "metaphorical word" will be used as an abbreviation for the more complex formulation "words exhibiting metaphorically motivated polysemy". Similarly, the terms "metonymy" and "metonymous word" will be used as an abbreviation for the formulation "words exhibiting metonymically motivated polysemy".

1. Is lexical ambiguity a homogeneous or a heterogeneous phenomenon depending on the type of ambiguity?
2. Are ambiguous words with multiple unrelated meanings (i.e., homonymous words) processed differently from ambiguous words with multiple related senses (i.e., metonymic and metaphorical polysemous words)?
3. What type of lexical ambiguity is producing the so-called "ambiguity advantage" effect?
4. If relatedness in meaning produces the processing advantage, is this advantage found for all types of polysemous words (i.e., both metaphorically and metonymically motivated polysemy)?

4.1. Psycholinguistic Studies on Homonymy and Polysemy

Before introducing the different experiments designed to investigate the processing patterns of homonymy and polysemy, it is worth mentioning briefly some of the psycholinguistic terminology used. Psycholinguistic (as well as neurolinguistic) experiments can use either a "simple" or a "priming" experimental design. In a simple experimental design, there is only one stimulus (i.e., the target) presented, either auditorily through headphones or visually on the computer screen. In a priming experimental design, two stimuli are presented, the one after the other (the first stimulus is known as the prime while the second stimulus is the target). The prime can be a single word or a sentence, and it can have different degrees of relatedness with the target (from closely related, for example *doctor – nurse*, to completely unrelated, for example, *doctor – truck*). Generally, it has been shown that a target word is recognized faster when it is preceded by a related than an unrelated prime word. Typically, after a stimulus (or a pair of stimuli) is presented, participants are expected to make a judgment about the target. All the experiments discussed in the present chapter, both simple and priming, used the lexical decision task in which participants are asked to judge whether the target presented to them was a real word or not in their language.

In order to begin exploring the processing differences of the three types of lexical ambiguity, a cross-modal sentence priming experiment[4] was designed that directly compared homonymous and polysemous words (Klepousniotou 2002). This study investigated whether the meanings of various types of ambiguous words are accessed differentially and whether they are stored differently in the mental lexicon. In accordance with the linguistic descriptions of lexical ambiguity, it was predicted that the participants' reaction times will be affected by the type of ambiguity. In particular, greater priming effects were expected for polysemous words relative to homonymous words based on the fact that the meanings/senses of polysemous words are interrelated which should lead to a processing advantage. Furthermore, differential processing was expected within polysemy, between metonymy and metaphor, with metonymous words

[4] The term "cross-modal" refers to an experimental design in which the prime and the target are presented in two different modalities (i.e., auditory and visual). Usually, the first stimulus (i.e., the prime) is presented auditorily (especially when it is a sentence), while the second stimulus (i.e., the target) is presented visually.

showing greater priming effects than metaphors, based on the assumption that metaphorical senses tend to be more lexicalized and unsystematic than metonymic senses.

Sentences that biased either the dominant or the subordinate meaning of ambiguous words were presented auditorily. Three types of ambiguous words were used, namely homonymous words (e.g. *pen* which means 'a writing device' and 'an enclosure'), polysemous words with metaphorical extensions (e.g. *lip*: 'part of the body' → 'edge of a vessel') and polysemous words with metonymic extensions (e.g. *rabbit*: 'kind of animal' → 'meat of that animal'). Homonymous words were chosen from standardized lists of ambiguous words (e.g. Gilhooly & Logie 1980; Nelson, McEvoy, Walling & Wheeler 1980; Twilley, Dixon, Taylor & Clark 1994), while metonymous and metaphorical words were chosen to exhibit specific relations between their two senses as documented in the theoretical linguistics literature (e.g. Nunberg 1979; Pustejovsky 1995), given that there are no standardized lists of polysemous words.

Immediately following the sentence primes (at 0 ms ISI[5]), a target was visually presented for lexical decision. Targets were the homonymous or polysemous words, two types of unrelated control words (matched for ambiguity type or frequency of occurrence) or non-words. Given that this was the first study investigating the processing of the different types of lexical ambiguity (i.e., homonymy and polysemy), two types of control words were used because of the peculiarities of ambiguous words. In particular, the frequency of ambiguous words in standardized lists is collapsed across meanings and does not reflect the real frequency of each meaning separately. Furthermore, previous studies have indicated that words with multiple (or many) meanings are accessed differentially from words with one (or few) meaning(s) (e.g. Forster & Bednall 1976; Jastrzembski 1981; Millis & Button 1989; Rubenstein et al. 1971). Thus, by using only frequency-matched control words, printed frequency would be controlled, but not meaning frequency and number of meanings. Therefore, it was important to include a second set of control words that matched the critical ambiguous words for ambiguity type and meaning frequency/familiarity (for the assessment of which a separate familiarity/frequency judgement task, administered to a different group of subjects, was designed).

Each of the three target word conditions was presented in two meaning bias conditions, one biasing the dominant interpretation and the other biasing the subordinate interpretation of the ambiguous word target. The sentence primes were constructed so that word associates[6] of the ambiguous words were excluded; in other words, the whole context biased/primed one of the meanings of the ambiguous target words. To exemplify, a set of sentences biasing the dominant and subordinate meanings/senses of the ambiguous words used in the experiment followed by the three types of target words are given below:

---

5 The term ISI, which is an acronym for the term "Inter-Stimulus Interval", indicates the period of time (i.e., the delay) between the end of the first stimulus and the onset/beginning of the second.

6 The term "word associate" refers to words that participants rate as being associated to a given word. There are published ratings of word associates (e.g. Nelson, McEvoy & Schreiber 1998) which are obtained by asking participants to list the first word (or sometimes the first 2 or 3 words) that comes to their mind when they encounter a specific word. For example, what is the first word that comes to mind when you hear the word *doctor*?

Prime		Target Ambiguous word/Ambiguity control/Frequency control
Homonymy		
Dominant bias	*He goes to every football game.*	fan/lap/lamp
Subordinate bias	*This room is very hot.*	fan/lap/lamp
Metaphorical Polysemy		
Dominant bias	*I bit myself by accident.*	lip/nose/rod
Subordinate bias	*The cup is chipped.*	lip/nose/rod
Metonymic Polysemy		
Dominant bias	*The hunter killed one.*	rabbit/plum/violin
Subordinate bias	*The chef made a stew.*	rabbit/plum/violin

Table 1

As expected, because of the 0 ms ISI delay between primes and targets, no dominance differences were observed. In other words, there was comparable biasing for both the dominant and subordinate meanings of the ambiguous word targets (unlike previous studies in which longer delays resulted in stronger and longer-lasting priming effects for dominant meanings; e.g. Simpson & Krueger 1991). Importantly, it was found that for the metaphor and metonymy conditions, ambiguous words showed significantly faster reaction times than the frequency control and ambiguity control words. In the homonymy condition, there was a significant difference only between ambiguous words and ambiguity control words, while no such difference was found between ambiguous words and frequency control words.

The priming effects were further explored by analysing the difference scores between the ambiguity control words and the critical ambiguous words, as well as between the frequency control words and the critical ambiguous words for all the conditions (i.e., homonymy, metaphor and metonymy). The priming effect was defined as the difference of the control word (ambiguity or frequency) minus the critical ambiguous word, divided by the control word. Between the ambiguity control and the ambiguous words, there were: for homonymy, a 6% difference (mean drop 35.5 ms); for metaphor, a 6.6% difference (mean drop 40.8 ms); and for metonymy, a 13.6% difference (mean drop 91.3 ms). Planned comparisons revealed that there were significantly greater priming effects for metonymy than homonymy. The difference in priming between metonymy and metaphor approached significance, while there was no significant difference between homonymy and metaphor.

Similarly, between the frequency control and the ambiguous words, there were: for homonymy, a 2.3% difference (mean drop 14.7 ms); for metaphor, a 10.5% difference (mean drop 65.1 ms); and for metonymy, a 19% difference (mean drop 128.2 ms). Planned comparisons revealed that there were significantly greater priming effects for metonymy than both homonymy and metaphor. Furthermore, there were significantly greater priming effects for metaphor than homonymy. Thus, although priming effects were observed for all types of ambiguous words relative to the control words, significantly more priming was observed for metonymically motivated polysemous words than both homonymous and metaphorically motivated polysemous words. In addition, comparisons among the three ambiguity types (i.e., homonymy, metaphor, and metonymy) only for word targets revealed significant differences between homonymy and metonymy, further supporting the assumptions of differential processing for these two types of lexical ambiguity. On the other hand, no such differences were found between homonymy and metaphor or metaphor and metonymy.

Overall, then, this study (Klepousniotou 2002) showed that polysemous words with metonymic extensions received significantly more priming and were processed significantly faster than homonymous words. Based on these results, it was concluded that there seems to be a dichotomy in the nature of mental representations, depending on the type of ambiguity that the words exhibit. Homonymous words appear to have several distinct representations in the mental lexicon – one for each meaning. Since two or more meanings of a homonymous word are competing for activation, the process of activation will possibly be compromised by the process of ambiguity resolution. Polysemous words, on the other hand, and in particular metonymies, appear to have a single mental representation. This representation would be specified for the basic/core sense of the polysemous word giving it a general semantic value. Having a single representation, metonymous words avoid any issues of ambiguity resolution that might compromise the activation process. Since only one meaning is stored, there is no competition among meanings for activation. As a result, the activation process is not compromised by extra processing that is caused by the necessity of selecting a single meaning of the ambiguous word when more than one has been activated (Simpson 1994). Thus, metonymous words were indeed expected to be processed faster than control words as well as homonymous words. Finally, with respect to metaphor, it seems to fall somewhere between homonymy and metonymy (which is assumed to represent "pure" polysemy), justifying the theoretical linguistic assumption of a lexical ambiguity continuum (e.g. Apresjan 1974).

In order to further investigate the effects of having multiple unrelated meanings (i.e., homonymous words) versus the effects of having multiple related senses (i.e., polysemous words) on word processing, another set of experiments (an auditory and a visual simple lexical decision) were designed (Klepousniotou & Baum, in press). For this set of experiments, target words represented four distinct types of lexical ambiguity, namely unbalanced homonymous words[7] (e.g. *coach*) (i.e., one meaning is more frequent (i.e., dominant) than the other meaning (i.e., subordinate)); balanced homonymous words (e.g. *panel*) (i.e., both meanings are equally frequent); metaphorical words (e.g. *mouth*); and metonymous words (e.g. *rabbit*), as well as one set of relatively unambiguous frequency-matched control words (e.g. *cigar*), given that no substantial differences were found between frequency-matched control and ambiguity-matched control words in the earlier study (Klepousniotou 2002). The same set of words was presented in both the auditory and visual experiments.

---

7 The terms "balanced" and "unbalanced" refer to the relative frequency/dominance of the two meanings of homonymous words. Frequency/dominance is determined by presenting participants the ambiguous word in question (for example the word *panel*) and asking them to give a definition of its meaning. If there is a clear preference for one interpretation, then the word is classified as an unbalanced homonym; otherwise, if either definition is given equally often, the word is classified as a balanced homonym.

As in the previous experiment (Klepousniotou 2002), unbalanced and balanced homonymous words were chosen from standardized lists of ambiguous words. Metonymous and metaphorical words were chosen to exhibit several relations between their two senses in an attempt to make these categories of words as heterogeneous as possible and, thus, match them as much as possible to the heterogeneity exhibited by homonymous words. In particular, metonymous words exhibited the following types of metonymic relations: the count/mass relation (e.g. *rabbit*); the container/containee relation (e.g. *bottle*); and the figure/ground reversals relation (e.g. *cage* referring to the 'aperture' sense and the 'physical object used to frame this aperture' sense of the word). Similarly, metaphorical words exhibited three types of metaphorical relations: the body part/object relation (e.g. *mouth*), the animal/human characteristic relation (e.g. *fox*), and the object/human characteristic relation (e.g. *star*). Finally, all experimental words (both ambiguous and control) were matched for frequency of occurrence (Francis & Kucera 1982), syllable and letter length, and grammatical category.

So, the experimental paradigm consisted of a single stimulus (either a real word or a non-word) which was presented, for 500 ms, to participants (either visually on the computer screen for the visual experiment or auditorily through headphones for the auditory experiment). Participants had to decide whether the presented stimulus was a real word or a non-word. For example, for the auditory experiment, the presentation of the stimuli had the following format:

	ISI	Auditory target	Response
Unbalanced Homonymy	100 ms	coach	yes
Balanced Homonymy	100 ms	panel	yes
Metaphorical Polysemy	100 ms	fox	yes
Metonymic Polysemy	100 ms	rabbit	yes
Frequency Control	100 ms	cigar	yes
Non-word	100 ms	viodin	no

Table 2

For the visual experiment, the stimuli presentation had the following format:

	Fixation point	ISI	Visual target	Response
Unbalanced Homonymy	##### (500 ms)	200 ms	port	yes
Balanced Homonymy	##### (500 ms)	200 ms	pupil	yes
Metaphorical Polysemy	##### (500 ms)	200 ms	pig	yes
Metonymic Polysemy	##### (500 ms)	200 ms	oak	yes
Frequency Control	##### (500 ms)	200 ms	noon	yes
Non-word	##### (500 ms)	200 ms	plazet	no

Table 3

Thus, similar to earlier studies (e.g. Jastrzembski 1981; Rubenstein et al. 1970), for this set of experiments, there was no biasing information priming the meanings/senses of the ambiguous words used. Participants recognized and activated the experimental ambiguous words without specifying which meaning/sense they accessed in particular.

It should be noted here that although it is possible that the ambiguous words had more than two meanings/senses (and in fact noun/verb alternations and metaphorically motivated interpretations may accompany most nouns), they served as instances/examples of their broader ambiguity group (i.e., unbalanced homonymy, balanced homonymy, metaphorically motivated polysemy and metonymically motivated polysemy). Thus, although it is possible that most words could exhibit additional nuances/senses, they predominantly and most clearly exhibited one type of lexical ambiguity and they were accordingly classified as such. In addition, the fact that most, if not all, nouns may exhibit metaphorically motivated interpretations and verb/noun alternations acted as a controlling mechanism in the sense that any differences in processing could not be attributed to these factors (since all the words exhibit them), but rather to differences in ambiguity type.

This set of experiments (Klepousniotou & Baum, in press) aimed to clarify in particular the so-called "ambiguity advantage" effect (i.e., ambiguous words are processed faster than unambiguous words) reported in previous simple lexical decision studies (e.g. Jastrzembski 1981; Rubenstein et al. 1970), as well as to further investigate the processing patterns of the different types of ambiguous words. Based on the hypothesis that the processing advantage observed for ambiguous words is produced by "sense-relatedness", it was predicted that, in general, ambiguous words with multiple related senses (i.e., polysemous words) would be processed faster than unambiguous control words matched for frequency. Nevertheless, as in Klepousniotou (2002), it was expected that differences might emerge within polysemy (between metonymy and metaphor), with metonymous words showing more robust processing advantage effects relative to metaphorical words. Finally, no such processing advantage was expected for ambiguous words with multiple unrelated meanings (i.e., homonymous words) relative to unambiguous control words.

For the auditory simple lexical decision experiment, it was found that reaction times were significantly faster for metaphorical and metonymous ambiguous words than unambiguous control words. On the other hand, no significant differences were found between balanced and unbalanced homonymous words and unambiguous control words. In addition, both types of polysemous words (i.e., metaphors and metonymies) were also processed significantly faster than both types of homonymous words (i.e., balanced and unbalanced homonymous words). Thus, consistent with the hypothesis that "sense-relatedness" produces the processing advantage that is observed in lexical decision studies with ambiguous words, only polysemous words (both metaphors and metonymies) showed faster reaction times than unambiguous control words, while homonymous words (both balanced and unbalanced) did not show any facilitation effects.

For the visual simple lexical decision experiment, it was found that reaction times were significantly faster only for metonymous ambiguous words relative to unambiguous control words. No significant differences were observed between ambiguous words and unambiguous control words in the metaphor, balanced-homonymy and unbalanced-homonymy conditions. Similar to the auditory experiment and consistent with the hypothesis that "sense-relatedness" produces the processing advantage that is observed in lexical decision studies with ambiguous words, again only polysemous words showed faster reaction times than unambiguous control words. However, in this experiment, differences emerged within polysemy as well; namely, the processing advantage which was observed for metonymous words was lost in metaphors (although the data pattern was in the expected direction). Thus, it seems that the extent to which the secondary/subordinate senses are lexicalized possibly plays a more crucial role in visual word recognition. The most important finding of this set of studies, however, was that in both the auditory and the visual task there was no indication of the so-called "ambiguity advantage" effect for homonymous words that had been previously reported; on the contrary, there was a slight disadvantage for homonymous words compared to unambiguous control words, which did not reach significance.

Overall, then, the results of the psycholinguistic studies discussed above provide evidence for differential processing among the different types of lexical ambiguity (i.e., homonymy and polysemy). In addition, differences also seem to emerge within polysemy (i.e., between metaphor and metonymy), providing further support for the notion of a lexical ambiguity continuum. These processing differences are taken as evidence for differences in the nature of the mental representation of ambiguous words, depending on whether their meanings/senses are considered to be related or distinct and unrelated.

4.2. Neurolinguistic Studies on Homonymy and Polysemy

Turning to neurolinguistics, a great deal of research has focused on the neural substrates underlying the processing of ambiguous words. Most studies with brain-damaged populations (both left-hemisphere damaged (i.e., LHD) aphasic patients and right-hemisphere damaged (i.e., RHD) patients) on lexical ambiguity, however, have only included homonymous or metaphorical words. On the other hand, the question of whether the theoretical distinctions and psychological differences found in normal populations among the three types of lexical ambiguity are differentially affected by brain damage has not yet received a great deal of attention. Following a brief review of the neurolinguistic research on lexical ambiguity, two studies discussed in some detail below (Klepousniotou & Baum 2005a; Klepousniotou & Baum 2005b) address exactly this question.

Early off-line studies (e.g. Brownell 1988; Brownell, Potter, Michelow & Gardner 1984; Brownell, Simpson, Bihrle, Potter & Gardner 1990; Schmitzer, Strauss & DeMarco 1997; Winner & Gardner 1977) identified the linguistic deficits of patients with right-hemisphere damage (RHD) with respect to lexical ambiguity and indicated that secondary or subordinate (i.e., non-literal, connotative) meanings are much less salient when the right hemisphere is dysfunctional. Based on these findings, as well as on later studies on lexical ambiguity processing by both normal and brain-damaged populations, two theories have been proposed to account for the lexical-semantic deficits observed in RHD individuals, namely the "suppression deficit" and the "coarse semantic coding" hypotheses. According to the "suppression deficit" hypothesis, RHD patients' deviant performance with ambiguous words may be due to problems with suppressing interpretations that are initially activated, but eventually become irrelevant or incompatible with the context due to the fact that the suppression mechanism operates less effectively in individuals with RHD than in normal individuals (Tompkins & Lehman 1998). The large majority of investigations of the processing of lexical ambiguity in context by individuals with RHD has supported the "suppression deficit" hypothesis (e.g. Tompkins, Baumgaertner, Lehman & Fossett 1997; Tompkins, Baumgaertner, Lehman & Fassbinder 2000). In general, these studies have shown that RHD patients seem to be impaired in the appreciation of context which leads them to the ineffective use of contextual cues to eventually suppress inappropriate (or irrelevant) meanings (Tompkins et al. 2000).

The other major hypothesis concerning RH processing abilities has been proposed by Beeman (1993), and is known as the "coarse semantic coding" hypothesis. Beeman (1993, 1998) based his hypothesis on evidence from both normal participants and brain-damaged individuals which shows that the intact RH may sustain multiple interpretations of ambiguous words (Burgess & Lund 1998; Burgess & Simpson 1988) and distant semantic relations (Beeman et al. 1994; Chiarello, Burgess, Richards & Pollock 1990), whereas the LH selects close associations and a single interpretation. It should be pointed out here that the terms "close" and "distant semantic relation" are not used in the linguistic semantics sense. In particular, in psycholinguistics (and neurolinguistics), words are considered to be closely related if there is a strong association between them (e.g. *bee – honey*) or if they are related via both semantic category and association (e.g. *doctor – nurse*). On the other hand, a distant semantic relation is considered to exist in words that are categorically related only (e.g. *deer – pony*). So, according to the "coarse semantic coding" hypothesis, during word processing, the LH is most selective, strongly activating small semantic fields[8], while the RH diffusely activates large semantic fields (Beeman 1998). A number of studies primarily using the divided visual field paradigm, as well as with brain-damaged populations, have been interpreted in light of the "coarse semantic coding" hypothesis (e.g. Abernethy & Coney 1993; Anaki, Faust & Kravetz 1998; Beeman et al. 1994; Burgess & Simpson 1988; Chiarello et al. 1990; Faust & Gernsbacher 1996; Koivisto 1997; Titone 1998). In general, it has been shown that even though irrelevant meanings are suppressed in the LH, no suppression or limited suppression effects are observed in the RH.

Although a large corpus of studies has provided evidence in favour of either the "suppression deficit" or the "coarse semantic coding" hypotheses, it is not always easy to compare their results and formulate a unified account of the lexical-semantic abilities of the RH and the deficits observed after RH damage, due to major methodological differences across the investigations. In particular, the studies that supported the "suppression deficit" hypothesis included brain-damaged populations, while the vast majority of studies that provided evidence in favour of the "coarse semantic coding" hypothesis mainly used the divided visual field methodology in young non-brain-damaged individuals. Thus, to date, experiments have been unable to unequivocally support one hypothesis over the other. The two studies discussed below were designed in

---

[8] The term "semantic field" refers to the abstract space where words, and the relations among them, are found. So, in the case of a small semantic field, only very closely related words are activated, whereas in a large semantic field, words with more loose relations will also be activated.

an effort to further address this issue, by carefully controlling the types of lexical ambiguity under investigation.

Interestingly, exploiting the theoretical linguistic distinction of lexical ambiguity into homonymy, metaphorical polysemy (i.e., metaphor) and metonymic polysemy (i.e., metonymy) enables us to contrast the predictions of the "suppression deficit" and the "coarse semantic coding" hypotheses. In homonymy, a word form carries two (or more) distinct and unrelated meanings. Therefore, no strong feature overlap exists between its meanings, and there is only a distant semantic relation at best. In metonymy, on the other hand, a single lexical item has several different but related senses, resulting in strong featural overlap between its senses, and a close semantic relation. In concert with the notion of a continuum from "pure" homonymy to "pure" polysemy (i.e., metonymy), metaphor seems to be somewhere between the two end-points. Although the multiple meanings may be somewhat related through analogy, they may not have strong feature overlap, and thus be closer to homonymy. Based on the nature of homonymy and metonymy, the "suppression deficit" and the "coarse semantic coding" hypotheses, in their strongest forms, make different predictions.

Despite the evidence from psycholinguistic studies (e.g. Klepousniotou 2002; Klepousniotou & Baum, in press; Rodd et al. 2002) that have shown differential processing for homonymous and polysemous words, the "suppression deficit" hypothesis does not make specific differential predictions depending on the type of lexical ambiguity. Therefore, the purest version of the "suppression deficit" hypothesis would predict that individuals with RHD should exhibit similar performance (i.e., an inability to suppress alternative meanings/senses) for all types of lexical ambiguity. On the other hand, the "coarse semantic coding" hypothesis in its purest version would predict differential performance depending on the type of ambiguity the lexical items exhibit. In homonymy, the alternative meanings are unrelated and there is very weak feature overlap (which could merely be phonological and/or orthographic), whereas in polysemy, and in metonymic polysemy in particular, the alternative senses are interrelated and there is strong feature overlap. Since the RH processes semantically distant relationships, while the LH processes close semantic relationships, individuals with RHD should be differentially impaired at accessing alternative meanings of homonymous and possibly metaphorical words, but not of metonymous words.

In order to investigate the effects of the strength of the semantic relations that hold between the different meanings or the different senses of ambiguous words, and test the "suppression deficit" and the "coarse semantic coding" hypotheses, two auditory priming lexical decision studies were conducted, a single-word priming study (Klepousniotou & Baum 2005a) and a sentence priming study (Klepousniotou & Baum 2005b), in which the site of lesion (LH, RH), the type of ambiguity (i.e., homonymy, metaphor, metonymy), the length of the interstimulus interval (100 ms or 1000 ms ISI), and for the sentence priming study, the type of context (dominant- or subordinate-meaning biasing) were controlled.

For both the single-word and the sentence priming experiments, the experimental stimuli consisted of prime-target pairs representing three distinct types of lexical ambiguity which were constructed in the following way. Three types of ambiguous words were selected as primes: 1) unbalanced homonymous words (e.g. *bank*); 2) metaphorical words (e.g. *mouth*); and 3) metonymous words (e.g. *rabbit*) following the same method as in the psycholinguistic experiments discussed above (Klepousniotou 2002; Klepousniotou & Baum, in press).

The primes were paired with four types of auditory targets: 1) a word associate related to the dominant meaning/sense of the ambiguous word prime; 2) a word associate related to the subordinate meaning/sense of the ambiguous word prime; 3) a control word unrelated to the ambiguous word prime; or 4) a legal non-word. As in the psycholinguistic experiment (Klepousniotou 2002) discussed above, word associates were chosen from a standardized list with word association norms (e.g. Nelson, McEvoy & Schreiber 1998). Both prime and target words were matched for frequency of occurrence, syllable length, concreteness, and grammatical category. Target non-words were constructed respecting the phonotactic rules of English and they were presented following primes (either single-word or sentence, depending on the experiment) that had the same characteristics as the experimental prime words (e.g. ambiguity type, syllable length, grammatical category, etc.), but were not part of the experimental prime word groups.

So, for the single-word priming experiment, the ambiguous word primes were presented in isolation followed by the different types of targets. Note here that each prime was presented three times, once followed by a word associated to the dominant meaning, once followed by a word associated with the subordinate meaning, and once followed by an unrelated control word. For example:

	Auditory prime	Auditory target Dominant/Subordinate/Unrelated
Unbalanced Homonymy	file	drawer/carpenter/trumpet
Metaphorical Polysemy	lip	chap/rim/swamp
Metonymic Polysemy	potato	spud/mash/claw

Table 4

For the sentence priming experiment, the same set of ambiguous word primes was incorporated in sentences that biased either the dominant or the subordinate meaning/ sense of the ambiguous lexical item which always appeared in the sentence-final position. Sentence primes were constructed with the restriction that word associates of the ambiguous words were not included in the sentences, so that the whole context, rather than an individual word, biased the meanings. Sentence primes were matched for length (5-8 words) and syntactic complexity (only active voice sentences). For example:

	Auditory prime	Auditory target Dominant/Subordinate/Unrelated
Unbalanced Homonymy		
Dominant bias	*He kept all the photographs in a file.*	drawer/carpenter/trumpet
Subordinate bias	*He smoothed the edges with a file.*	drawer/carpenter/trumpet
Metaphorical Polysemy		
Dominant bias	*While chewing, she bit her lip.*	chap/rim/swamp
Subordinate bias	*She accidentally chipped the vase's lip.*	chap/rim/swamp
Metonymic Polysemy		
Dominant bias	*At the supermarket, she chose a big potato.*	spud/mash/claw
Subordinate bias	*For lunch, she only had some potato.*	spud/mash/claw

Table 5

Thus, this sentence priming experiment differed significantly from the sentence priming psycholinguistic experiment (Klepousniotou 2002) that was discussed earlier. In particular, the psycholinguistic experiment (Klepousniotou 2002), which used the ambiguous lexical items as targets, was designed to measure the effect of having multiple meanings, as opposed to multiple senses, on the activation process. The present experiment (Klepousniotou & Baum 2005b), which, in contrast, used the ambiguous lexical items as primes, was designed to measure whether and how ambiguous word primes can facilitate access to dominant and subordinate meaning/sense related word associates. In other words, the neurolinguistic sentence priming experiment was not designed to assess the cost of having multiple meanings or senses, but rather whether participants can access the multiple meanings/senses of ambiguous words in the presence of sentential context.

For both the single-word and sentence priming experiments, each trial consisted of the auditory presentation of an ambiguous prime (either single-word or sentence, depending on the experiment) followed by a target (either word or non-word). Participants (LHD, RHD, as well as normal control, NC, individuals) were asked to make lexical decisions on the targets. All trials were presented at both ISIs (100 ms and 1000 ms delay between the end of the prime and the beginning of the target) for both the single-word and the sentence priming experiments.

Overall, in the single-word priming study (Klepousniotou & Baum 2005a), it was found that, at both the short (100 ms) and the long (1000 ms) ISI, there were no differences across the three subject groups (i.e., LHD, RHD, NC). In particular, both dominant- and subordinate-related targets were processed significantly faster than unrelated targets for the homonymy and metonymy conditions. In contrast, for the metaphor condition, only targets related to the dominant meaning were facilitated. The results of the single-word priming study thus provide evidence that, in the absence of context, the impaired brain (i.e., LHD non-fluent aphasic and RHD patients) can appreciate semantic relations and exhibit performance parallel to that of normal age-matched (i.e., older) control subjects at least at the single-word level.

On the other hand, the sentence priming study (Klepousniotou & Baum 2005b) revealed crucial differences among the three subject groups (i.e., LHD, RHD, NC). In particular, for all three types of ambiguous words, both the effects of context and ISI were obvious in the performance of normal control subjects, who showed multiple meaning activation at the short ISI, but eventually, at the long ISI, contextually appropriate meaning selection. Largely similar performance was exhibited by the LHD nonfluent aphasic patients as well. In contrast, RHD patients showed limited effects of context, and no effects of the time-course of processing. In particular, for the homonymy and metonymy conditions, for both ISIs, RHD patients showed activation for both dominant- and subordinate-related targets relative to unrelated targets. For the metaphor condition, however, RHD patients had difficulties activating the subordinate meanings, regardless of context bias and interstimulus delay, suggesting a selective problem with figurative meanings (see also Brownell 1988; Brownell et al. 1984; Brownell et al. 1990; Schmitzer, Strauss & DeMarco 1997; Winner & Gardner 1977).

Although these findings failed to support the strongest versions of either the "suppression deficit" or the "coarse semantic coding" hypotheses, they are viewed as being more consistent with the former, given that RHD patients were shown to have difficulties selectively activating the appropriate meaning of ambiguous words, and ultimately, inhibiting inappropriate meanings, while they also seem to have a specific impairment in the appreciation of figurative meanings. In addition, the findings of this set of studies address a number of issues regarding lexical ambiguity processing and resolution with respect to neurolinguistics, psycholinguistics, and theoretical linguistics. In particular, the findings for the normal control subjects contribute to our understanding of the importance of the semantic relations between the multiple meanings/senses of ambiguous words. The present findings indicate that when homonymous and metonymous ambiguous words appear as primes, either in isolation or in sentential contexts, there are no processing differences between their two meanings/senses (i.e., the strength of the semantic relation among their multiple meanings/senses does not seem to play a crucial role in the activation process). Although psycholinguistic studies have provided evidence that homonymous and polysemous words are processed differentially and, thus, may be stored differently in the mental lexicon (e.g. Frazier & Rayner 1990; Klepousniotou 2002; Klepousniotou & Baum, in press; Rodd, Gaskell & Marslen-Wilson 2002; but cf. Klein & Murphy 2001, 2002), the present neurolinguistic studies did not find differential processing for homonymous and metonymous words. As mentioned earlier, though, there are crucial differences in the methodology of the present neurolinguistic experiments as compared to such psycholinguistic studies. In particular, studies that have shown differential processing for homonymous and metonymous words have used the ambiguous lexical items as targets, thus measuring the effect (or cost) of having multiple meanings, as opposed to multiple senses, on the activation process. The present studies used the ambiguous lexical items as primes, measuring whether and how they can facilitate access to word associates that are related to their dominant or subordinate meanings/senses. Therefore, the present studies were not specifically designed to assess the cost of having multiple meanings or senses, but rather whether participants can access the multiple meanings/senses of ambiguous words when they appear both in and out of context. The findings of the present studies suggest that when the ambiguous words serve as primes, there are no differences in the activation patterns for their multiple meanings/senses.

The most interesting finding, though, was the fact that contrary to the normal control subjects and the LHD non-fluent aphasic patients, in the sentence priming study, RHD patients did show differential effects for metaphorically ambiguous words, for which only the dominant meaning was facilitated, regardless of biasing context and interstimulus interval. This finding, which is consistent with earlier off-line studies by Brownell and colleagues (e.g. Brownell et al. 1984; Brownell et al. 1990), supports the contention that RHD patients may have a particular problem activating the subordinate figurative meanings of metaphors. Crucially, then, the results of the present set of studies provide further support that metaphor is treated differently from homonymy and metonymy, which is largely consistent with the findings of the psycholinguistic studies discussed above. In particular, the findings of the single-word priming study suggest that subordinate meanings of metaphors require contextual support to be triggered, and even when they appear in context, they are harder to activate (especially after RH damage). Interestingly, these findings are also consistent with the theoretical linguistics literature that has argued that metaphorical polysemy (i.e., metaphor) is quite unconstrained and irregular in nature, in the sense that the referent of the subordinate meaning is not always predictable (e.g. Apresjan 1974; Copestake & Briscoe 1995; Nunberg 1979; Pustejovsky 1995). Thus, there is a loose relation between the meanings/senses of metaphorically polysemous words. Due to this loose connection between the dominant and subordinate meanings/senses, it seems that subordinate meanings of metaphors need a highly specific context situation to be triggered and they are more susceptible to RH damage.

5. General Discussion

As mentioned above, the majority of research on lexical ambiguity has focused on homonymy, making this the most understood type of lexical ambiguity. Polysemy continues to be under scrutiny about the actual processing and representation of multiple related senses (i.e., whether each sense is stored independently, like the meanings of homonymous words are, or whether senses are actively processed from a core meaning/sense representation). A number of studies described in this chapter were designed to investigate from different angles this most interesting aspect of lexical semantics and word processing.

In particular, the studies discussed here addressed the issue of whether all lexical ambiguity is represented and processed in a similar manner or whether representation and processing differs depending on the type of ambiguity. Overall, the results of the psycholinguistic studies discussed (Klepousniotou 2002; Klepousniotou & Baum, in press) supported the hypothesis that, depending on the type of ambiguity, differential processing is involved in the mental lexicon. In particular, in these studies, faster reaction times and greater priming effects were observed for metonymous words than for homonymous words, indicating different processes in the recognition of ambiguous words depending on the type of ambiguity. Furthermore, within polysemy, there were also differences in the processing of metonymy and metaphor in that there was a tendency for metonymous words to be processed faster and receive more priming than metaphors, as there was also a tendency for metaphors to be processed faster and receive more priming than homonyms.

Along similar lines, the findings of Klepousniotou and Baum (in press) supported our hypothesis of a "sense-relatedness advantage" effect, as opposed to an "ambiguity advantage" effect, in that a processing advantage (i.e., faster reaction times) was found when ambiguous words with multiple related senses (i.e., polysemous words) were presented (either aurally or visually), but not when ambiguous words with multiple unrelated meanings (i.e., homonymous words) were presented for lexical decision, further supporting the distinction between homonymy and polysemy.

Crucially, then, the findings of these studies (Klepousniotou 2002; Klepousniotou & Baum, in press) are consistent with our initial hypothesis that there is a lexical ambiguity continuum, comprised of homonymy at one endpoint and polysemy at the other endpoint. Furthermore, if homonymy and metonymy are assumed to be at the two ends of the lexical ambiguity continuum (i.e., from separately stored meanings to a basic/core meaning representation), then the findings of the studies suggest that metaphorically motivated polysemy seems to lie somewhere in the middle. In some cases, the multiple meanings of metaphorical words are felt to be quite related, whereas in other cases, they are further apart and the relatedness in meaning is not so obvious. These results are consistent with the observations made by Apresjan (1974) that metaphorically motivated polysemy, unlike metonymically motivated polysemy, seems to be quite unconstrained. Metaphorical words seem to be in a transition phase from generated senses to separately stored senses. In the former case, the representation of metaphorical words would resemble the representation of metonymous words. In the latter case, their representation would resemble the representation of homonymous words. In fact, metaphor seems to show the most variability among the three types of lexical ambiguity and is possibly comprised of words that are in different stages of representation. This heterogeneity in the nature of mental representations among the words that exhibit metaphorically motivated polysemy is probably reflected in the results of the studies discussed in this chapter. In particular, it may not be the case that there is a third type of mental representations (in addition to separately stored meanings and basic/core meaning representations) that is instantiated in the case of metaphor, but rather that some instances (or subdivisions) of metaphor show one pattern, while other words show another pattern, leading to the observed variability in the results.

The two neurolinguistic studies discussed in this chapter (Klepousniotou & Baum 2005a; Klepousniotou & Baum 2005b) provide further support to the existence of the subdivision within polysemy by showing that only metaphor is differentially affected by right hemisphere damage. In particular, the neurolinguistic studies revealed that context may be necessary to trigger access to the subordinate meanings of metaphors only (when they appear as primes). Furthermore, even in the presence of context, processing of the subordinate meaning of metaphor is disrupted in the face of RH brain damage, possibly indicating that the processes involved in the computation of figurative meaning differ substantially from the processes involved in the computation of literal interpretations (as in the case of homonymous and metonymous subordinate meanings/senses).

5.1. Implications for the Nature of Mental Representations of Ambiguous Lexical Items

Given the observed processing differences of the various types of lexical ambiguity (i.e., homonymy and polysemy), it seems that the results of the present studies point towards a dichotomy in the nature of the mental representations that cannot be accounted for by approaches which hold that each meaning of an ambiguous word must be stored separately in the mental lexicon. Rather, the results of the present set of studies seem to be mostly consistent with approaches that allow for differential representation of homonymy and polysemy in the mental lexicon.

In particular, polysemous words were found to show differential processing with respect to homonymous words, revealing a processing advantage relative to unambiguous words. These findings suggest that, for polysemous words, only a basic/core sense, which has general specifications about the meaning of the word, may be assumed to be stored in the lexicon. Polysemous words thus have a single, semantically rich representation in the mental lexicon. The extended senses, which are closely related to the basic sense, are generated (presumably on-line) from the basic/core sense that is stored in the lexicon (possibly by means of lexical rules). Having a single representation in the mental lexicon, polysemous words (and in particular metonymous words which are assumed to represent "pure" polysemy) avoid any issues of ambiguity resolution that might compromise the activation process. Since only one meaning is stored, there is no competition among meanings for activation, as might happen in the case of homonymous words. As a result, the activation process is not compromised by extra processing that is caused by the necessity of selecting a single meaning of the ambiguous words when more than one has been activated. Thus, no processing disadvantage should emerge for polysemous words relative to unambiguous words. Furthermore, given that they are assumed to have a single, semantically rich representation in the mental lexicon, this would further contribute to processing rates by facilitating meaning/sense activation relative to unambiguous words.

On the other hand, as Klepousniotou (2002) discussed, homonymous words have been assumed to have several distinct mental representations, one for each of their multiple and unrelated meanings (e.g. Jastrzembski 1981; Joordens & Besner 1994; Klepousniotou 2002; Rubenstein et al. 1970). Homonymous words seem to have a single phonological/orthographic representation in the mental lexicon which is associated with multiple semantic representations; and possibly with different further word forms which are derived when morphological and syntactic properties linked to each semantic representation take place (e.g. a noun-noun homonym may not have identical morphosyntactic properties for both its meanings, in that one interpretation/noun may belong to one nominal inflection class, the other to a different one). Thus, homonymous words have their different meanings represented separately in the lexicon, and are, therefore, understood by selecting their intended meaning from a (presumably exhaustive) list of potential meanings. Thus, homonymy requires the process of sense selection. In homonymy, the ambiguity is already established and the different meanings (i.e., the semantic representations) of the word pre-exist and are stored separately in the mental lexicon from where they are selected when required. Thus, when a homonymous word is encountered, its multiple unrelated meanings are competing for activation, slowing down the word recognition process. The results of the present set of studies suggest that the fact that homonymous words have separate representations eliminates the processing advantage that is observed for polysemous words, and, in particular, metonymous words.

5.2. Implications for Models of Lexical Processing

The results of the present set of studies also have important implications for models of lexical processing. In particular, in concert with the assumptions discussed above about the nature of the mental representations of homonymy and polysemy, the findings are mostly consistent with models of lexical processing that allow for differential representation of homonymy and polysemy (e.g. Pustejovsky 1995). As a result, the present findings pose an important challenge to traditional views of how lexical ambiguity affects the recognition of words presented in isolation. Previous studies on lexical ambiguity processing did not distinguish between the different types of ambiguous words (i.e., homonymy, metaphor, and metonymy), interpreting their findings as showing a processing advantage for ambiguous words relative to unambiguous words, known as the "ambiguity advantage" effect (e.g. Jastrzembski 1981; Rubenstein et al. 1970). Models of lexical access have tried to accommodate such findings, but most simulations have failed to produce the so-called "ambiguity advantage" effect (e.g. Balota, Ferraro & Connor 1991; Besner & Joordens 1995; Borowsky & Masson 1996; Hino & Lupker 1996; Joordens & Besner 1994; Kawamoto, Farrar & Kello 1994; Piercey & Joordens 2000; but cf. Rodd et al. 2004). Yet, this failure to simulate the so-called "ambiguity advantage" effect is not surprising given that previous behavioural data were based on sets of ambiguous words which tended to conflate homonymous and polysemous words. Given the findings discussed in this chapter that clearly distinguish between the two types of lexical ambiguity (homonymy and polysemy), a re-evaluation of models of word recognition is necessary, so that the advantage found for polysemous words (i.e., words with multiple related senses), but not for homonymous words (i.e., words with multiple unrelated meanings), can be accommodated.

In general, distributed models of word recognition assume that words are represented as patterns of activation across a set of nodes which are subdivided into groups that represent the various layers of information (e.g. orthography, phonology, semantics) of any given word (e.g. Gaskell & Marslen-Wilson 1997; Joordens & Besner 1994; Kawamoto et al. 1994; Pexman & Lupker 1999). In addition, a feedforward/feedback type of activation is typically assumed to hold between orthography/phonology and semantics. Such models can account for the lack of a processing advantage for homonymous words simply by assuming competition among the semantic representations of the different unrelated meanings within the component or layer of semantics. In particular, an intra-level mechanism (which is considered to be an inhibition only mechanism; e.g. McClelland 1987; McClelland & Rumelhart 1981; Rumelhart & McClelland 1981; Rumelhart & McClelland 1982) affects the recognition process by impeding the activation of neighbouring features that exist within the same level, when they are inconsistent with each other. In the case of homonymy, where the multiple meanings of an ambiguous word are unrelated (i.e., inconsistent with each other), the inhibition mechanism results in competition (i.e., inhibition) among the semantic units that represent the multiple meanings of the ambiguous word which, in turn, results in compromised processing times for homonymous words compared to unambiguous words.

On the other hand, the same intra-level inhibition mechanism (or rather the inactivity of it) could account for the processing advantage that has been found for polysemous words. In particular, since the senses of polysemous words (and in particular metonymous words) are related, it is assumed that they have richer semantic representations than unambiguous words (i.e., they have a considerable number of core semantic units/features in common). Thus, activation of one sense of a polysemous word would entail the activation of the common core features. Since the senses of polysemous words are related (i.e., they have semantic features that suggest each other's existence), there would be no competition among their semantic features but rather synergy (i.e., the intra-level inhibition mechanism would be inactive, in contrast to what would happen with homonymous words). As a result, activation of one sense would spread the activation to all the other related senses, resulting in a processing advantage in the recognition of polysemous words relative to unambiguous words.

6. Conclusion

To conclude, then, the studies discussed in this chapter investigated the processing patterns of different types of lexical ambiguity (i.e., homonymy, metaphor and metonymy). Collectively, the findings provide experimental support to the theoretically motivated differentiation of lexical ambiguity into homonymy and polysemy, which is further subdivided into metaphor and metonymy. They provide evidence that homonymy and polysemy rely on distinct underlying processing mechanisms that reflect differences in the nature of their mental representations. Homonymy seems to rely on the process of sense selection whereby the different meanings of the word are activated by being chosen from a pre-existing, exhaustive list of meanings. In other words, the findings of the studies discussed here suggest that the distinct and unrelated meanings of homonymous words are stored separately in the mental lexicon and they compete for activation. Polysemy, on the other hand, and metonymy in particular, seems to rely on the process of sense creation, whereby the extended senses are created on-line from a basic/core sense/meaning representation which is stored in the mental lexicon. In other words, the present findings suggest that polysemous (and in particular metonymous) words have a single, rich mental representation of their core meaning/sense and their related senses do not compete for activation, but rather exist in synergy facilitating, thus, the word recognition process.

References

Abernethy, M. & Coney, J. (1993): Associative priming in the hemispheres as a function of SOA. *Neuropsychologia* 31, 1397-1410.

Anaki, D., Faust, M. & Kravetz, S. (1998): Cerebral hemispheric asymmetries in processing lexical metaphors. *Neuropsychologia* 36, 691-700.

Apresjan, J. (1974): Regular polysemy. *Linguistics* 142, 5-32.

Azuma, T. & Van Orden, G.C. (1997): Why SAFE is better than FAST: The relatedness of a word's meanings affects lexical decision times. *Journal of Memory and Language* 36, 484-504.

Balota, D.A., Ferraro, R.F. & Connor, L.T. (1991): On the early influence of meaning in word recognition: A review of the literature. In: Schwanenflugel, P.J. (ed.) (1997): *The psychology of word meanings*. Hillsdale, NJ: Erlbaum, 187-222.

Beeman, M. (1993): Semantic processing in the right hemisphere may contribute to drawing inferences from discourse. *Brain and Language* 44, 80-120.

Beeman, M. (1998): Coarse semantic coding and discourse comprehension. In: Beeman, M. & Chiarello C. (ed.) (1998): *Right hemisphere language comprehension*. Mahwah, NJ: Lawrence Erlbaum Associates, 255-284.

Beeman, M., Friedman, R.B., Grafman, J., Perez, E., Diamond, S. & Lindsay, M.B. (1994): Summation priming and coarse semantic coding in the right hemisphere. *Journal of Cognitive Neuroscience* 6, 26-45.

Besner, D. & Joordens, S. (1995): Wrestling with ambiguity – Further reflections: Reply to Masson and Borowsky (1995) and Rueckl (1995). *Journal of Experimental Psychology: Learning, Memory, and Cognition* 21, 515-519.

Borowsky, R. & Masson, M.E.J. (1996): Semantic ambiguity effects in word identification. *Journal of Experimental Psychology: Learning, Memory and Cognition* 22, 63-85.

Brownell, H.H. (1988): Appreciation of metaphoric and connotative word meaning by brain-damaged patients. In: Chiarello, C. (ed.) (1988): *Right hemisphere contributions to lexical semantics*. Berlin: Springer-Verlag, 19-31.

Brownell, HH., Potter, H.H., Michelow, D. & Gardner, H. (1984): Sensitivity to lexical denotation and connotation in brain-damaged patients: A double dissociation? *Brain and Language* 22, 253-265.

Brownell, H.H., Simpson, T.L., Bihrle, A.M., Potter, H.H. & Gardner, H. (1990): Appreciation of metaphoric alternative word meanings by left and right brain-damaged patients. *Neuropsychologia* 28, 375-383.

Burgess, C. & Lund, K. (1998): Modeling cerebral asymmetries in high-dimensional space. In: Beeman, M. & Chiarello, C. (ed.) (1998): *Right hemisphere language comprehension*. Mahwah, NJ: Lawrence Erlbaum Associates, 215-244.

Burgess, C. & Simpson, G.B. (1988): Cerebral hemispheric mechanisms in the retrieval of ambiguous word meanings. *Brain and Language* 33, 86-103.

Chiarello, C., Burgess, C., Richards, L. & Pollock, A. (1990): Semantic and associative priming in the cerebral hemispheres: Some words do, some words don't ... sometimes, some places. *Brain and Language* 38, 75-104.

Clark, H.H. & Gerrig, R.J. (1983): Understanding old words with new meanings. *Journal of Verbal Learning and Verbal Behavior* 22, 591-608.

Conrad, C. (1974): Context effects in sentence comprehension: A study of the subjective lexicon. *Memory and Cognition* 2, 130-138.

Copestake, A. & Briscoe, T. (1995): Semi-productive polysemy and sense extension. *Journal of Semantics* 12, 15-67.

Cruse, D.A. (1986): *Lexical semantics*. CUP.

Duffy, S.A., Morris, R.K. & Rayner, K. (1988): Lexical ambiguity and fixation times in reading. *Journal of Memory and Language* 27, 429-446.

Faust, M.E. & Gernsbacher, M.A. (1996): Cerebral mechanisms for suppression of inappropriate information during sentence comprehension. *Brain and Language* 53, 234-259.

Fodor, J.A. (1983): *The modularity of mind*. MIT Press.

Forster, K.I. & Bednall, E.S. (1976): Terminating and exhaustive search in lexical access. *Memory and Cognition* 4, 53-61.

Francis, W.N. & Kucera, H. (1982): *Frequency analysis of English usage: Lexicon and grammar.* Boston: Houghton Mifflin.

Frazier, L. & Rayner, K. (1990): Taking on semantic commitments: Processing multiple meanings vs. multiple senses. *Journal of Memory and Language* 29, 181-200.

Frisson, S. & Pickering, M.J. (1999): The processing of metonymy: Evidence from eye movements. *Journal of Experimental Psychology: Learning, Memory and Cognition* 25, 1366-1383.

Gaskell, M.G. & Marslen-Wilson, W. D. (1997): Integrating form and meaning: A distributed model of speech perception. *Language and Cognitive Processes* 12, 613-656.

Gilhooly, K.J. & Logie, R.H. (1980): Meaning-dependent ratings of imagery, age of acquisition, familiarity, and concreteness for 387 ambiguous words. *Behavior Research Methods & Instrumentation* 12, 428-450.

Glucksberg, S., Kreuz, R.J. & Rho, S.H. (1986): Context can constrain lexical access: Implications for models of language comprehension. *Journal of Experimental Psychology: Learning, Memory, and Cognition* 12, 323-335.

Hino, Y. & Lupker, S.J. (1996): Effects of polysemy in lexical decision and naming: An alternative to lexical access accounts. *Journal of Experimental Psychology: Human Perception and Performance* 22, 1331-1356.

Jastrzembski, J.E. (1981): Multiple meanings, number of related meanings, frequency of occurrence, and the lexicon. *Cognitive Psychology* 13, 278-305.

Joordens, S. & Besner, D. (1994): When banking on meaning is not (yet) money in the bank – explorations in connectionist modelling. *Journal of Experimental Psychology: Learning, Memory and Cognition* 20, 1051-1062.

Kawamoto, A.H., Farrar, W.T. & Kello, C.T. (1994): When two meanings are better than one: Modelling the ambiguity advantage using a recurrent distributed network. *Journal of Experimental Psychology: Human Perception and Performance* 20, 1233-1247.

Kellas, G., Ferraro, F.R. & Simpson, G.B. (1988): Lexical ambiguity and the timecourse of attentional allocation in word recognition. *Journal of Experimental Psychology: Human Perception and Performance* 14, 601-609.

Kempson, R.M. (1977): *Semantic theory.* CUP.

Kintsch, W. & Mross, E.F. (1985): Context effects in word identification. *Journal of Memory and Language* 24, 336-349.

Klein, D.E. & Murphy, G.L. (2001): The representation of polysemous words. *Journal of Memory and Language* 45, 259-282.

Klein, D.E. & Murphy, G.L. (2002): Paper has been my ruin: conceptual relations of polysemous senses. *Journal of Memory and Language* 47, 548-570.

Klepousniotou, E. (2002): The processing of lexical ambiguity: Homonymy and polysemy in the mental lexicon. *Brain and Language* 81, 205-223.

Klepousniotou, E. & Baum, S.R. (2005a): Unilateral brain damage effects on processing homonymous and polysemous words. *Brain and Language* 93, 308-326.

Klepousniotou, E. & Baum, S.R. (2005b): Processing homonymy and polysemy: Effects of sentential context and time-course following unilateral brain damage. *Brain and Language* 95, 365-382.

Klepousniotou, E. & Baum, S.R. (in press): Disambiguating the ambiguity advantage effect in word recognition: An advantage for polysemous but not homonymous words. *Journal of Neurolinguistics.*

Koivisto, M. (1997): Time course of semantic activation in the cerebral hemispheres. *Neuropsychologia* 35, 497-504.

Lucas, M.M. (1987): Frequency effects on the processing of ambiguous words in sentence contexts. *Language and Speech* 30, 25-46.

Lyons, J. (1977): *Semantics.* Vol. 1-2. CUP.

Masson, M.E.J. & Freedman, L. (1990): Fluent identification of repeated words. *Journal of Experimental Psychology: Learning, Memory and Cognition* 16, 355-373.

McClelland, J.L. (1987): The case for interactionism in language processing. In: Coltheart, M. (ed.) (1987): *Attention and performance XII: The psychology of reading.* Lawrence Erlbaum Associates, 1-36.

McClelland, J.L. & Rumelhart, D.E. (1981): An interactive activation model of context effects in letter perception: Part 1. An account of basic findings. *Psychological Review* 88, 375-407.

Millis, M.L. & Button, S.B. (1989): The effect of polysemy on lexical decision time: Now you see it, now you don't. *Memory and Cognition* 17, 141-147.

Neill, W.T., Hilliard, D.V. & Cooper, E. (1988): The detection of lexical ambiguity: Evidence for context-sensitive parallel access. *Journal of Memory and Language* 27, 279-287.

Nelson, D.L., McEvoy, C.L. & Schreiber, T.A. (1998): *The University of Florida word association, rhyme and word fragment norms*. http://w3.usf.edu/FreeAssociation/.

Nelson, D.L., McEvoy, C.L., Walling, J.R. & Wheeler Jr., J.W. (1980): The University of South Florida homograph norms. *Behavior Research Methods and Instrumentation* 12, 16-37.

Nunberg, G. (1979): The non-uniqueness of semantic solutions: polysemy. *Linguistics and Philosophy* 3, 143-184.

Nunberg, G. (1995): Transfers of meaning. *Journal of Semantics* 12, 109-132.

Oden, G.L. & Spira, J.L. (1983): Influence of context on the activation and selection of ambiguous word senses. *Quarterly Journal of Experimental Psychology* 35A, 51-64.

Onifer, W. & Swinney, D. A. (1981): Accessing lexical ambiguity during sentence comprehension: Effects of frequency of meaning and contextual bias. *Memory and Cognition* 9, 225-236.

Pacht, J.M. & Rayner, K. (1993): The processing of homophonic homographs during reading: Evidence from eye movement studies. *Journal of Psycholinguistic Research* 22, 251-271.

Pexman, P.M. & Lupker, S.J. (1999): Ambiguity and visual word recognition: Can feedback explain both homophone and polysemy effects? *Canadian Journal of Experimental Psychology* 53, 323-334.

Piercey, C.D. & Joordens, S. (2000): Turning an advantage into a disadvantage: Ambiguity effects in lexical decision versus reading tasks. *Memory and Cognition* 28, 657-666.

Pustejovsky, J. (1995): *The generative lexicon*. MIT Press.

Rayner, K., Binder, K.S. & Duffy, S.A. (1999): Contextual strength and the subordinate bias effect: Comment on Martin, Vu, Kellas, and Metcalf. *The Quarterly Journal of Experimental Psychology* 52, 841-852.

Rayner, K. & Duffy, S.A. (1986): Lexical complexity and fixation times in reading: Effects of word frequency, verb complexity, and lexical ambiguity. *Memory and Cognition* 14, 191-201.

Rayner, K. & Frazier, L. (1989): Selection mechanisms in reading lexically ambiguous words. *Journal of Experimental Psychology: Learning, Memory and Cognition* 15, 779-790.

Rayner, K. & Morris, R.K. (1991): Comprehension processes in reading ambiguous sentences: Reflections from eye movements. In: Simpson, G.B. (ed.) (1991): *Understanding word and sentence*. Elsevier Science Publishers, 175-198.

Rayner, K., Pacht, J.M. & Duffy, S.A. (1994): Effects of prior encounter and global discourse bias on the processing of lexically ambiguous words: Evidence from eye fixations. *Journal of Memory and Language* 33, 527-544.

Rodd, J., Gaskell, G. & Marslen-Wilson, W. (2002): Making sense of semantic ambiguity: Semantic competition in lexical access. *Journal of Memory and Language* 46, 245-266.

Rodd, J.M., Gaskell, M.G. & Marslen-Wilson, W.D. (2004): Modelling the effects of semantic ambiguity in word recognition. *Cognitive Science* 28, 89-104.

Rubenstein, H., Garfield, L. & Millikan, J.A. (1970): Homographic entries in the internal lexicon. *Journal of Verbal Learning and Verbal Behavior* 9, 487-494.

Rubenstein, H., Lewis, S.S. & Rubenstein, M.A. (1971): Homographic entries in the internal lexicon: Effects of systematicity and relative frequency of meanings. *Journal of Verbal Learning and Verbal Behavior* 10, 57-62.

Rumelhart, D.A. & McClelland, J.L. (1981): Interactive processing through spreading activation. In: Lesgold, AM. & Perfetti, C.A. (ed.) (1981): *Interactive processes in reading*. Lawrence Erlbaum Associates, 37-60.

Rumelhart, D.A. & McClelland, J.L. (1982): An interactive activation model of context effects in letter perception: Part 2. The contextual enhancement effect and some tests and extensions of the model. *Psychological Review* 89, 60-94.

Schmitzer, A.B., Strauss, M. & DeMarco, S. (1997): Contextual influences on comprehension of multiple-meaning words by right hemisphere brain-damaged and non-brain-damaged adults. *Aphasiology* 11, 447-459.

Schreuder, R. & Flores d' Arcais, G.B. (1989): Psycholinguistic issues in the lexical representation of meaning. In: Marslen-Wilson, W. (ed.) (1989): *Lexical Representation and Process*. MIT Press, 409-436.

Seidenberg, M.S., Tanenhaus, M.K., Leiman, J.M. & Bienkowski, M. (1982): Automatic access of the meanings of ambiguous words in context: Some limitations of knowledge-based processing. *Cognitive Psychology* 14, 489-537.

Simpson, G.B. (1981): Meaning dominance and semantic context in the processing of lexical ambiguity. *Journal of Verbal Learning and Verbal Behavior* 20, 120-136.

Simpson, G.B. (1984): Lexical ambiguity and its role in models of word recognition. *Psychological Bulletin* 96, 316-340.

Simpson, G.B. (1994): Context and the processing of ambiguous words. In: Gernsbacher, M. A. (ed.) (1994): *Handbook of psycholinguistics*. San Diego: Academic Press, 359-374.

Simpson, G.B. & Kang, H. (1994): Inhibitory processes in the recognition of homograph meanings. In: Dagenbach, D. & Carr, T.H. (ed.) (1994): *Inhibitory processes in attention, memory and language*. San Diego, CA: Academic Press, 359-381.

Simpson, G.B. & Krueger, M.A. (1991): Selective access of homograph meanings in sentence context. *Journal of Memory and Language* 30, 627-643.

Swinney, D.A. (1979): Lexical access during sentence comprehension: (Re)consideration of context effects. *Journal of Verbal Learning and Verbal Behavior* 18, 645-659.

Swinney, D.A. (1991): The resolution of indeterminacy during language comprehension: Perspectives on modularity in lexical, structural and pragmatic process. In: Simpson, G.B. (ed.) (1991): *Understanding word and sentence*. Elsevier Science Publishers, 367-385.

Tabossi, P. (1988): Accessing lexical ambiguity in different types of sentential contexts. *Journal of Memory and Language* 27, 324-340.

Tabossi, P., Colombo, L. & Job, R. (1987): Accessing lexical ambiguity: Effects of context and dominance. *Psychological Research* 49, 161-167.

Tabossi, P. & Zardon, F. (1993): Processing ambiguous words in context. *Journal of Memory and Language* 32, 359-372.

Tanenhaus, M.K., Leiman, J.M. & Seidenberg, M.S. (1979): Evidence for multiple stages in the processing of ambiguous words in syntactic contexts. *Journal of Verbal Learning and Verbal Behavior* 18, 427-440.

Titone, D. (1998): Hemispheric differences in context sensitivity during lexical ambiguity resolution. *Brain and Language* 65, 361-394.

Tompkins, C.A., Baumgaertner, A., Lehman, M.T. & Fassbinder, W. (2000): Mechanisms of discourse comprehension impairment after right hemisphere brain damage: Suppression in lexical ambiguity resolution. *Journal of Speech, Language, and Hearing Research* 43, 62-78.

Tompkins, C.A., Baumgaertner, A., Lehman, M.T. & Fossett, T.R.D. (1997): Suppression and discourse comprehension in right brain-damaged adults: A preliminary report. *Aphasiology* 11, 505-519.

Tompkins, C.A. & Lehman, M.T. (1998): Interpreting intended meanings after right hemisphere brain damage: An analysis of evidence, potential accounts, and clinical implications. *Topics in Stroke Rehabilitation* 5, 29-47.

Twilley, L.C., Dixon, P., Taylor, D. & Clark, K. (1994): University of Alberta norms of relative meaning frequency for 566 homographs. *Memory and Cognition* 22, 111-126.

Van Petten, C. & Kutas, M. (1987): Ambiguous words in context: An event-related potential analysis of the time course of meaning activation. *Journal of Memory and Language* 26, 188-208.

Weinreich, U. (1964): Webster's third: A critique of its semantics. *International Journal of American Linguistics* 30, 405-409.

Williams, J.N. (1992): Processing polysemous words in context: Evidence for interrelated meanings. *Journal of Psycholinguistic Research* 21, 193-218.

Winner, E. & Gardner, H. (1977): The comprehension of metaphor in brain-damaged patients. *Brain* 100, 719-727.

Parsimony and the Psychological Representation of Polysemous Words*

Gregory L. Murphy

Department of Psychology, New York University
6 Washington Place, New York, NY 10003
E-mail: gregory.murphy@nyu.edu

1. Introduction

Although the study of polysemy has been a long-standing one within linguistics, it has never had much popularity in psycholinguistics. Indeed, an examination of psycholinguistics textbooks and review articles would show little if any discussion of polysemy. Instead, psychologists have focused much attention on lexical "ambiguity", which generally means homonymy (although many experiments have mixed polysemous words and homonyms together without distinction). Because polysemy is a much more widespread phenomenon, and indeed, a more difficult problem, it deserves greater attention than it has hitherto received from psychologists. Fortunately, there has been a recent increase in experimental studies of polysemy, and there is some hope that the phenomenon will make its way into the psycholinguistic mainstream.

A major goal of this chapter is to contrast the psychological study of polysemy with the linguistic approach. The interface of these fields is ever ripe for misunderstandings and lack of communication. I cannot pretend to describe the framework within which linguists study polysemy, and indeed there seems to be more than a single one. However, I think it is important to explain the underlying assumptions behind a psychological approach to polysemy, because some of the questions and conclusions arising from this field seem to be at variance with linguistic conclusions. As will be seen, I attribute some of these differences to the difference between the questions "what meanings should a theory of grammar represent in the lexicon?" and "what meanings do speakers represent in their mental lexicons?"

However, a second goal of this chapter is to perform the complementary function of bringing to the attention of psychologists the arguments and conclusions of linguists. Many psycholinguistic studies of polysemy do not describe their underlying as-

* The writing of this chapter was supported by NIMH grant MH41704. Its publication was supported by the Research Group for Theoretical Linguistics of the Hungarian Academy of Sciences at the Universities of Debrecen, Pécs and Szeged. I thank the reviewers and editors for helpful comments on a draft of the chapter.

sumptions of how polysemous words are represented. But insofar as one can infer them, many studies seem to assume that all senses are explicitly listed in the lexicon. As we shall see, this assumption is not in fact very popular within linguistics. But as we shall also see, there may be more validity to that assumption than is often thought within linguistic theorizing.

Polysemy is a rich topic with many interesting aspects, and this chapter will focus on the specific question of how polysemous words are represented in the mental lexicon. A complete theory of polysemy would also explain how polysemy arises in a language, cross-linguistic commonalities and differences in polysemy, children's acquisition of polysemous words, and so on. Of course, all these issues are interconnected, and my hope is that making progress on the representation of polysemy in the lexicon will illuminate these other issues as well.

In the next section, I begin by outlining the goals of a psycholinguistic theory of polysemy. I also provide my own assumptions regarding the nature of word meaning, which form the basis for my later discussion. Then, I consider basic proposals for how polysemous words might be mentally represented. In this section of the chapter, some readers may find my conclusions to be overly obvious and others to be obviously wrong. However, I do not apologize for either. I think that it can be helpful to bring new evidence to support widely agreed conclusions, because it serves to confirm the methods and reasoning of earlier investigations, as well as their conclusions. I also think that the conclusions that seem obviously wrong (to someone) are important in raising questions about the underlying assumptions that led to the disagreement. In discussions with linguists, I have sometimes found that they have very strong feelings about the nature of the lexicon, polysemic senses, the representation of meaning, and so on, which they believe are beyond question – but which in fact are not universally held, certainly not universally held by psychologists. Understanding these conflicts is an important step in developing a unified theory of polysemy.

Finally, a theme throughout the chapter is to question the role of parsimony as a principle in analyzing polysemy. I will point out that although parsimony in scientific theories is a universal goal (so far as I know), parsimony in the lexicon does not follow from this goal. And although parsimony in linguistic description is a nearly universal desideratum of linguists, there is much evidence showing that human memory is not as parsimonious as psychologists once thought. This fact has important implications for theorizing about the lexicon.

2. The Mental Representation of Meaning

Within most contemporary psycholinguistic theory, word meaning is thought to be represented as a relationship between word forms and conceptual representations. Something like a *lemma* (a node that connects the phonological, orthographic, syntactic and semantic representations) is linked to a structure within conceptual knowledge in order for people to know when to use a particular word and what to think when they hear the word (e.g., Levelt 1989). Other approaches to word meaning, such as referential semantics or purely linguistic semantic markers, simply cannot do the job that word meanings are supposed to do in controlling people's behavior. That is, when one sees a dog, one must know to say *dog*, and when one hears *Watch out for the dog*, one must know what to watch out for. Because concepts form our knowledge representations of the world, words must be connected to conceptual representation in order for us to know what to look out for and to know what word to say when we encounter something. Approaches to word meaning that are not conceptual may provide useful ways of analyzing how meaning works (e.g., referential semantics might provide a way of understanding how truthful information is communicated), but they generally do not refer to plausible psychological representations and cannot be taken as theories of mental representation. See Murphy (1991) and Murphy (2002: ch. 11) for much more detailed discussion of this point, as well as considerable empirical evidence showing that word meanings are built out of concepts. I mention this assumption because everything else in the chapter relies on it, if only implicitly. Unfortunately, addressing the general issue of meaning in more depth is impossible here, as it is one of the most complex questions in cognitive science, and it cannot be done justice as part of a chapter.

Saying that word meaning is represented as a relation between a word form and conceptual structure does not get us very far, however. The exact relationship must be worked out, and the way that relationship is used in language understanding and production must be discovered. This is the goal of a psychology of word meaning, and it has not been achieved yet, by any means. Complicating matters, we cannot assume that each word is linked directly to a single, simple concept, nor can we assume that our prelinguistic concepts map perfectly onto the word meanings of our language (Murphy 2002: ch. 11). Concepts must sometimes develop and change in response to learning the weird meanings that our particular language has. And cross-linguistic differences in lexical structure show that word meanings do not always pick out a single, most natural conceptual structure, but that the particular structures encoded in one's language must be learned and encoded (Malt, Sloman, Gennari, Shi & Wang 1999; Slobin 1996). Thus, the relationship between words and concepts is to some degree a two-way street.

Finally, I should point out that I assume that conceptual structure is very rich and highly interconnected. This allows us to have the best of both worlds in the dictionary/encyclopedia question of what is in the lexicon. It is possible that a lexical item picks out a fairly small, circumscribed section of conceptual structure (i.e., the core aspects of the word's meaning), but because this piece of conceptual structure is embedded in related knowledge and memories, one's encyclopedic knowledge can be used in interpreting words. This situation may accommodate the warring intuitions that our knowledge of the world is heavily involved in interpreting meaning and that the meaning of a word does not include everything we know about the referents of that word.

This perspective gives a simple answer to how the meaning of unambiguous words and homonyms are mentally represented. If there is such a thing as a word with a simple meaning, then its meaning is represented by a link between the word form and a piece of conceptual substructure. This substructure might be fairly complex and gerrymandered, if the meaning is very particular. If there is such a thing as a homonym with only two simple meanings, then it is fairly clear how this must be represented as well. Most likely, there are two separate lexical entries (words), each of which is linked to independent conceptual substructures, with no obvious relation between them. (Alternatively, homonyms could be considered the same lexical item with two different meanings. That possibility is not the concern of this chapter, but it is worth noting that there is neurolinguistic evidence against it; Pylkkänen, Llinás & Murphy 2006.)

2.1. Mental Representations of Polysemy, in Particular

If there is little argument over the representation of homonyms and unambiguous words, the same cannot be said about polysemous words. As most readers know, polysemous words have multiple meanings that are related in some way. Often, the different senses are related via a rule or productive pattern that can be found in other words, such as the animal-meat pattern (*A chicken/salmon/lamb went past; I ate some chicken/salmon/lamb.*) or the representational object/content pattern (*I dropped the book/film/CD; The book/film/CD was boring.*). Other senses are related but not through any productive pattern, such as *glasses* meaning drinking vessels and spectacles.[1]

Drawing on standard linguistic analyses of polysemy (Cruse 1986; Lyons 1977; Ruhl 1989), one can specify the following possible ways of mentally representing these different senses within the same word. First, the word could be **vague**, with a single general sense that covers the specific uses. For example, the word *glasses* might have the sense 'things typically made out of glass', which would thereby include both the spectacles and drinking vessel senses. So, in spite of appearing to have multiple senses, polysemous words would be associated to a single, but abstract conceptual substructure.[2] Vagueness is in a sense a denial of polysemy, because it suggests that the different uses of a word in fact reflect a common property, even though they intuitive-

1 A reviewer pointed out that the example of *glasses* is complex. In the drinking vessel sense, the word is simply a plural of *glass*, which also can refer to a drinking vessel (*She handed me a glass.*). Presumably, the plural inherits any polysemy found in the singular. However, the eyeglasses sense of *glasses* in conventionally pluralized and hence may have its own lexical entry. If so, *glasses* may not technically be polysemous, because there are two different lexical entries involved. If I had not already used this example on almost every page of the chapter, I admit I would have changed it just to avoid controversy. However, I do not believe the reviewer's analysis is correct. The eyeglasses sense of *glasses* could be the same lexical entry as *glass*, along with a convention that eyeglasses should be **conceived of** as plural. Note that *spectacles, bifocals, goggles,* and *binoculars* are referred to in the plural as well, suggesting that this is a general convention. Furthermore, the meaning of *glasses* is clearly derived from the earlier meaning of *glass* referring to the substance – just as the drinking vessel sense is – following a standard pattern of polysemy. So, the plural word is not independent of the singular by any means. In my view, the best account of these data is that both uses derive from the basic lexical item *glass*, plus the convention of thinking of glasses and similar objects as plural. In fact, the *OED* reports that the singular *glass* was earlier used to refer to spectacles, confirming that the plural version is derived from it. However, if the fastidious reader wishes to translate all my *glasses* (spectacles) examples to *glass* meaning a mirror or barometer instead, I certainly have no objection, and all my arguments will stand as written, mutatis mutandis.

2 Note that *glasses* does not simply pick out the material concept of glass, but rather must be something more like 'things made of glass', which is why I am using the term **conceptual substructure** rather than simply **concept**, which implies a pre-existing, simple concept that is connected to the word.

ly appear to us to be distinct. If the different uses can in fact be represented by a single concept, then these are not different meanings.

A second approach to polysemy is to list the senses of the word, presumably within the same lexical item. Thus, a word like *chicken* is connected to (at least) two concepts to indicate its two separate senses. The question of whether senses are mentally represented this way is essentially identical to the question in linguistic theory about whether to list senses or allow them to be derived. However, I will argue below that the evidence within cognitive psychology may provide a different answer than the one that is often arrived at in linguistic theory.

A third approach to polysemy is to rely on **rules** to generate the senses, thereby obviating the need to list them in the mental lexicon. This approach can be taken for forms of polysemy that follow productive patterns (like *chicken* and *book*), but cannot be taken for idiosyncratic examples that follow no established rule. Psychologists have not addressed the issue of semantic rules very much (though see Caramazza & Grober 1976), but this issue is quite analogous to a general issue in semantic memory first raised by Smith (1978) about whether knowledge is **prestored** or **computed**. There is a tradeoff between storage and process in cognition such that the more information that is stored in memory, the less that needs to be derived later. And correspondingly, the stronger the reasoning processes that can draw inferences about intended word meanings, the less information there needs to be in the lexicon to guide processing. Thus, the tension between generating senses and listing them within linguistics is matched by a similar tension in the psychological literature.

Finally, it should be noted that it is possible, and indeed very likely, that each of these options occurs somewhere in the lexicon. Perhaps some words that appear polysemous are in fact just vague and have a single, coherent semantic representation; others may have distinct senses; and some senses may be computed by rules whereas others are listed. However, such a possibility should not lead us to give up the hope of a general explanation. Instead, it should lead us to recognize that different meanings may lead to different forms of representation, and to attempt to discover the factors that determine when a word's senses are represented in each way.

One reaction to these possibilities has been to characterize polysemy as including one of these alternatives but not the others. For example, it is quite common for writers to distinguish vagueness from polysemy. Certainly, there are cases that everyone agrees are not ambiguous, which should be treated as lexical underspecification (e.g., *neighbor* does not have two senses, one for each gender of neighbor), but other cases, such as *glasses*, are not so obvious. Although drinking vessels and spectacles can both be thought of as items (traditionally) made (largely) of glass – i.e., fitting a common abstract description – they are not like the male and female neighbors, who differ only in one property that is largely irrelevant for the word's meaning. Clearly, eyeglasses and drinking vessels differ in important ways that would be relevant in almost any context. Nonetheless, such cases might be rejected as being really polysemous, because they can be treated as being vague: Perhaps *glasses* means things made largely of glass, and it is simply unspecified as to what the shape and function of such an object is. Therefore, it is not polysemous and need not be addressed in our investigation of how polysemy is represented.

In my view, it is wrong to make such distinctions in a psychological account at this stage. The analysis of *glasses* as vague may well be right. But it is an empirical question, for which we have very little evidence. To decide prior to empirical investigation exactly what is and is not polysemous, especially in difficult cases, could have the effect of making distinctions where there are none in terms of mental representations. Although it might be correct to distinguish vague words from senses derived from productive rules, for example, we cannot simply assume that the mental representations of these two forms of ambiguity are different. Certainly, dictionaries do separately list the different senses of *glasses*, and for all we know, people do so too, even if they could be represented by a single abstract definition. One reason I say this is because my own guess about what senses are explicitly represented in the lexicon depends on factors that are not as theoretical as the polysemy-vagueness distinction. If one ignores some aspects of lexical ambiguity because they are "not true polysemy", then one is cutting off empirical evidence that could either bolster that distinction (showing that true polysemy is distinct) or call it into question (finding similar principles operating in the two cases).

Thus, I am going to consider many different cases that might be called *polysemy* without being too fussy about discriminating polysemy from related notions. With further empirical evidence, such discriminations may well be called for.

3. Proposed Representations of Polysemy

In this section I am going to consider different ways of representing polysemous words, starting from the simplest and working my way to the most complex. My discussion will draw freely on the linguistic literature, psychological studies of polysemy (such as there are), and also more general claims about cognitive processing. The last source is obviously speculative, as it is difficult to draw specific conclusions from general principles. But given our current level of understanding of semantic representation, such general principles must guide our thinking until more specific data are available.

3.1. Monosemy and the Parsimony Principle

The simplest way to represent polysemy is to deny that the phenomenon, as usually conceived of, exists. Instead, apparent cases of polysemy are almost all cases of vagueness – abstract meanings that apply to all the uses of a word. For example, although *chicken* seems intuitively to have at least two different senses, referring to the animal and the meat, one could argue that there is a single meaning, perhaps of a chicken-essence, which would fit both of these uses equally well. Although most writers do argue that some words are only vague (see Cruse 1986 for standard discussion), the only author I know of who argues that this is the way to analyze almost all polysemy is Ruhl (1989). Indeed, Ruhl's book is so useful in its presentation of this hypothesis that if it did not exist, we would have to invent it. I am going to spend more time on this proposal than one might expect, given its unpopularity, because the issues that it raises are relevant for evaluating all theories of polysemy.

Ruhl's basic argument is based on two main claims. First, as a methodological rule, we should propose the simplest lexicon possible, in keeping with the general principle of Occam's Razor in all scientific investigation. This is **the parsimony principle**, which is shared by a large number of authors writing on polysemy (though not usually taken to such an extreme). Second, Ruhl proposes that there is a single, abstract meaning that is common across the different uses of almost every word. In combination, these assumptions result in the theory that most word meanings are represented as abstract concepts. The notion that *glasses* has two rather different senses is an illusion. *Glasses* may mean something like objects constructed primarily in glass, which picks out both eyeglasses and drinking vessels. But the fact that these two different things can be called *glasses* is not in fact stored in the lexicon. This illusion is caused when we (linguists et al.) think "what do we call *glasses*?" and then retrieve these different examples from memory. We have much conceptual knowledge about what eyeglasses and drinking glasses are, and we mistakenly import that conceptual knowledge into our analysis of the word meaning. But in fact, the lexicon per se does not include knowledge of drinking glasses and spectacles.

Ruhl analyzes in detail a number of words to attempt to show a common thread running through their use. The resulting common meaning turns out to be extremely vague and abstract, if indeed the reader can discern such a meaning at all. For the verb *bear*, Ruhl cannot provide a paraphrase or explicit account of the meaning, although he believes that there is in fact a commonality running through its uses, one that is probably unconscious. (This result is problematic, however, in that it makes it difficult to do semantics if one cannot specify what the meaning of a word is. Even if Ruhl's account were correct, in order to make progress in understanding meaning, we would have to provide some kind of explicit analysis of individual words.) One might point out that people often interpret sentences quite specifically. For example, in reading *Lee hit Chris*, one might interpret the hitting as a punch, even though the word *hit* is consistent with a wide variety of contacts, major and minor, direct and indirect, metaphorical and literal. But Ruhl argues that our specific interpretations are not primarily linguistic ones, based on the meaning of *hit*, but rather are stereotypical world knowledge. People start with the very abstract word meanings and then build up the sentence meaning from their more general knowledge. So, *I picked up the glasses and put them on my nose* is consistent only with the spectacles sense of *glasses*, because that is the only object made predominantly of glass that I am likely to put on my nose. Ruhl suggests that we have been overly promiscuous in putting that kind of knowledge into the lexicon, where it has no business being.

Ruhl's book is quite interesting, addressing a number of theoretical and methodological issues that often seem to be assumed rather than argued for, and so it is worth reading independently of this particular hypothesis. His monosemy proposal, however, has some severe problems. First, the inability to specify the very abstract meanings of words limits the theory's testability. Second, the meanings are so abstract that it is not clear that they can do the job Ruhl asks of them, to interact within a sentence to narrow down the intended meaning. He argues that *bear* refers only to an abstract sense of movement (which may be nonphysical), but that richer interpretations such as bearing young, bearing a load, bearing in a given direction, bearing out an idea, and so forth can be identified through constraints from the other words in the sentence. This proposal requires that we have interpreted the other words in the sentence, so that they can restrict the sense of *bear*. But the other words in the sentence are just as abstract, as they are also polysemous, and so they also have only very vague meanings. How is it that these extremely vague meanings combine to produce extremely concrete interpretations of a sentence?

A third problem is that a number of senses of a word cannot be predicted from general meanings (Rice 1992). One cannot use general inferential procedures to get from the meaning of *bear* 'abstract motion in a particular direction' to the conventional sense 'give birth to'. Well, one could infer such a meaning for *bear*, I suppose, but then one would also have to infer meanings such as to throw, to drive, to plant, to dive, to conclude, and any other meaning involving (perhaps abstract) motion. But these other meanings are not in fact picked out by *bear*, and there is no obvious way to generate the actual meanings while not generating the wrong ones – unless one lists some of them in the lexical entry of *bear*.

In conceptual terms, the monosemy argument is reminiscent of the so-called Classical Theory of Concepts, which claimed that concepts could be defined by necessary and sufficient features (see Rosch 1978; Smith & Medin 1981). This theory, which was famously disconfirmed by Eleanor Rosch's seminal research, also failed to explain the detailed knowledge that we have of the world. If one seeks a classical concept of dogs, one must not include properties such as barking, having four legs, having fur, eating meat, and so on, because there are exceptions to all such properties – they aren't necessary and sufficient to define the category of dogs. Instead, a classical concept of dogs must be based on a very abstract property such as 'canine', which (aside from its gross circularity) provides no obvious information about what dogs are, how one would identify them, and how one would reason about them. Thus, these concepts would be useless (Murphy 2002: ch. 2). The Classical View fell out of favor in part when researchers realized that properties such as 'canine' were vacuous, and therefore unable to account for actual concepts; the monosemy view suffers from a similar problem. Although one may argue that words have common, extremely abstract meanings, it is simply not clear what such very abstract meanings are good for.

This parallel leads to another point about the monosemy view, namely that the rejection of word knowledge from the lexicon may be simplistic. It is an example of what I call **borrowed parsimony**. Ruhl argues that the lexicon should not include encyclopedic knowledge of what glasses are, that drinking vessels are often made of glass, and so on. Instead, the lexicon should include the abstract meaning of *glasses* and leave the rest to some other cognitive component. This use of the principle of parsimony does have the effect of keeping the lexicon as simple as possible, but when applied to a psychological model of word meaning, it is in fact not more parsimonious. Since we know that people do know what eyeglasses are like and what drinking vessels are made of, and in fact know hundreds of facts about each of these, and since Ruhl admits that such knowledge is involved in interpreting sentences with the word *glasses*, parsimony is not possible. Any simplification that takes place in the lexicon must be balanced by knowledge that is placed elsewhere in the comprehension system so that it can have the desired effect on interpretation. Borrowed parsimony must eventually be paid back. Moving knowledge from the lexicon to the conceptual system or vice versa does not make any gain in overall parsimony, and so has no motivation in a model of language use.

This conclusion is related to findings in the psychology of concepts that background knowledge is used in learning concepts, and that such knowledge cannot be kept separate from the basic learning mechanisms themselves (Kaplan & Murphy 2000; Murphy & Medin 1985). Although some authors have argued that it is simpler to keep concept-learning models separate from such knowledge, since we know that people do in fact have and use such knowledge, this separation only moves the complexity elsewhere – it does not reduce it.

In summary, monosemy does not seem to be an adequate account of polysemy and word meaning in general. This will not be a shock to most readers, who likely have not taken this proposal seriously. However, we will see that some of the arguments and phenomena described here reappear in more controversial questions to be discussed later.

3.2. Prototype-based Monosemy

Perhaps the main problem with Ruhl's (1989) monosemy proposal is that the meaning is so abstract as to be virtually useless. One possible way to salvage the proposal is to take advantage of more modern thinking in the psychology of concepts and give up the notion that a concept has defining features that are present in every member. Rather than look for a mysterious, abstract dog essence that is present in every dog, psychologists would argue that one's concept of dog consists of a large number of properties that vary in their frequency and salience. None of these properties may be necessary for category membership, but they all characterize dogs to some degree. Thus, Rosch's notion of a prototype might be able to form the basis of a rich monosemic word meaning (Rosch & Mervis 1975).

This proposal has not received careful attention in the linguistic literature, so far as I know. Certainly, there have been discussions of "prototype semantics" (Coleman & Kay 1981), though not usually applied to the problem of polysemy. Furthermore, references to Roschian prototypes in polysemy have usually assumed that there are multiple senses (e.g., Lakoff's 1987 radial categories). In contrast, the present proposal is that *bear* and *glasses* have a single representation consisting of features that are typical of the entities (events and objects) called by these names. The features may not even be completely consistent with one another (e.g., 'drink from' and 'see through' for *glasses*). However, that is not a problem so long as when the word is interpreted in context, the features that are incorporated into the interpretation are themselves coherent. In *She poured whiskey into the glasses*, the other words help select the correct features so that 'see through' is not incorporated into the interpretation, but 'drink from' is.

This proposal then preserves monosemy's simplicity of single representations for polysemous words but not the extreme abstraction of Ruhl's version. Because the prototype structure is so rich, it can contain properties associated with all the senses of the word, thereby including all aspects of meaning that are necessary to understanding.

Unfortunately, this proposal will not quite make it either. One problem involves hyperonymic polysemy, when a single word refers to a specific and a general concept, such as *dog* referring to the species of dog and to male dogs in particular (in contrast to *bitch*). The solution of the prototype view would be to list the features of the most specific meaning (male canine) and then allow the irrelevant features to be canceled by context when appropriate. For example, in *The dogs are smaller than the bitches*, the feature of maleness would be retained. But in *Dogs have a spleen*, this feature would be canceled, because there is no reason to think that the predicate applies to only male dogs in particular. Thus, by representing only the most detailed sense, one can have an efficient lexical representation that permits more general interpretations through inference. The problem is that if the general sense is not represented, how does one know which general senses are permitted? Why is the gender feature canceled and not other features, such as hair, number of legs, or behavioral properties? Why can *dog* refer to canines but not to mammals or to any animal that barks or has four legs? After all, there is nothing in *Dogs have spleens* to suggest that the predicate does not apply to mammals in general, just as there was nothing to suggest that it only applies to male dogs. It seems that in order to know that one particular feature (e.g., male) but not others can be canceled, one must represent this fact explicitly. And then one is representing the different senses of *dog* rather than just one prototype.

Another problem is that for polysemous words with diverse senses, the resulting prototype is not a coherent object but is a mishmash. How is this mishmash of features sorted out to result in specific coherent interpretations? If most words in a sentence are polysemous, we again have the problem that we cannot always count on the "other" words to select out the correct features, because there are no "other" words that have only one interpretation. The other words have the exact same problem. Some properties of distinct senses are not logically inconsistent, and so there is no way to prevent them from co-occurring. For example, there is nothing incoherent about a drinking glass having a frame, but in fact that property is found in eyeglasses and not in drinking glasses. If one does not have separate representations of eyeglasses and drinking glasses, it is not at all clear how the features of only one of them would be retrieved from the *glasses* prototype when the word is interpreted.

Of course, one might argue that in addition to this prototype, one also knows perfectly well what eyeglasses and drinking glasses are, and so that world knowledge is what helps to correctly segregate the properties of the word *glasses*. But if one is going to assume this, then one can simply get rid of the lexical prototype and instead link the word directly to the concepts of eyeglasses and drinking glasses, since they are going to have to do the work of disambiguation anyway. The monosemic representation does not seem necessary to account for understanding on this view, and so there is no clear argument for proposing it.

3.3. Complete Listing

Veering from one extreme to the other, I now shift to the proposal that "every" sense is completely listed in the mental lexicon. This is the logical opposite of the previous two positions that polysemous words have a single, unified representation. Instead, the claim here is that every different sense is listed separately, meaning that each sense is a separate link from the lemma to a different conceptual substructure.

I put "every" in scare quotes above to immediately raise the question of determining just how many senses there are for a word. Caramazza and Grober (1976) analyzed the words *line* and *run* and found 26 and 40 senses for the two of them, respectively.[3] But it seems certain that if others did a study of the same words that they would come up with different numbers of senses (see Tyler & Evans 2001). A persistent problem in the study of polysemy is the inability to say for certain exactly what the senses are of a given word. There are no accepted methodology and data base that can be consulted to give a firm answer of what different uses of words there are and which uses count as different senses.

This kind of problem can stifle research if one dwells on it for too long. Although it may seem a major limitation that we cannot specify the senses of a word for certain, in fact, many studies only require us to be fairly sure that two uses of a word are or are not exemplars of the same sense. We do not need to be able to decide every hard case in order to study the cases that are not hard and make progress on them.

That said, if we propose that every sense of a word is listed in the mental lexicon, we must add some kind of criterion by which word senses are distinguished. Do we mean that any perceivable difference in the referent of a word must be distinguished? That every shade of meaning must be distinguished? Proponents of this view must provide at least an operational definition of how to decide which senses are different, or otherwise the proposal is untestable. Unfortunately, the standard tests of polysemy are not particularly reliable and do not always give what seems to be the right answer (Geeraerts 1993; Tuggy 1993). Nonetheless, proponents may finesse the difficulty by saying something like "However people decide which senses are different, they then list each of them separately in their mental lexicons." Thus, I leave aside this difficult question for the moment and consider the proposal as best I can in the absence of a complete answer.

I divide this proposal into two different subtypes. The first version claims that complete listing is required because there is no other way for people to identify the intended sense of the word. Contextual and rule-based interpretation do not actually allow people to understand polysemous senses, and so the precise meaning must be stored. The second version does not make this claim but instead argues that people store all the senses for reasons of processing efficiency.

---

3 They included senses in different syntactic categories in their counts, which is controversial. Some researchers exclude word uses with syntactic differences from polysemy, because a different lemma must be involved. However, there were still plenty of senses within each syntactic category in their analyses.

3.3.1. Complete Listing, Version 1

On this view, people must store the specific senses of *chicken* or *glasses* because there is no way to accurately derive the senses based on knowing a core meaning or the other senses. Of course, it is well known that some polysemies follow a pattern like animal/meat, representational object/content, or container/amount contained. But these patterns are not concrete and productive enough to allow speakers to generate actual senses. Instead, these patterns describe conventions within the language community, perhaps operating diachronically, but they are not rules known by individual speakers.

I have investigated this possibility in a number of studies in which I introduced people to novel words, within a story format in which it was natural to introduce new entities. By using novel words, I was able to maintain control over which senses people had experienced and which ones they had not. In the first set of studies (Murphy 1997), people read passages involving the new word and then rated the acceptability of other passages using the words in different ways. One experiment revealed that if a new use of a word was similar (but not identical) to a previous use, it was rated as more acceptable than if it was not similar to a previous use. (Across subjects, the same uses served in the similar and dissimilar conditions, so the difference in acceptability cannot be explained by properties of the sense itself.) In another experiment, I found that novel uses of a word that followed known patterns like animal/meat were rated as more acceptable than novel uses that did not follow such a pattern.

In an unpublished study with Rebecca Singer, we measured how long people spent reading sentences with polysemous words used in novel ways, as part of a story. There we also found that if the new use followed a known pattern, it was read more quickly than if it did not. However, once the word was encountered with a given sense, then this difference disappeared. That is, even unpredictable forms of polysemy could be understood once they had been encountered.

These results show that the assumptions underlying this proposal are not correct. Individual language users are able to comprehend novel uses of words that they have never encountered. (And, in fact, it is hard to explain how language learners could gain the experience that this view assumes if they could not understand words used in new ways.) Thus, it is not necessary to list every sense of a word in order for it to be understood.

3.3.2. Complete Listing, Version 2

The second version of the complete listing proposal does not argue that complete listing is necessary for people to be able to understand polysemous uses of words. But it argues that people do in fact list all the senses in order to quickly process meaning. By explicitly listing *chicken* as meaning both an animal and the edible flesh derived from that animal, people can easily understand both uses without having to go through an unconstrained inference process of attempting to derive one sense from the other. And the experiment with Rebecca Singer in fact did provide evidence that people learned from their first experience with novel senses, such that they later could understand those uses even if they did not follow a lexical rule. Previous exposure even aided comprehension of senses that could be rule-generated. Also, listing is presumably necessary to represent cases such as *iron*, meaning a wedge-shaped device with a flat bottom used to remove wrinkles from clothing. Although this sense may be consistent with a lexical pattern (material/object made from that material), that pattern grossly underspecifies this specific meaning (Lehrer 1990): An iron is not any object made from iron. Thus, in order to correctly use the word in this way, speakers must encounter irons, form a concept of them, and link it to the word *iron*.

Such examples are not controversial in principle: If the precise sense cannot be predicted on general principles, then it obviously must be learned. (However, it is not really known what properties of senses **can** be adequately predicted based on general lexical rules.) What is controversial is whether cases that could be explained on general principles are nonetheless learned and explicitly listed in the lexicon, as this proposal suggests. To address this issue, I first introduce the final theoretical position to be considered, the limited listings approach, as it contrasts with complete listing exactly on this point.

3.4. Limited Listings and the Return of Parsimony

Although many writers do not explicitly describe their theory of how polysemy is represented in general, to the degree that one can infer one through their practice, the **limited listings** approach seems to be the most popular. By this I mean the notion that some polysemic senses are listed, but not all of them. For example, Rice (1992: 93), studying polysemous prepositions, proposed

> a more constrained polysemic [as opposed to monosemic] account in which each preposition is attributed with a small set of canonical meanings which over time can engender additional meanings that may be either highly schematic or specific in character.

Common to examples of this approach are two main assumptions. First, a monosemic representation simply will not work, for the reasons discussed above. Second, although there must be multiple senses, it is important to limit the number of proposed senses to the minimum necessary. Thus, Rice emphasizes "constrained polysemy" and proposes a small set of core meanings. Tyler and Evans (2001), analyzing the word *over,* take as their main goal the elimination of unnecessary senses proposed in past analyses, so that the resulting representation will be as efficient as possible. Like Ruhl (1989), they argue that previous proposals for different senses of *over* have imported world knowledge into the lexicon, and that lexical representations could be much sparser, once one allows extralexical knowledge to augment them.

Other writers who do not explicitly adopt this overall approach seem to be sympathetic to its goals. For example, many authors argue that vague terms should not be considered polysemic, apparently based on the assumption that the number of senses in a lexical representation should not be multiplied beyond what is necessary. Nunberg (1979: 153) argues that various problems

> vanish the moment we assume that words like *newspaper* and *window* have only one conventional use, with the other normal uses generated pragmatically.

I take this also to reflect the assumption that lexical senses should be minimized. Fellbaum (2000: 53) takes the minimalist assumption as representing a psychological principle:

> Dictionaries that aim to be parsimonious, *or mirror the mental lexicon,* would include only non-predictable readings of polysemous words, along with the rules underlying regular polysemy. [emphasis added]

Although his overall approach to polysemy does not fit clearly into any of the categories I've formed here, Pustejovsky (1995) also argues against the **sense enumeration lexicon** in which all senses of a word are listed.

Thus, even though we have rejected monosemy, we are back to the principle of parsimony as an organizing force in our theory of polysemy. Indeed, monosemy would clearly be the preferred theory of the lexicon, if only the lexicon were not so inconveniently messy. Too many senses are unpredictable or based on historical relations that are no longer transparent, and so such senses must be explicitly listed. But predictable senses do not need to be listed, and so analysis of polysemous words involves identifying what uses there are, figuring out if they are predictable based on the other senses and world knowledge, and then arriving at a lexical representation that includes only the remaining senses (e.g., Tyler & Evans 2001: 731-2). This all seems to be fairly straightforward linguistic practice, and (except for Ruhl) most authors who embrace it do not give a detailed defense of these assumptions. After all, parsimony is accepted as a goal of linguistic theory, and no one defends multiplying the number of senses beyond what is needed.

However, I will in fact argue that the principle of parsimony does not have the same force when applied to the question of what is in the mental lexicon. To begin, I think that everyone will agree that the issue of what is in the mental lexicon is ultimately an empirical one. If the lexicon is parsimonious, then our model should reflect that; if the lexicon is unparsimonious, redundant, or otherwise messy, then our model should reflect that. It is important not to confuse parsimony of our theory – a metatheoretical goal – with parsimony inside people's heads – a psychological claim. It is an empirical question as to whether people are parsimonious in representing word senses, and it must be settled by data rather than by an assumption made before the investigation.

What reason do we have to believe, then, that people will be parsimonious in their lexical entries? Is there good psychological reason to imagine that the senses listed will be the minimal number necessary, so as to avoid listing predictable senses? I argue that psychological evidence suggests that the lexicon will not be parsimonious.

First, we need to understand that the mental lexicon exists in order to be acted upon by the cognitive processes involved in language understanding and production. The purpose of the lexicon is to allow fast and accurate language use, and so it is adapted for that purpose. When people hear the word *chicken*, they need to know what the speaker intends by this word as quickly as possible. And when they are talking about spectacles, they need to be able to retrieve and produce the word *glasses* quickly. These tasks involve both a long-term representation (of the meaning and syntactic properties of each word) and processes that retrieve and make use of the information in that representation. As noted above, these two components of cognition – representation and processing – trade off with one another. Efficiency of representation comes at a cost of more processing being required. On the other hand, extremely powerful processing allows less information to be stored in the representation.

In the case of polysemy, this tradeoff is easily stated. If a lexical item contains only a core or prototype meaning from which other senses are derived, then during language processing, considerable work must be done in order to effect that derivation. For example, if one has stored only the sense of *chicken* referring to a farm animal, when the word occurs in a culinary context, one must go through Gricean reasoning something like the following: "Clearly, the speaker is not intending to suggest that a live (or even dead) chicken will be served here, as that would be unusual and disgusting. Since words for animals can often be used to refer to salient products of the animal, including their meat, and given that we are discussing eating, it seems most likely that the person is referring to the edible flesh of a chicken, cooked." Although reasoning can be quite fast, such a chain of inference is clearly not trivial.

In contrast, imagine that the lexical entry for *chicken* included at least the following two listings: $chicken_1$: bird often found on farms, raised for food, lays eggs, has beak, ...; $chicken_2$: meat of $chicken_1$, usually cooked, derived from breast and legs, lacking strong taste, ... Now when an interlocutor utters *chicken* in a culinary context, the contextual features will match the representation of $chicken_2$, which refers to meat, cooking, eating, and so on. Thus, this sense is immediately retrieved as the correct sense, without much work. Because the two interpretations of *chicken* were prestored in the lexicon, savings in processing are possible.

If we compare these two ways of understanding the meat sense of *chicken*, we can see that **the principle of parsimony in lexical representation comes at the cost of greater complexity elsewhere in the language-processing system** (i.e., it is another example of borrowed parsimony). Thus, arguments for a parsimonious lexicon, either based on metatheoretical goals or psychological principles, are incomplete at best. In order to show that a lexicon with the minimal number of senses is in fact parsimonious, one must consider the inference processes that would be required to derive the unlisted senses and then compare those processes to the cost of the additional representations. I don't know how to make that comparison, and I have never seen a serious attempt at making it. But unless one can show that the entire lexical **system** (representation and process) is more efficient with a parsimonious lexicon, then one simply does not know what is parsimonious and what is not.

An analogy can be made with a different aspect of lexical processing, namely the orthographic representation of English. It is agreed that one way by which people read is to translate the written word into a phonological representation, which then accesses the lemma using the processes of speech perception. We know that people know the letter-sound translation rules, because they can read novel words and jabberwocky words that do not have pre-existing orthographic representations. Thus, it would be "parsimonious" to suggest that using such spelling rules is the way that people read all words that follow the normal spelling rules of English. However, there is considerable evidence that in fact people redundantly represent the orthographic representations of regular words when they are highly frequent. For example, they may represent that the word *the* is spelled T-H-E, and then access this word when they see these three letters, even though they could access the word via the spelling-sound rules. Indeed, violating parsimony even more, they may well do **both** processes simultaneously, and the fastest one wins (see Balota 1994).

The reason for this redundancy is that the spelling-sound rules for English are not that simple, whereas the direct association between T-H-E and the word *the* would provide a fast, direct route to recognizing the word, even if such a route is not strictly speaking necessary. Returning to polysemy, one might note that the sense-generation rules for polysemic forms are also not very simple (see below), and that it might be faster to store some senses and directly retrieve them, even if a speaker could use the rules to derive the intended meaning (eventually).

For example, consider the animal/meat form of polysemy used in *chicken* and elsewhere. This seems to be an example of a more general and productive producer/product rule, accounting for uses such as *oak* referring to a type of wood, *beaver* referring to pelt, or *wheat* referring to the grain of the plant. This also seems to be the rule covering the general grinding senses exemplified by *There was dog all over the road.* If one has not stored the fact that *chicken* is a type of meat, then one must apply this producer/product rule (as well as other rules) in order to try to derive a sense of the word that fits the context better than the core meaning. But the rule does not specify that *chicken* refers to the edible meat and not to undifferentiated chicken substance, not to the skin of the chicken, and not to a specific salient part (because the rule does produce those interpretations in some cases). Thus, all these interpretations must be generated, and the correct one selected. That seems an onerous process. Now, if one objects that "everyone knows that meat of the chicken is often eaten", and so selecting which version of the rule to apply is in fact fairly simple, one has snuck in the information that was supposed to be eliminated by not listing senses. If we assume that people have a representation of the culinary form of chicken, then we have assumed exactly the information necessary to represent the meat sense of *chicken*, and we cannot gain any parsimony by suggesting that this sense is not listed in the lexicon. Indeed, the only thing that is required is to link this representation to the word *chicken* and take advantage of it. It would be peculiar to say that people know this fact about chickens, that they often talk about chickens this way, but they do not take advantage of this fact by linking it to the word *chicken*... instead they go through an inference process to discover that this is a possible meaning.

Finally, it is worth noting that a whole class of psychological models argue that people represent specific information, like word senses, because doing so speeds processing. For example, Logan's (1988) theory of attention argues that rule-based processing is eventually supplanted with memories of specific instances that follow the rule, because retrieving those instances is faster than applying the rule. For example, as people improve on a novel task with practice, their improvement is strongest for the specific items they have practiced on and is weaker for novel items that also follow the task's rule but that are not in memory (Logan 1988). Logan's argument is that storage in the brain is cheap, and so people will remember specific items and what response was made to them, in order to speed later responding. Within the field of category learning, there is also a class of **exemplar models** that claim that people learn the identity of individual instances, even when the category could be represented by a broader generalization (Medin & Schaffer 1978; see Murphy 2002: ch. 4). So, the argument I am making about polysemy is by no means original or even controversial within cognitive psychology.

One might take the above discussion to mean that I am proposing a complete listing view, but in fact I have made no specific proposal. Instead, what I have done is to point out that the logic of the parsimony principle (contra complete listing) is not very strong. First, I argued that minimalism in the lexicon often has to be made up by information stored elsewhere, and so our complete theory of language processing is not necessarily more parsimonious when the lexicon is assumed to be parsimonious. Second, I pointed out that there are good psychological reasons for believing that specific senses could be represented even when they are perfectly predictable. Thus, in a psychological model, the **assumption** of parsimony is a questionable one at best. However, that does not mean that parsimony is wrong (although I am dubious about it) or that senses are fully enumerated. What it means is that it is an open question as to just how often senses are listed, which ones are listed and which ones are not, and what principles determine that choice. So we need to investigate this possibility rather than simply assume it or rule it out (see next section).

One might counter the above conclusion by saying that in a linguistic theory, one should still hold to the assumption of parsimony and not list senses that are predictable. After all, the issues of processing efficiency, learning of instances, and the like are all matters of performance and have nothing to do with the abstract description of a language in a grammar. I specifically began this chapter by stating the goals and assumptions of a psycholinguistic model of the lexicon exactly so that I would make clear that performance is exactly the issue. The question of the mental representation of word meaning is a question about how people actually store this information, and not a question about an abstract description of language structure. I acknowledge that there may be other enterprises in which parsimony could still be a guiding principle and issues of processing speed and the like do not enter. That said, I must also confess that I don't actually understand what questions about the lexicon could be about if they are not questions about how people actually represent and use lexical information. An abstract description of lexical information can serve any number of uses and be organized any number of ways, and if one does not have the constraint of developing a description that is functionally equivalent to what people actually do, then I don't see how one can choose among different accounts. There is no particular reason an abstract description of the lexicon must be parsimonious or complete or efficient or anything else. If I wish to claim that the lexicon is organized by the properties of the third phoneme in each word, there seems no way to argue against this proposal other than to point out that it is ridiculous in terms of the tasks speakers and hearers must carry out with the lexicon. Of course, one might have theory-internal constraints on the lexicon, as lexical information interacts with the grammar's phonological and syntactic processes. But such constraints cannot provide much help with psychological modeling until there is greater agreement on a theory of grammar.

4. Principles Counteracting Parsimony

Lexical parsimony is intuitively a natural state of affairs (why represent more than one has to?), so it is natural to ask under what circumstances it is overridden. Do people represent the meat sense for the words *chicken, salmon, dog, muskrat, robin* and *worm*, or only for some of them? If only some of them, how do we predict which senses will get their own listing and which will not?

My own thinking on this matter was greatly influenced by Alan Kawamoto's (1993) computational model of lexical access for ambiguous words. Although the model focused primarily on homonymy, at the end of his article, Kawamoto also addressed polysemy. Kawamoto thinks of semantic structure as a multidimensional space in which each dimension indicates the presence of a property or related set of properties (e.g., size, hue, behavioral disposition, etc.).[4] A word's meaning is a mapping from its form to locations in this space. Words with similar meanings can be thought of as occupying nearby locations in semantic space (i.e., they have overlapping properties). Homonyms occupy two distinct locations in semantic space (i.e., they map onto two distant semantic representations). Polysemous words, in his view (pp. 511-2), map word forms into multiple adjacent locations in the semantic space. If a word is used in two different ways that are very similar to one another, then the meanings form a continuous distribution with no clear demarcation between the two. In this case, polysemy is simply a broadening of the semantic space such that a wider range of features is associated to the word. If the word senses are more distinct, then they will form two distinct mappings that do not overlap. However, unlike homonyms, these mappings will be close to one another, sharing some but not all properties. (It is not clear that all polysemous senses do share some properties, as Kawamoto appears to assume – see Klein & Murphy 2002. But then the senses will be functionally like homonyms, which the model also accommodates.)

In such a system, two main factors lead to separate representation of senses. The first is semantic distance. If a new word use is not similar to the previous uses (i.e., does not share many properties), then the old mappings from form to meaning will not evoke the new use, and a new mapping must be learned. That mapping competes with the others when the word is used, and context usually serves to pick out the intended sense. The second factor is frequency. As an associative learning system, this model represents some mappings very strongly and others more weakly, based on their frequency. And indeed the literature on ambiguity shows that the most frequent mean-

---

4 This is basically just a feature representation. However, the multidimensional space metaphor helps to explain the model's workings. (My assumption is that "features" are just simple concepts, which themselves follow the principles of concepts such as typicality. Eventually some features may be cashed out as perceptual, motor, or emotion primitives, thereby avoiding a completely vicious circle. However, that question is independent of polysemy, and my discussion does not depend on this assumption.)

ings of a homonym are activated more quickly (Duffy, Morris & Rayner 1988). My guess is that these two factors are not independent. When two word uses are quite similar, people may not clearly distinguish them, and the represented sense may be a broad one that embraces both. But if these similar senses are quite frequent, then the speaker has many chances to learn the distinguishing details of the two and then to explicitly represent them as separate senses. In contrast, if two uses are very different, it does not take many trials and learning of details to represent them separately. If they do not overlap at all, then any properties learned about the two uses will serve to distinguish them. Thus, frequency is probably important, but it is most important in distinguishing very similar senses; and semantic distance is important, but it is most important when the senses are infrequent.

Note that this theory provides a unified treatment of homonymy and polysemy (as regards the issue of meaning representation). Homonyms will always have separate representations, on this theory, because their meanings are essentially non-overlapping. Polysemous senses will sometimes be explicitly represented and sometimes not, depending in part on just how distant a given sense is from other, established senses. Thus, the same mechanism can account for the difference between homonyms and (some) polysemous senses. Homonyms simply sit on one end of the semantic distance continuum, whereas polysemous senses are distributed more evenly across this continuum. The model does not explicitly distinguish these two classes of words, but its use of semantic distance serves to separate the two classes.

On this view, what is the role of lexical rules in the establishment of senses? Recall that some writers rely on lexical rules as being the determining factor in representation. For example, Ruhl (1989) and Fellbaum (2000) both argue that only unpredictable information should be listed in the lexicon. Implicitly, they are arguing that no matter how frequent a given word sense is, if it is predictable from a core meaning (or previously known sense), then it will not be represented. On the view I am describing, rules have no direct bearing on whether a sense will be mentally represented; this is largely determined by whether the sense has been experienced before, and how often. What rules are important for is understanding **novel** uses of words, which by definition are not prestored in the lexicon. When someone first said to me, *I saw a great DVD last night*, I was immediately able to understand the use of the word *DVD* to refer to the content of the disk (and not to its beautiful shape), because this novel use followed the familiar pattern of *CD, record, film, book, magazine*, and so on, in which words for representation-containing objects refer to both the object and its representation. No doubt this pattern aided my understanding and use of this word the first few times I heard and used it this way. But by now, this usage is no longer novel, and I strongly suspect that I have encoded this sense with the term *DVD* in my mental lexicon, even though it is perfectly predictable by this rule.

In short, the fact that lexical rules or patterns allow us to understand certain word uses does not entail that such uses are not explicitly represented. That would only follow if 1) use of the rule were easier and faster than retrieving the specific sense, and 2) there were some way for the rule to block the normal rules of associative learning by which people learn how words are used. Although we might think that there is "no need" to learn a predictable sense, so far as I know, no one has proposed a word-learning mechanism that turns itself off when there "is no need" for it to acquire information. (For example, Logan 1988: 493 argues that "encoding into memory is an obligatory, unavoidable consequence of attention".) Indeed, the recent history of implicit memory research has shown that we learn all kinds of material that seems pointless to the task (e.g., the typeface in which words are written, the characteristics of a voice reading a list of words to be recalled, the arbitrary sequences of stimuli in an experiment, etc. – see Church & Schacter 1994; Roediger & Blaxton 1987).

And, finally, I think that Lehrer (1990) provides convincing evidence that the rules of polysemy are filled with exceptions. Often one can understand why the exception exists (preemption of the meaning by another word, possible ambiguity that would result, etc.), but the point remains that one cannot generally just learn the rule and then rely on it. Rules would have us call an oven a *baker* and say *I smell that something wonderful is going to happen* and *I boated the package to the shore*. And, as I commented earlier, once one starts to list the words that each rule applies to, one is essentially listing the senses of each word.

What I am suggesting, then, is that the importance of lexical rules is primarily in constructing novel senses, both at the level of the language community, and at the level of the individual language learner. When new words (like *DVD*) enter the language, speakers can use the lexical rules to create new senses for the word, which are easily understood by other speakers even though they are novel. And when a language learner encounters a word that is new for him or her, the predictable senses of this word can be easily constructed. The rules do not, however, determine which senses are represented in the mental lexicon, either by adding new senses that are predictable (after learning a new word that is subject to the rule), nor by blocking the listing of encountered senses that are predictable. Use of such rules is slower and less accurate than retrieving a previously stored meaning and so will be overridden when a sense is frequently encountered.

I hope it is clear that this proposal is not questioning the usefulness of lexical rules or, more generally, of linguistic analyses of why words have some senses and not others and where those senses come from. For example, the research program of Pustejovsky (1995; also Copestake & Briscoe 1995), which attempts to explain how rule-based polysemies of the *church* or *chicken* sort come about, may well be an accurate account of how new senses enter the language or how a speaker generates a new sense of a word. But I would not take such theories as telling us which senses are represented in the lexicon (the senses that can't be generated by the theory) and which senses aren't mentally represented (the senses that the theory generates).

5. Psycholinguistic Studies

From the perspective of the issues discussed in this chapter, there are a number of important psycholinguistic investigations that should be done on the topic of polysemy. For the most part, those investigations have not yet been done. Therefore, rather than comprehensively review past work and attempt to squeeze it into the present framework, I will end this chapter with a more forward-looking prospectus of what research might be interesting to pursue.

One serious problem in the psychological research on polysemy is that there is no well-accepted way by which we can tell what senses are mentally represented. There is no obvious dependent measure that can be used to tell us exactly which senses are in the lexicon and which are not. For example, consider standard measures of comprehension, as measured by eye movements during reading, reading comprehension time, or semantic judgments. If a word is understood easily when used in one sense, can't one assume that its sense must have been stored in the lexicon? No, because the interpretation of the word could have been quickly inferred from the context. Furthermore, to draw a conclusion from fast comprehension, we would need to be sure that the reader did in fact interpret the word in that sense, while reading it – instead of, for example, making no particular commitment to an interpretation (as suggested by Frazier 1999; Frazier & Rayner 1990).

One result that seems to prove listing of an entry was described by Klein and Murphy (2001). We found that when a polysemous word is used in one sense (e.g., *tasty chicken*) and then used in a different sense (e.g., *loud chicken*), processing of the second sense was interfered with, that is, was slower (compared to a control – see Klein & Murphy 2001 for details). We argued that such interference entails separate listing. That is, the meat sense of *chicken* selected in the first phrase then inhibited the animal sense of *chicken*, making it slower to be retrieved when it was necessary to do so. If the second sense had not been listed, then there would have been nothing to inhibit. That is, there is no obvious way that choosing one sense could have a negative effect on another sense that is not mentally represented but that might possibly be encountered later on – there is nothing to inhibit. As Pylkkänen et al. (2006) pointed out, inhibition of representations is a well-known phenomenon in attention and psycholinguistics, whereas inhibition of processes (constructing a new sense) is not. Thus, this result gives evidence of listing of different senses. However, it has not been carried out systematically on a word-by-word basis with different sorts of polysemy (see below), and so it has not yet been used to distinguish forms of polysemy that are and are not represented.

Searching for interference cannot answer every question that we have about how polysemy is represented, however. We still need to know how different senses are selected or constructed in different sorts of sentence contexts, and here it seems likely that a piecemeal attack on the problem will be necessary. For example, if one is interested in lexical rules, one can look at cases in which we know that rules must be used and then examine the variables that influence comprehension (as in Murphy 1997, and my unpublished work with Rebecca Singer). If one believes that frequency is important in establishing a lexical sense (as suggested by Kawamoto's theory), then one can examine the importance of frequency of senses in comprehension (Foraker & Murphy 2005; Frisson & Pickering 1999). If semantic distance is important to the establishment or comprehension of senses, one can look at what happens when one switches from one sense to a close or distant sense of the same word (Klein & Murphy 2001; Murphy 1997). The totality of these studies will, one hopes, eventually result in a complete picture of polysemic representation and processing.

Another goal for psychological research will be to carefully consider different classes of polysemy that may be represented differently. For example, there might be some difference between polysemy that can be generated by rule vs. polysemy that is idiosyncratic. This question cannot be settled unless we compare different classes of polysemy within a single paradigm. Alternatively, it might be important to compare examples of polysemy based on how frequent they are, or how similar they are to another sense.

Such comparisons have not been done in the psycholinguistic literature. Either different types of polysemy have been lumped together (as in my own work, I must confess, where I have primarily contrasted polysemy as a whole with homonymy), or else a single type of polysemy has been studied. As an example of the latter, Frisson and Pickering (1999, Experiment 1) studied place/institution polysemies such as *church* and *school*. Although this does not mix together different types of polysemy, neither does it provide a basis for comparing theoretically different forms of polysemy.[5] As results from the polysemy literature do not seem entirely consistent across studies, it will probably be necessary in the future to more carefully choose and compare different classes of polysemy, to discover whether they produce similar results.

Finally, studies need to make more explicit their assumptions about the structure of the lexicon. Psycholinguistic theories have often failed to say exactly what is supposed to be in the lexicon, and individual studies have attributed different information to the lexicon depending on their specific results (Gerrig 1986). Recent studies on the processing of polysemy have provided a welcome spotlight on this topic, but they have largely focused on how the correct senses are selected, without stating very clearly which senses are listed in the lexicon and which are not (e.g., Pickering & Frisson 2001). I think this is because the authors of these studies assume that these senses must be listed in the lexicon and have not considered other possibilities in detail. However, part of the goal of this chapter is to show that in fact there is considerable debate on which senses are listed (from almost none, to the minimum necessary, to all), and there is almost no psychological evidence to decide what the correct situation is. Therefore, even researchers who focus on the processing, rather than representation, of polysemy must make a clear statement about their representational assumptions, so that they can be tested along with any processing proposal.

6. Conclusion

I hope that this sketch of the different proposals of polysemous representation serves the function of spurring further research into the different possibilities as well as making researchers more aware of the challenges facing each proposal as a psychological hypothesis. Finally, I hope that the chapter has had the effect of showing that the assumptions that often drive linguistic reasoning about the lexicon may not apply to the

---

5 Also, there is a methodological problem with presenting large numbers of a single kind of polysemy in an experiment, as subjects may become sensitized to this particular form of polysemy and adopt strategies designed to interpret it in particular, which would not be representative of normal discourse.

mental lexicon as studied by psychology, given that issues of processing efficiency and memory must influence what is represented in the mental lexicon, even if they are not a critical part of the description of a grammar.

References

Balota, D.A. (1994): Visual word recognition: The journey from features to meaning. In: Gernsbacher, M.A. (ed.): *Handbook of psycholinguistics*. San Diego: Academic Press, 303-358.
Caramazza, A. & Grober, E. (1976): Polysemy and the structure of the subjective lexicon. In: Rameh, C. (ed.): *Georgetown University roundtable on languages and linguistics. Semantics: Theory and application*. Washington, DC: Georgetown University Press, 181-206.
Copestake, A. & Briscoe, T. (1995): Semi-productive polysemy and sense production. *Journal of Semantics* 12, 15-67.
Church, B.A. & Schachter, D.L. (1994): Perceptual specificity of auditory priming: Implicit memory for voice intonation and fundamental frequency. *Journal of Experimental Psychology: Learning, Memory, and Cognition* 20, 521-533.
Coleman, L. & Kay, P. (1981): Prototype semantics: The English word *lie*. *Language* 57, 26-44.
Cruse, D.A. (1986): *Lexical semantics*. Cambridge: Cambridge University Press.
Duffy, S.A., Morris, R.K. & Rayner, K. (1988): Lexical ambiguity and fixation times in reading. *Journal of Memory and Language* 27, 429-446.
Fellbaum, C. (2000): Autotroponomy. In: Ravin, Y. & Leacock, C. (eds.): *Polysemy: Theoretical and computational approaches*. Oxford: Oxford University Press, 52-67.
Foraker, S. & Murphy, G.L. (2005): *Polysemy in sentence comprehension: Effects of meaning dominance*. Manuscript in preparation.
Frazier, L. (1999): *On sentence interpretation*. Dordrecht: Kluwer.
Frazier, L. & Rayner, K. (1990): Taking on semantic commitments: Processing multiple meanings vs. multiple senses. *Journal of Memory and Language* 29, 181-200.
Frisson, S. & Pickering, M.J. (1999): The processing of metonymy: Evidence from eye movements. *Journal of Experimental Psychology: Learning, Memory, and Cognition* 25, 1366-1383.
Geeraerts, D. (1993): Vagueness's puzzles, polysemy's vagaries. *Cognitive Linguistics* 4, 223-272.
Gerrig, R.J. (1986): Process and products of lexical access. *Language and Cognitive Processes* 1, 187-195.
Kaplan, A.S. & Murphy, G.L. (2000): Category learning with minimal prior knowledge. *Journal of Experimental Psychology: Learning, Memory, and Cognition* 26, 829-846.
Kawamoto, A.H. (1993): Nonlinear dynamics in the resolution of lexical ambiguity: A parallel distributed processing account. *Journal of Memory and Language* 32, 474-516.
Klein, D.E. & Murphy, G.L. (2001): The representation of polysemous words. *Journal of Memory and Language* 45, 259-282.
Klein, D.E. & Murphy, G.L. (2002): Paper has been my ruin: conceptual relations of polysemous senses. *Journal of Memory and Language* 47, 548-570.
Lakoff, G. (1987): *Women, fire, and dangerous things: What categories reveal about the mind*. Chicago: University of Chicago Press.
Lehrer, A. (1990): Polysemy, conventionality, and the structure of the lexicon. *Cognitive Linguistics* 1, 207-246.
Levelt, W.J.M. (1989): *Speaking: From intention to articulation*. Cambridge, MA: MIT Press.
Logan, G.D. (1988): Toward an instance theory of automatization. *Psychological Review* 95, 492-527.
Lyons, J. (1977): *Semantics*. Cambridge: Cambridge University Press.
Malt, B.C., Sloman, S.A., Gennari, S., Shi, M. & Wang, Y. (1999): Knowing versus naming: Similarity and the linguistic categorization of artifacts. *Journal of Memory and Language* 40, 230-262.
Medin, D.L. & Schaffer, M.M. (1978): Context theory of classification learning. *Psychological Review* 85, 207-238.

Murphy, G.L. (1991): Meaning and concepts. In: Schwanenflugel, P. (ed.): *The psychology of word meaning*. Hillsdale, NJ: Erlbaum, 11-35.
Murphy, G.L. (1997): Polysemy and the creation of new word meanings. In: Ward, T.B., Smith, S.M. & Vaid, J. (eds.): *Creative thought: An investigation of conceptual structures and processes*. Washington, DC: American Psychological Association, 235-265.
Murphy, G.L. (2002): *The big book of concepts*. Cambridge, MA: MIT Press.
Murphy, G.L. & Medin, D.L. (1985): The role of theories in conceptual coherence. *Psychological Review* 92, 289-316.
Nunberg, G. (1979): The non-uniqueness of semantic solutions: Polysemy. *Linguistics and Philosophy* 3, 143-184.
Pickering, M.J. & Frisson, S. (2001): Processing ambiguous verbs: Evidence from eye movements. *Journal of Experimental Psychology: Learning, Memory, and Cognition* 27, 556-573.
Pustejovsky, J. (1995): *The generative lexicon*. Cambridge, MA: MIT Press.
Pylkkänen, L., Llinás, R. & Murphy, G.L. (2006): The representation of polysemy: MEG evidence. *Journal of Cognitive Neuroscience* 18, 97-109.
Rice, S.A. (1992): Polysemy and lexical representation: The case of three English prepositions. In: *Proceedings of the Fourteenth Annual Conference of the Cognitive Science Society*. Hillsdale, NJ: Erlbaum, 89-94.
Roediger, H.L., III & Blaxton, T.A. (1987): Effects of varying modality, surface features, and retention interval on priming in word fragment completion. *Memory & Cognition* 15, 379-388.
Rosch, E. (1978): Principles of categorization. In: Rosch, E. & Lloyd, B.B. (eds.): *Cognition and categorization*. Hillsdale, NJ: Erlbaum, 27-48.
Rosch, E. & Mervis, C.B. (1975): Family resemblance: Studies in the internal structure of categories. *Cognitive Psychology* 7, 573-605.
Ruhl, C. (1989): *On monosemy: A study in linguistic semantics*. Albany: SUNY Press.
Slobin, D.I. (1996): From "thought and language" to "thinking for speaking". In: Gumperz, J.J. & Levinson, S.C. (eds.): *Rethinking linguistic relativity*. Cambridge: Cambridge University Press, 70-96.
Smith, E.E. (1978): Theories of semantic memory. In: Estes, W.K. (ed.): *Handbook of learning and cognitive processes*, Vol. 6. Potomac, MD: Erlbaum, 1-56.
Smith, E.E. & Medin, D.L. (1981): *Categories and concepts*. Cambridge, MA: Harvard University Press.
Tuggy, D. (1993): Ambiguity, polysemy, and vagueness. *Cognitive Linguistics* 4, 273-290.
Tyler, A. & Evans, V. (2001): Reconsidering prepositional polysemy networks: The case of *over*. *Language* 77, 724-765.

Identifying, Specifying and Processing Metaphorical Word Meanings*

Raymond W. Gibbs, Jr./Julia E. Lonergan

University of California, Santa Cruz, Dept. of Psychology
Santa Cruz, CA 95064, USA
E-mail: gibbs@ucsc.edu

The metaphorical nature of many word meanings poses several distinct challenges for cognitive theories of polysemy. Consider several expressions that contain metaphorical word meanings:

(1) *I don't see the point of your argument.*
(2) *John couldn't stand working for his boss.*
(3) *John has to elevate his game now that his team was in the championship.*
(4) *John has a bright future.*
(5) *John is a bulldozer.*

Each of these expressions are centered around a lexical item that is not used in a strictly literal sense. In (1) the person's message is not about his inability to visually perceive something because an argument is inherently unseeable. Instead, the word *see* refers to the idea of knowing something, or being able to understand it. Thus, in (1) the speaker is metaphorically conceiving of knowing as seeing, which in contemporary cognitive linguistics reflects the primary metaphor KNOWING IS SEEING.

The speaker in (2) does not mean that John was unable to remain upright on two feet while working for his boss. Instead, the speaker metaphorically conceives of a psychological process (i.e., being able to cope with working for his boss) in terms of being able to persist in a viable physical position (i.e., standing).

In (3), the word *elevate* does not have a literal, physical, or spatial meaning, because the idea of 'his game' has a more abstract quality, such that *elevate his game* implies that John must improve his performance, or to continue with the metaphorical reading, push it to a higher dimension. Similarly, the speaker in (4) employs a word often used to convey something about visual luminance to refer to the abstract idea of a person's future promise. The use of *bright* in this case is presumed to be derived from the metaphorical mapping of the more basic source domain of visual experience onto the less coherent domain of a person's future life. This metaphorical mapping

* Publication of the present paper was supported by the Research Group for Theoretical Linguistics of the Hungarian Academy of Sciences at the Universities of Debrecen, Pécs and Szeged.

fleshes-out the abstract idea to give it a more concrete metaphorical meaning for *bright*. Expressions (1) through (4), then, refer to common bodily activities as source domains for conceiving of and talking about more abstract target domains.

The metaphorical meanings of *see*, *stand*, and *bright* are conventional parts of the wide range of senses typically associated with these polysemous words. But it is less clear whether the metaphorical meaning of *bulldozer* in (5) (e.g., John is persistent, single-minded, insensitive) is an established sense. Thus, understanding that (5) refers to human qualities, as opposed to machine characteristics, may be done through access of a sense already part of the word's lexical representation, inferentially derived given a metaphorical mapping of machines onto people, or inferentially derived via rich pragmatic knowledge.

These different examples of metaphorical word meaning raise several interrelated questions about metaphor in a cognitive theory of polysemy. What defines a particular sense of a word as metaphorical? Do people recognize metaphorical word meanings? Are metaphorical word meanings derived from more concrete, possibly embodied, source domain knowledge? Are metaphorical meanings accessed from entrenched lexical representations or derived via pragmatic knowledge in context? Is it even possible to enumerate the meanings of a polysemous word?

Our aim in this chapter is to consider these questions in light of research on lexicography, cognitive linguistics, and psycholinguistics. We will argue (a) that it may be quite difficult to distinguish a metaphorical word meaning from overly abstract senses that also incorporate so-called literal senses of a word, (b) that it is still, nonetheless, quite difficult to articulate what constitutes the abstract, core meaning for a polysemous word, (c) that dictionaries provide relatively poor models for how people typically conceptualize of metaphorical word meanings, (d) that it may be impossible to enumerate or count the meanings of polysemous words, (e) that psycholinguistic studies do not necessarily show that metaphorical word meanings are derived after some initial core, nonmetaphorical meaning is first examined, and, most generally (f) that good reasons exist to doubt whether mental lexicons possess detailed semantic content. We alternatively suggest that people create appropriate meanings for polysemous words, including those thought to be metaphorical, on-the-fly through appeal to complex conceptual/embodied knowledge rather than merely picking out these meanings from a structured list or network of entrenched senses.

Identifying Metaphorical Meanings

Defining what constitutes a metaphorical meaning for a word is a terribly difficult task for polysemy scholars. Although many metaphor researchers claim to have reasonably well-formed intuitions about what is "metaphorical", these intuitions often differ within and across individuals, which often has important consequences for proposed theories of metaphor and metaphor understanding. Consider again the statement in (3) *John had to elevate his game now that his team was in the championship.* Does the word *elevate* have a metaphorical meaning, or can we concretely, and literally, talk about elevation in the context of a nonspatial idea, such as in reference to one's athletic performance?

Metaphor scholars give very different answers to this question. Many traditional linguists and philosophers suggest that a metaphor exists whenever there is some comparison or similarity established between a word or expression and the concept to which it refers. Under this view, the word *elevate* is used to draw a comparison between what John has to do to improve his performance and the idea of making something spatially higher to denote its better quality. This metaphorical comparison, therefore, implies that the word *elevate* in (3) is indeed metaphorical. In the same way, an expression like *We've come to a crossroads in our relationship* is judged to be metaphorical in some scholars' opinion, perhaps rooted in the widespread conceptual metaphor LOVE RELATIONSHIPS ARE JOURNEYS.

A different perspective claims that the above account represents how speakers may have initially conceived of *elevate* in relation to abstract idea (e.g., athletic performance where no real spatial motion is involved), but that over time the metaphorical sense of *elevate*, meaning 'to make better', has become conventional and exists as a literal sense in individuals' lexical representations for the word *elevate*. Under this view, understanding the non-spatial sense of *elevate* only requires a search through the established senses of this polysemous word to find the one that fits best in context. There is no need to construct any cross-domain mapping or metaphorical inference to determine what *elevate* means in a sentence context like (3). In the same way, an expression like *We've come to a crossroads in our relationship* is seen as nonmetaphorical, despite its possible metaphorical origins, and is understood as expressing a literal meaning.

Underlying both these accounts is the assumption that some basic, standard, literal sense of *elevate* is elaborated upon to create a metaphorical meaning. Thus, many dictionaries list different senses of polysemous words in an order starting with the literal meanings (although these senses are not labelled "literal"), with established metaphorical senses subsequently listed. For instance, consider the definition of *elevate* in the *American Heritage Dictionary* (3rd edition):

Elevate, v.
1. To move something to a higher place or position from a lower one, lift.
2. To increase the amplitude, intensity, or volume of.
3. To promote to a higher rank.
4. To raise to a higher moral, cultural, or intellectual level.
5. To lift the spirits of; elate.

The first listed sense seems literal as it appears to apply most directly to cases where there is concrete, physical upward motion as in *Bob had to elevate the ceiling of his living room by six inches*. The final sense of *elevate* appears to be metaphorical given that feelings and moods are not concrete entities that can be physically moved in a vertical direction to a higher place or position. One easily gets the impression that there is a metaphorical mapping of the first literal sense (i.e., the source domain) onto the more abstract target domain (e.g., feelings and moods) to create a metaphorical meaning of *elevate* in (3) that captures the idea of 'John having to improve his game by moving it to a new, higher dimension'.

There are two problems with this proposal. First, the first literal sense defined for *elevate* is general enough to capture both the physical and non-physical uses of the word. After all, when John wishes to 'elevate his game' in a metaphorical sense, he moves to a higher place or position. A cognitive linguistic analysis suggests that this metaphorical construal of the first literal sense of *elevate* is motivated by two entrenched conceptual metaphors: STATES ARE LOCATIONS and GOOD IS UP/DOWN IS BAD. In this way, the putative literal sense of *elevate* may itself be understood metaphorically, or may be general enough to simultaneously capture the literal and metaphorical meanings of the word.

Dictionaries clearly differ in the extent to which their primary definition for a polysemous word refers solely to physical, concrete entities and actions (e.g., *see* as visual perception, and *stand* as being upright on two feet), as opposed to providing highly general, abstract definitions that encompass a range of literal and metaphorical uses. But we suspect that in many instances, the first listed definition in most dictionaries is intended to be literal, but unwittingly also is applicable to metaphorical meanings, precisely because the definition provided can itself be easily interpreted in a metaphorical manner. Of course, dictionaries tend not to explicitly state whether a given word meaning is literal, metaphorical, or whatever. For instance, Moon (2004) acknowledges that there is little scholarship and notation of metaphor identification, analysis and representation in the many literary-based dictionaries. She writes:

> Most dictionaries contain the metaphorical senses, but the acknowledgment of the metaphor in its handling and notation has been relegated to second status. Dictionaries do not usually say anything about the relationship between word senses. There are no clearly represented links between polysemous words in most dictionaries. The word divisions into parts-of-speech and sequential lists of senses is a manifestation of the dominant and traditional view of knowledge lexicalization. (Moon 2004: 8)

A second problem with the assumption that metaphorical word meanings are derived in some manner from an initially understood core sense is that it is often unclear what constitutes the basic, core, concrete, or literal sense of any polysemous word. Consider the numerous things to which the word *cell* may refer (Nunberg 1979). There are cells of the body, battery cells, prison cells, communist cells, photocells, the cells of a matrix, and so on. Each of these uses may possibly be members of a single "fuzzy" or "vague" extension, for example, the uniform constitutive parts of a large structure. But, people speak of single celled organisms. Moreover, speakers use *cell* to refer to political organizations only when they are secret. Prisons and monasteries may have cells, but not libraries, dormitories, or cruise ships, which are divided into compartments. It is not clear, then, that one sense of any polysemous words can be defined as primary and the others as secondary (Nunberg 1979).

These problems identifying the metaphorical meanings of a word from a derived sense have important implications for psychological and cognitive linguistic work on polysemy. For example, cognitive linguistic research has advanced three broad proposals about polysemy (Croft & Cruse 2004). First, the multiple meanings of polysemous words are related to one another according to a variety of cognitive principles (e.g., metaphor, metonymy, generalization) such that the meanings of polysemous words are, at least, partly motivated. Second, the meanings of polysemous words can be organized into prototype structures, family resemblance structures or lexical networks, which are constructed beginning with a core, or central, sense that is elaborated upon using the different cognitive principles. Third, the study of polysemy shares many characteristics with the study of categorization for both linguistic and non-linguistic concepts (e.g., Lakoff 1987; Taylor 1995). Most generally, cognitive linguists argue that the lexical organization of polysemous words is not a repository of random, idiosyncratic information, but is structured by general cognitive principles that are systematic and recurrent throughout the lexicon. These principles partly arise from our phenomenological, embodied experience.

A good example of a radial category for a polysemous word has been given for the preposition *over* (Brugman & Lakoff 1988). Consider some of the senses for the word *over*.

The plane is flying over the hill.
The wall fell over.
Sam is walking over the hill.
She spread the tablecloth over the table.
The play is over.
Look over my corrections, and don't overlook any of them.
You've made over a hundred errors.

These different senses are motivated by a small number of relations that are principled, systematic, and recurrent throughout the lexicon. For example, the two sentences *Sam walked over the hill* and *Sam lives over the hill* exemplify a single relationship between two senses of *over*. The first sentence expresses the shape of a path relative to a reference location, and collocates with a motion verb. The second sentence expresses a stative location that is understood to be the endpoint of a path of the same shape as that coded by the motion sense of the preposition. The systematicity of this relationship between the two senses justifies the hypothesis of a single principle relating path-focus to end-of-path focus (Brugman & Lakoff 1988).

The same principle that relates path-focus to end-of-path focus for spatial uses of prepositions can also apply to metaphorical uses. For example, the sentence *He's finally over the most difficult part of the job* exemplifies a metaphorical projection of the end-of-path schema to include two fundamental conceptual metaphors CONTROL IS UP and LACK OF CONTROL IS DOWN that map one domain of experience (e.g., control) in terms of a different domain (e.g., space). The person who had completed the most difficult part of a job is now in control of the task and can metaphorically be thought to be "over" it. Other metaphorical projections motivate other figurative uses of *over*. For instance, the MORE IS UP metaphorical mapping applies to the stative sense of *over* to yield a quantity sense of the word as in *Our sales were over $20 million last year*.

Cognitive linguistic analyses of polysemy are impressive for their detailed suggestions about the ways different senses of words are linked together in non-arbitrary ways. Nonetheless, these studies typically begin by positing a single core, or central sense from which all other senses are inferentially derived. For example, Brugman and Lakoff begin their analysis by claiming that the central sense of *over* combines the ideas of above and across as in *The plane flew over the hill.* An expression like *Sam walked over the hill* is derived from the central sense by having the further specification of contact. Other senses within the complex radial category for *over* are extended from these initial, schematic interpretations. But once again, what determines which sense is most basic, primary, or core? Why is the above and across senses of *over* more central than those associated with expressions like *Bill lives over the hill* or *The house fell over*? With only one or two exceptions (see Evans 2003), cognitive linguists have not offered principled reasons for identifying what constitutes a core sense in analyses of polysemous meaning. Furthermore, all linguistic studies suffer from the related problem of having been conducted by individual analysts, and several commentators have questioned whether the resulting complex of lexical relations are really in the mind of the analyst or the minds of ordinary language users (Sandra & Rice 1995).

The cognitive linguistic studies stand in contrast with other linguistic and psychological accounts that propose that there really is an abstract sense that is an invariant part of all established, and newly created, senses for a polysemous word, including those deemed literal and metaphoric. This abstract sense, which may be the only thing coded in the lexical representation for a word, is subsequently fleshed out using different pragmatic principles to provide a contextually appropriate meaning. Consider the word *line* in the sentences *The shortest distance between two points is a straight line* and *They came to different conclusions using the same line of reasoning*. The "abstractionist view" of word meaning assumes that there is a single, very general, and abstract concept 'line' that is neutral between the spatial meaning of *line* and the form of reasoning meaning of *line*. Both sentences contain special cases of the same abstract concept. Some experimental findings suggest that the many different uses of *line* all share the common semantic feature of EXTENSION (Caramazza & Grober 1976), although this conclusion was not directly seen in the data, but inferred by the researchers from their examination of students' intuitions about the different uses of *line*.

A related theory claims that all multiple meanings of a polysemous word are mapped onto some psychologically primitive concept (Rakova 2003). This "no polysemy" view argues that the literal-metaphorical distinction in classifying word senses does not apply to conceptual structure, given that one meaning of a polysemous word (e.g., the metaphorical use of *line*) is not derived or accessed from a more basic, experiential concept (e.g., the geometrical sense of *line*). This no polysemy view does not claim that speakers can not distinguish between different word meanings (e.g., the geometrical vs. the metaphorical meanings of *line*), only that there is one primitive concept associated with a polysemous word. To give another example, the concept of 'bright light' is different from 'bright future', because the property of brightness is instantiated differently in the visual and psychological domains (Rakova 2003). It may be true that one's concept for *bright* is primarily grounded in embodied, visual experience, yet this does not imply that our understanding of the word *bright* in *John has a bright future* is itself embodied. In this way, the no polysemy view provides an alternative to thinking about the relationship between different literal and metaphorical word meanings and between word meanings and conceptual structure.

Although some linguists have attempted to specify the very abstract senses of certain polysemous words (Groefsema 1995), other advocates of this abstractionist, or monosemy, view claim that underspecified senses are so abstract as to be semantically unspecifiable (Ruhl 1989). The failure to specify the abstract, underspecified sense of a polysemous word makes it difficult to empirically test the abstractionist view as a psychological account of linguistic processing (but see below). Furthermore, most cognitive linguists reject the underspecification view precisely because they have failed to discover senses that are rich enough to capture the wide range of meanings (up to 100 for some polysemous words) many words possess (Gibbs 1994; Sweetser 1986).

The problem of defining what constitutes a metaphorical use of a word has been recently tackled by an interdisciplinary group of scholars titled "Pragglejaz" (Steen 2002). The scholars in Pragglejaz have struggled to provide a set of reliable criteria for metaphor identification. Although this project still relies on individual analysts' intuitions, it aims to provide a set of constraints that may be followed to reliably select metaphorically used words in discourse. Quite reasonably, the scope of this work is limited to providing criteria that "experts" may use in conducting empirical and theoretical studies of realistic discourse. Our present proposal is that analysts may use the following set of steps to reasonably identify, with a significant degree of consistency, the metaphorically used words in texts.

1. Read the entire text (i.e., written text or talk transcript) to establish a general understanding of the discourse.
2. Determine the lexical units in the text.
3. For each lexical unit in the text, check metaphorical use:
  (a) Establish the meaning of the lexical unit in context (i.e., how it applies to an entity, relation in the situation evoked by the text (contextual meaning). You should take into account what words are before and after the lexical unit.
  (b) Determine if the lexical unit has a more basic current/contemporary meaning in other contexts than the one in the given context. For our purposes, basic meanings tend to be:
    – more concrete; what they evoke is easier to imagine, see, hear, feel, smell and taste
    – related to bodily action
    – more precise (as opposed to vague)
    – historically older.
  Basic meanings are not necessarily the most frequent meaning of the lexical unit.
4. If the lexical unit has a more basic current/contemporary meaning in other contexts than

- the given context, decide whether the contextual meaning can be understood by comparison or
- contrast with the basic meaning.

If yes, mark the lexical unit as metaphorical

Repeat steps 1-4 for each lexical unit.

This procedure has been shown to be reasonably reliable, although a great deal of variability still exists both within and across individual analysts (Steen 2002). Not surprisingly, one problem that Pragglejaz scholars have faced in trying to establish criteria for metaphor identification is seen in Step 2 where an analyst must determine a lexical unit's basic, current meaning in other contexts. We have frequently struggled with how to describe this specific step, and resisted calling this a search for a word's literal meaning, precisely because calling something "literal" was quite unsuccessful in getting analysts to agree on what that essence was for each word. However, we believe that some basic meaning may be identified through a collection of symptoms, including a word's concrete, imageable, related to bodily action, more precise, and historically older meanings, while at the same time not necessarily a word's most frequent meaning. Once again, these hints as to what makes a particular word meaning "basic" are helpful in establishing the reliability of the Pragglejaz procedure for metaphor identification. But even if there may be a reliable process by which experts may agree on whether a word is metaphorical, it is not at all clear that ordinary speakers and listeners engage in similar processes during normal language use. Speakers may sometimes deliberately employ a word in a metaphorical way, yet this conscious realization may be a special, infrequent event. The fact that a group of metaphor experts struggle to articulate their own metaphor identifications is testimony to a problem that most individual scholars ignore when they present their own linguistic analyses of metaphor and polysemy.

A different method for identifying metaphorical word meanings is to conduct corpora analyses. Corpora work demonstrates that patterns of word use often differ from ordinary speakers' intuitions about metaphorical word meanings, and whether these are best viewed as conventional or novel. For example, consider two texts used in a series of psycholinguistic experiments looking at people's understanding of conventional and novel metaphors (Keysar, Shen, Glucksberg & Horton 2000).

1. *As a scientist, Tina thinks of her theories as her children. She is a prolific researcher, conceiving an enormous number of new findings each year. Tina is currently weaning her latest child.*
2. *As a scientist, Tina thinks of her theories as her children. She is a fertile researcher, giving birth to an enormous number of new findings each year. Tina is currently weaning her latest child.*

Keysar et al. argued that the opening sentence of each story established an explicit metaphorical mapping. But the second line in each story differs in that the first contains conventional phrases (e.g., "prolific" and "conceiving"), while the second contains novel metaphors (e.g., *fertile* and *giving birth*). The final sentence of each story presents the same novel metaphor (e.g., *weaning her latest child*). Keysar et al. claimed that their assumption about the conventionality of each phrase was supported by a rating study in which undergraduate students were asked to judge the conventionality of each phrase.

However, it is not clear that assessing people's intuitive judgments best reflects natural language patterns (a lesson psychologists already know from the different data on people's familiarity with words and actual word frequency from corpora studies-see Gernbacher 1990). In fact, Deignan (in press) performed a corpora analysis of the different items in the above texts and discovered something different from what Keysar et al. claimed to be the case. For instance, there were 365 cases of *fertile* in the corpora, 210 referring to lands that bear crops, and 97 referring to people, animals, and plants. However, 61 of the 97 citations of *fertile* referring to people were metaphorical, such as *For me, the artist's fertile imagination failed him*. This data suggests, then, that *fertile* is not a novel metaphor, contrary to what was claimed by Keysar et al.

An analysis of *wean*, in reference to *weaning* in the last sentence of each text, showed that it, and its affiliates, appeared 188 times in the corpus. But only 5 citations had *weaning* followed by a direct object (e.g., *weaning her latest child*). All of these were used specifically in discussing the feeding of children (e.g., *She didn't experience any trouble weaning her daughter*). In this way, Keysar et al are correct that *weaning* in this context was a novel metaphor, at least in terms of this exact lexico-grammatical form. But *wean* like *fertile* has various metaphorical meanings that are closely related to the meaning conveyed in the experimental texts, such as *wean people away from exclusive reliance on the automobile*. As suggested by research in processing polysemy during online text comprehension (Williams 1992), it is quite likely that these closely related metaphorical senses may be accessed during reading. This fact could have led experimental participants in Keysar et al's reading-time studies to treat *weaning* as a conventional, and not novel, metaphor.

Finally the term latest child in the texts' final sentence appears on the surface to be ambiguous between a literal and metaphorical reading. Yet corpus analysis shows that a metaphorical interpretation is strongly favored, because the collocation *latest* + *child* almost never occurs (compared to words like *youngest* which appears frequently with *child*). This result suggests that the collocation *latest child* would suggest a non-conventional meaning of *child*, because it reflects an atypical language pattern, regardless of the previous context.

This corpora analysis raises questions about the stimuli employed by Keysar et al, especially in the way they classified different phrases as having literal or metaphorical, and conventional or novel metaphorical, meanings. Thus, people's raw intuitions about whether a given word or expression has metaphorical meaning, and the extent of its metaphoricity, may differ from how words are actually employed in real discourse.

An analogy is useful in thinking about how anyone may go about identifying any word as having "literal" or "metaphorical" meaning (Gibbs 2005). Trying to identify metaphors from real-life discourse is analogous to walking down a crowded street and picking out those people who are ill with the common cold. For example, you first come across a person who has runny eyes, a nasty cough, and complains, when asked, of having a headache. Surely, this person can be marked as having a *cold*. Next, you find someone with a runny nose, who complains of having a headache and a sore throat. Once more, you identify this person as having a *cold*. The following person, however, has none of the symptoms experienced by the first two people, as this individual only has chest congestion. But again, this person seems to be suffering from some type of cold. Finally, the fourth person experiences a runny nose and a bad cough, and so, once more, you identified this person as someone who has a *cold*.

In everyday life, each of the four people you have encountered walking down the street appear to be good *cold* candidates. After all, they, in their various ways, seem to be experiencing all the classic symptoms associated with having a *cold*. But a moment's reflection makes you realize that none of these people experience the same *cold* symptoms, and that there is no single symptom that is common across all instances of these people with *colds*. So what then defines the category of things called *colds*?

Metaphors may be like colds in the sense that they have symptomatic, but not yet, defining features. Under this view, one may not be able to devise a set of criteria, or a procedure that applies these criteria in an orderly manner, to determine that something is, for certain, a metaphor or a metaphorically used word. But there may be a variety of clues that are symptomatic of some word have metaphorical meaning, including it expressing indirect meaning in context, having other more concrete, imageable, embodied, historically older meanings from which the metaphorical meaning is perhaps created. One implication of this alternative view is that the category "metaphorical", like that of "literal", is inherently unstable, with judgments of metaphoricity being influenced by a variety of personal (e.g., past attempts to identify metaphors) and contextual (e.g., oral vs. written language, knowledge of the speakers/writers, the genre) factors. Another possibility is that judgments of metaphoricity in words are given on-the-fly given some explicit or implicit context and are read from some predetermined list of metaphorical senses of a word's lexical representation.

Specifying Metaphorical Meanings

The difficulty with identifying whether some word is metaphorical or not represents just the first step in understanding a word used metaphorically. Thus, once one offers a judgment that a word may have metaphorical meaning, it is still unclear how best to articulate what that metaphorical meaning is. Metaphors, most generally, are notoriously difficult to paraphrase, especially given that these words and phrases are often seen as being "pregnant with meaning". For instance, the meanings of metaphorical statements are usually understood as conveying a lengthy list of correspondences (e.g., LIFE IS A JOURNEY from Lakoff & Johnson 1980). Many metaphor scholars question whether there are any constraints on the number and kind of meaning correspondences associated with a verbal metaphor, and also asked if people actually draw these many complex inferences when reading or hearing both conventional and novel metaphors. Some research show, nonetheless, that people have far more complex understandings of conventional metaphors in English, such as *blow your stack* than they do for putative literal definitions or paraphrases of these expressions (e.g., 'to get very angry') (Gibbs 1992). Thus, people infer that the cause of someone getting angry is internal pressure, that the expressions of anger is unintentional, and conveyed in a violent manner when they read *blow your stack*, but not when they read 'get very angry'. This complex set of metaphorical meaning inferences are directly related to the underlying conceptual metaphor ANGER IS HEATED FLUID IN A CONTAINER, which partly motivates the existence and continued use of verbal expressions like *blow your stack*.

The situation in regard to precisely defining what a metaphorical word means is similar to the problem of determining the meaning of metaphorical phrases. Consider, for example, a conversation where a doctor tells a cancer patient that the cancer that was in the bones is *dormant* (Semino, Heywood & Short 2004: 1283). This use of *dormant* may be understood in terms of at least two different conceptual metaphors:

> REMISSION PHASE OF CANCER IS BEING DORMANT
> The cancer corresponds to the hibernating animal/volcano.
> The period of remission of the cancer corresponds to the period in which the animal/volcano is dormant.
> The end of inactivity/remission corresponds to the volcano erupting or to the animal waking up.
>
> CANCER IS HIBERNATING ANIMAL/VOLCANO
> The period of remission of the cancer corresponds to the period in which the animal/volcano is dormant.
> The end of inactivity/remission corresponds to the volcano erupting or the animal waking up.

Which metaphor is most appropriate for the analysis of *dormant* in this case? One possibility is that the hibernating animal presents the best metaphorical mapping because it is linked with the animal reading of cancer "galloping away" in one of the participant's earlier utterances. Under this characterization, there is a superordinate conventional metaphor CANCER IS AN ANIMAL that has HORSE and (HIBERNATING) ANIMAL as basic-level categories, which give rise to the sub-mapping CANCER IS A HORSE and CANCER IS A HIBERNATING ANIMAL. But a different understanding of cancer links up with earlier use of *erupt* in the discourse suggests that *dormant* specifically refers to CANCER IS A VOLCANO metaphor.

Thus, it is not always possible to determine which metaphorical meaning a word has by appealing to context and what speakers said previously. Although listeners may understand *dormant* very simply to mean 'not active', perhaps through recognition of a simple psychological primitive for the concept 'dormant', people may nonetheless draw more elaborate metaphorical inferences about 'dormant' given one, as opposed to another, conceptual metaphor. For instance, thinking of 'dormant' in terms of an animal suggests the possibility that the cancer can continue to be trained and controlled. But thinking of the cancer as being like a volcano suggests a certain unpredictability in the way the cancer is understood and indeed experienced, especially the likelihood that the cancer may "erupt" again.

This example, and discussion, demonstrates additional difficulties in specifying the complex metaphorical meanings associated with polysemous words in context. Studies have not yet examined in great deal the specific complex meanings people ordinarily understand, both immediately and upon reflection, when reading or listening. As we show below, psycholinguistic studies too often simply compare access or creation of a single literal meaning against a single metaphorical meaning. The complex metaphoricity of many words has not been adequately examined in theories of linguistic processing.

It is not surprising that people's intuitions about whether a word has a metaphorical meaning are complex and variable. Research shows that both the literality or metaphoricity of any word is a judgment that anyone can make, but this determination is deeply inconsistent both within and across individuals (Gibbs, Buchalter, Moise & Farrar 1993). This situation is directly parallel to the work on concepts in cognitive psychology showing that individual concepts are not consistently-defined, pre-established mental entities, but may be created in the moment in different ways depending on the context and history of the person. For example, studies in which people had to provide definitions for categories, such as bachelor, bird, and chair, showed only 47% of the features in one person's definitions for a category existed in another person's definition (Barsalou 1995). A great deal of flexibility also exists within individuals when they are asked to provide definitions for concepts. When participants in the above study returned two weeks later and defined the same categories again, only 66% of the features noted in the first session were produced again in the second session. These results indicate that that substantial flexibility exists in how a person conceptualizes the same category on different occasions. This research from categorization studies suggests that people may not be accessing the same essence of a word each time they encounter it in discourse, The significant flexibility shown by many experiments on defining categories and word meanings arises not from differences in conceptual and linguistic knowledge, but from differences in the retrieval of this knowledge from long-term memory. On different occasions, different individuals retrieve different subsets of features from their extensive knowledge of a category, and its history of use.

Do people ordinarily understand the various contextual instances of a polysemous word as being related? Several psycholinguistic studies demonstrate the speakers can, under specific conditions, be consciously aware of the relationships between the different senses of polysemous words (Columbo & Flores d' Arcais 1984; Durkin & Manning 1989). For instance, Gibbs, Beitel, Harrington and Sanders (1994) showed that people systematically sorted different senses of the word *stand* together, a behavior that could be explained by an independent analysis of people's bodily experiences of different aspects of standing. Participants in these studies did not group physical senses of *stand* (e.g., *The clock stands on the mantle*, *He stood up tall*) together and metaphorical senses (e.g., *He couldn't stand his job*, *He stood up for justice*) together. Instead, physical and metaphorical senses of *stand* were often seen as being closely related, again, depending on the degree to which these were motivated by different patterns of bodily experiences (i.e., image schemas, such as VERTICALITY, RESISTENCE, and BALANCE). Similar work shows the embodied basis of people's understandings of the various meanings of the preposition *on* (Beitel, Gibbs & Sanders 2000).

Other psycholinguistic studies employed tasks that do not ask people to be consciously aware of the different senses of polysemous words, but use indirect methods, such as semantic priming and lexical decision, to see the degree to which various senses of words are related. These studies refute the simple monosemy view and imply that ordinary speakers are reasonably sensitive to the finer distinctions in meanings for polysemous words (Sandra & Rice 1995).

But an important qualification to these general findings is that people may not simply be judging the relations between the senses of individual polysemous words, but the possible contexts in which these senses may be used. For instance, studies show that when two words were similar in meaning, such as *car* and *automobile*, the contexts in which they could be used were frequently confused. But unrelated words never were seen in contexts that could be confused (Miller & Charles 1991). One possibility is that contextual representations are always associated with different word meanings, which specify how a word form can be used to express a particular meaning. Contextual representations are absent from dictionary definitions, which is one reason why dictionaries provide such a poor model of human word knowledge and use.

This later set of empirical results highlight the strong possibility that people's judgments about the relatedness of different senses of a polysemous word may derive from their in-the-moment imaginings of various contexts, as opposed to being generated from a simple list of meanings within mental lexicon. Thus, the intuition that some senses are similar in meaning is a momentary judgment and not a direct reflection of some enduring, purely linguistic representation. Research on human categorization provides support for this view. When people are asked to list instances of the category 'fruit', for instance, people often report imagining walking down an aisle in a grocery store, and simply naming the different fruits as they are encountered (Vallee-Tourangeau, Anthony & Austin 1997).

The contextual shaping of meaning for metaphorically used words also raises the question of whether the senses of a polysemous word are truly independent. For instance, in the Random House Dictionary, the word *stand* has over 60 different uses listed. Thus, #12 refers to the idea of 'remaining erect or whole, resisting change, decay, or destruction' as in *The ruins still stand*. But #6 'to remain steadfast as in to be set, placed, fixed, located' seems terribly similar to #12, as does #10 referring to 'remaining standing' as in *The bicycle stood in the basement all winter*. One can ask a similar question about the relations between various metaphorical meanings associated with *stand for justice* and *stand to reason*, both of which convey a sense of remaining steadfast to maintain some idea or principle. Clark (1983) has argued that words may have innumerable meanings because of the potentially infinite ways that they may contextually used. More generally, one problem in specifying metaphorical meanings is that these are often so related as to make it impossible in principle to differentiate between them, or to know where one meaning ends and another begins. Although lexicographers do their best to list numbers of senses for words, this kind of listing does not necessarily mean that ordinary speakers maintain such lists as their lexical representations for words. Once again, it may be likely that word meanings are always created in the context of their use and there may not be a process that abstract away from these contexts to form a mental lexicon.

Processing Metaphorical Word Meanings in Context

How do people process polysemous metaphorical word meanings in context? This question has been examined using various experimental techniques in studies on lexical ambiguity resolution and figurative language processing. There are far fewer studies on metaphorical word processing than exist for ambiguous word processing, although many of the studies on lexical ambiguity employ stimuli that may indeed be metaphorical (e.g., the word *bug* in reference to a spy device may be a metaphorical extension of the word *bug* used to refer to an insect – Swinney 1979). But the studies on metaphorical word processing, again, present a mixed picture of how people immediately deal with polysemous word meanings, some of which may be metaphorical. Part of the difficulty with this work is that scholars mostly compare processing of a single, yet unspecified, metaphorical word meaning to a single, but often broader, literal meaning. Few studies explore how the relationships between different metaphorical senses influence metaphorical word comprehension in context.

For instance, one research project examined comprehension of more or less familiar metaphorical expressions (Blasko & Connine 1993). Participants in these experiments heard different sentences and made lexical decisions at various times to visually presented word strings. For instance, as participants heard the sentence *The belief that hard work is a ladder is common to this generation*, they saw a letter string immediately after hearing the word *ladder*. The visually presented letter string was related to some aspect of the sentence's literal meaning (e.g., *rungs*), the sentence's metaphoric meaning (e.g., *advance*), or was a control word unrelated to the sentence (e.g., *pastry*). The results revealed that participants were equally fast in responding to the literal and metaphorical targets, both of which were faster than the controls. This was true both when participants made their lexical decisions immediately after hearing the critical word (e.g., *ladder*), and when the same decisions were made 300 msecs after hearing the critical word.

However, the findings differed when participants made these same types of lexical decisions to literal and metaphorical targets having heard less familiar expressions, such as *The thought that a good professor is an oasis was clung to by the entire class*. In this case, only literal targets were primed immediately after hearing the critical word (e.g., *oasis*), while responses to the metaphorical targets were facilitated only 750 msecs after the critical word. These findings generally imply that people can infer metaphorical meanings directly for familiar metaphors, but access some aspects of literal meaning when interpreting novel metaphors.

Although Blasko and Connine's conclusion seems reasonable, this type of experiment examines different aspects of meaning (word vs. phrasal) when it compares response times to literal (word) and metaphoric (phrasal) targets. The literal target 'rung' is a simple semantic associate of the word *ladder*, while the metaphoric target 'advance' relates to the general meaning of the entire expression. This makes it difficult to conclude anything about the time-course under which so-called literal and metaphorical meanings are processed. Furthermore, the words used as literal and metaphoric targets in these studies do not seem to reflect very distinctive literal and metaphoric meanings. The literal target 'rung', for instance, is related to the idea of advancing (i.e., the metaphoric target) given that climbing ladders, even literally speaking, is one kind advancing along some physical path. Once again, the so-called literal meaning may be broad enough to evoke metaphorical meanings. These confounds make it difficult to accept Blasko and Connine's study as a fair test of the primacy of literal versus metaphoric processing during metaphor understanding.

A different set of studies examined whether the language processor initially accesses an interpretation that can be compatible with both a word's literal and metaphoric meanings (i.e., the abstractionist or underspecification views). Consider the verb *disarmed* in *Mrs. Graham is quite certain that they disarmed about every critic who was opposed to spending more money on art*. The use of *disarmed* reflects its subordinate, metaphorical interpretation (as determined by pre-tests). The results of an experiment measuring readers' eye-movements suggests that the processing difficulty with the subordinate sense of *disarmed*, relative to when the word was used in a literal, dominant sense (e.g., *After the capture of the village, we disarmed about every rebel and sent them to prison*), did not emerge until after the critical verb was read (Pickering & Frisson 2001). Context appears to reduces processing difficulty, but the difference again did not emerge until much after the verb was seen.

This work suggests that people did not initially access either a specific sense or several senses for an ambiguous verb, but alternatively initially recovered a general, underspecified meaning for the verb and then created a further concrete instantiation of its meaning later on. According to the underspecification model, then, context does not operate to judge between different word meanings, but functions to change an underspecified, or highly general meaning, into a specific interpretation. In this way, the putative distinction between literal and metaphoric senses of a word is irrelevant, at least in terms of ordinary processing. As noted earlier, the underspecification model suffers from the problem of generally not being able to specify exactly what constitutes the abstract, underspecified meaning of a polysemous word. Moreover, even if such a meaning could be articulated, there is no direct evidence indicating that people ordinarily access this underspecified meaning during online language processing. The fact that processing times to read specific verbs (i.e., used in their dominate and subordinate senses) are equivalent does not imply that only an abstract meaning has been initially accessed.

A different model of metaphorical word processing assumes that the highly salient meanings of both words and phrases are automatically processed during the initial stages of metaphor comprehension, the graded salience hypothesis (Giora 2002). Salient meanings are those that are most typically associated with a word across contexts. Salient meanings are independent of embodied meaning, semantic meanings, accessible referential meanings, and literally-based minimal meanings, each of which include information that, strictly speaking, have little to do with the immediate accessibility of familiar, frequent meanings outside of context. One experiment, for example, used a word-fragment completion task (i.e., say the word that comes next) to see if reading familiar metaphors produce two salient meanings (i.e., a literal and metaphoric), while novel metaphors initially produce only one (i.e., a literal) (Giora & Fein 1999). Results showed that reading familiar metaphors in metaphorically biased contexts (e.g., *In order to solve the math problem, the student broke her head*) retained both the metaphor (i.e., 'great effort') and literal (i.e., 'wound') meanings, but that only a literal meaning was available when these same metaphors were read in context inducing a a literal meaning (e.g., *Because she was so careless when she jumped into the pool, the student broke her head*). Reading unfamiliar metaphors results in only a literal meaning being initially available in both types of contexts. These results were interpreted as showing that salience meanings for metaphorically used words are always activated regardless of context.

The graded salience hypothesis is similar to the underspecification model in that context has its effect only after some initial meaning is automatically accessed. This work is inconsistent with research supporting a constraint-based, context-sensitive account of lexical ambiguity resolution (Vu, Kellas, Metcalf & Herman 2000). Constraint satisfaction models of online processing propose that information from various sources, both linguistic and nonlinguistic, is used early on in the immediate processing of words in discourse (McCrae, Spivey-Knowlton & Tannenhaus 1998). As usual in the debates on lexical ambiguity, researchers argue about the stimulus materials (e.g., the strength of contexts) and methods used to examine the meanings initially accessed or constructed during online comprehension. We think it fair to say that there is little consensus in the psycholinguistic literature over whether some context-free meaning of a metaphorically used word is initially accessed during online processing.

Other studies, nonetheless, suggest that people's quick comprehension of metaphorical words in context may involve complex conceptual and embodied information. For instance, a series of reading-time studies examined people comprehension of fictive motion sentences, such as *The road runs along the coast*. Although fictive motion expressions communicate no explicit motion (i.e., roads do not literally run), people may understand these statements in terms of implicit, imaginary sensations of movement. Experimental studies show this is true (Matlock 2005). Participants read stories about protagonists traveling through spatial regions and then made speeded decisions about whether a fictive motion statement related to the story. Reading times in different experiments were faster when sentences followed stories depicting short distances, fast motion, and uncluttered terrains. People gave faster positive decisions to statements containing fast verbs, such as *The road runs along the coast*, than to expressions with slower verbs, such as *The road meandered along the coast*. None of these differences were found in control studies examining comprehension of nonfictive motion spatial sentences, suggesting that the fictive motion effects are not due to lexical priming. These findings imply that embodied simulation is critical to processing fictive motion, in that people may understand the metaphorical use of a polysemous word like *run* by "replaying" the movement, reconstructing a mental enactment of movement implicit in the sentence. People are not aware of these simulations, and so fictive motion processing is not dependent on deliberate thought about motion.

Matlock's data are not consistent with the idea that people understand a word like *run* as having some abstract meaning that is common to all possible contexts it may occur in. Instead, people's processing of metaphorical words is a creative process rather than one in which some pre-specified meaning is accessed and applied.

Do Mental Lexicons Contain Metaphorical (or any other) Meanings?

Most theories of word meaning and polysemy assume that the lexicon is the repository of all the knowledge needed to specify the meanings of words in sentences. Once a word's meaning, perhaps the literal meaning, is accessed from the lexicon, it is then passed to the conceptual system for further nonlinguistic interpretation. Yet determining whether some aspect of metaphorical word meaning is accessed or derived from linguistic or non-linguistic knowledge is problematic. Thus, the particular knowledge that one relies on to infer metaphorical meaning can be indeterminate between lexical and nonlexical.

Consider the following expression *Alpine France is dominated by new brutalist architecture: stacked rabbit hutches reaching into the sky* (Kilgarriff 2001). The phrase *rabbit hutch*, of course, does not refer to actually little hutches containing furry little animals, but to human residences that are rabbit-hutch-like being uncomfortably small. Thus, *rabbit hutch* is a collocation that can be understood based on general knowledge that buildings and rooms, when small and cramped, may be similar to rabbit residences. Moreover, the knowledge that both are small is similarly indeterminate between lexical and general knowledge because it is based on the definitions of hutch (lexical knowledge) or based on one's familiarity with pet rabbit residences (general knowledge). This example, among others, shows that there must also be a significant repository of specific knowledge about each word, the context it normally occurs in, and the different ways these norms have been exploited in the past.

In fact, many earlier theories of lexical semantics and language comprehension suggest that words serve as pointers or instructions to conceptual knowledge by which language is understood, as opposed to possessing context-free meanings on their own (Bransford, Barclay & Franks 1972; Winograd 1983). Contemporary connectionist models of word learning concretely demonstrate how word meaning need not be encoded in a mental lexicon that is separate from conceptual and experiential knowledge (Elman 2003).

Various psycholinguistic findings support the idea that a word's lexical representation simply points to a general-purpose conceptual system in which the meanings of words are retrieved and combined using both linguistic and non-linguistic (e.g., conceptual) information. To take one example, people in one series of experiments were asked to quickly judge whether a sentence was plausible both when one of its words was replaced with a picture, called a rebus sentence (e.g., a picture of a stool replaced *stool*), and when the sentence contained all its words (Potter, Kroll, Yachzel, Carpenter & Sherman 1986). Because a pictorial object is conceptually but not lexically equivalent to the corresponding noun, the ability to understand rebus sentences would support the hypothesis that a noun acts as a conceptual element. The logic of these experiments was to present sentences so rapidly that a delay in encoding the rebus pictures into the needed linguistic form would be highly disruptive. Difficulty with understanding a rebus sentence would support the hypothesis that a noun (e.g., *stool*) taps specific lexical information during composition of sentence meaning. However, the main result of these studies was that rebus sentences were not more difficult to understand, and later remember, than equivalent all-word sentences. These findings support the idea that a word's lexical representation simply points to a general-purpose conceptual system in which the meanings of words are retrieved and combined.

More recently, Carston (2002) considered the possibility that in utterance interpretation, (a) almost every concept has to be built ad hoc, and that (b) words are only pointers to conceptual spaces. Under this alternative view, linguistic elements such as words or phrases do not have a meaning per se, but only provide clues to conceptual spaces that can be narrowed down or loosened to conceptual elements in context. Consider, again, the expression in (5) *Robert is a bulldozer*. How does one go from *Robert is a bulldozer* to understanding that Robert is single-minded, persistent, insensitive, and so on? First, we can suppose that any metaphorical utterance appears in a communicative context that facilitates understanding of its meaning, precisely because of the communicative principle of relevance. Even if a speaker may not always succeed in creating the best utterance for a given situation, she will at least try to achieve this aim in ostensive communication. Second, ad hoc category construction assumes that words point to conceptual spaces that are partly structured as enduring metaphorical concepts. In fact, there is a great deal of linguistic and psychological evidence showing that people readily access rich metaphorical domains/concepts during many aspects of reasoning and immediate linguistic processing (Gibbs 2006; Gibbs & Tendahl 2006). With these two assumptions, in *Robert is a bulldozer*, the word *bulldozer* typically points to a set of familiar conceptual metaphors, such as PEOPLE ARE MACHINES, THE MIND IS A MACHINE, THINKING IS MECHANICAL ACTIVITY, and so on. In some instances, the link between a lexical concept and a specific conceptual metaphor may be so entrenched that a specific metaphorical concept is immediately accessed, and found to help establish a relevant reading of *Robert is a bulldozer*. In other cases, listeners will need to test various conceptual metaphors in order of their accessibility until finding one that creates an interpretation of *Robert is a bulldozer* which satisfies the expectation of optimal relevance. Not surprisingly, the more accessible a conceptual metaphor is given a lexical concept, the easier it will be to create an appropriate ad hoc concept and to understand a metaphorically used word.

Our suggestion that metaphorically used words, and indeed all words, need not have fully specified meanings listed in a mental lexicon that is separate from nonlinguistic knowledge is contrary to the belief held by many linguists and psycholinguists. Nonetheless, word meanings may be created on the fly given contextual information and past history of use. This does not imply that the meanings created for a metaphorical word will never have contextually inappropriate meanings being activated. After all, the process of creating meaning will travel along certain pathways in which so-called conventional, highly salient meanings may be accessed given, again, past histories of the words use for a speaker/listener. Yet the problems of identifying, specifying, and processing metaphorical words meanings are complex enough to cast doubts on traditional models of polysemy as structured entirely within individual mental lexicons.

References

American Heritage Dictionary, (3rd edition): New York: Houghton Mifflin.

Barsalou, L. (1995): Flexibility, structure, and linguistic vagary in concepts: Manifestations of a compositional system of perceptual symbols. In: Collins, A., Gathercole, S., Conway, M. & Morris, P. (eds.): *Theories of memory*. Hillsdale, NJ: L. Erlbaum.

Blasko, D. & Connine, C. (1993): Effects of familiarity and aptness on metaphor processing. *Journal of Experimental Psychology: Learning, Memory, and Cognition* 19, 295-308.

Bransford, J., Barclay, J. & Franks, J. (1972): Sentence memory: A constructive versus interpretive approach. *Cognitive Psychology* 3 193-209.

Brugman, C., & Lakoff, G. (1988): Cognitive typology and lexical networks. In Small, S., Cottrell, G. & Tannenhaus, M. (eds.): *Lexical ambiguity resolution*. Palo Alto, CA: Morgan Kaufman, 477-508.

Caramazza, A., & Grober, E. (1976): Polysemy and the structure of the subjective lexicon. In: Rameh, C. (ed.): *Semantics: Theory and application*. Washington, DC: Georgetown University Press, 181-206.

Carston, R. (2002): *Thoughts and utterances*. London: Blackwell.

Columbo, L. & Flores d'Arcais, G. (1984): The meanings of Dutch prepositions: A psycholinguistic study of polysemy. *Linguistics* 22, 51-98.

Croft, W. & Cruse, A. (2004): *Cognitive linguistics*. New York: Cambridge University Press.

Deignan, A. (in press): Metaphor and corpus linguistics. In Gibbs, R. (ed.): *Cambridge handbook of metaphor and thought*. New York: Cambridge University Press.

Durkin, K. & Manning, J. (1989): Polysemy and the subjective lexicon: Semantic relatedness and the salience of intraword senses. *Journal of Psycholinguistic Research* 18, 577-612.

Elman, J. (2004): An alternative view of the mental lexicon. *Trends in Cognitive Science* 5, 101-111.

Evans, Y. (2003): *The structure of time: Language, meaning and temporal cognition*. Amsterdam: Benjamins.

Gibbs, R. (1992): What do idioms really mean? *Journal of Memory and Language* 31, 485-506.

Gibbs, R. (1994): *The poetics of mind: Figurative thought, language, and understanding*. New York: Cambridge University Press.

Gibbs, R. (2005): Literal and nonliteral meanings are corrupt ideas: The view from psycholinguistics. In: Lewondoka, B. & Coulson, S. (eds.): *The literal and nonliteral continuum*. Berlin: Lang.

Gibbs, R. (2006): *Embodiment and cognitive science*. New York: Cambridge University Press.

Gibbs, R. & Tendahl, M. (2006): Cognitive effort and effects in metaphor comprehension: Relevance theory and psycholinguistics. *Mind & Language* 21, 329-403.

Gibbs, R., Beitel, D., Harrington, M. & Sanders, S. (1994): Taking a stand on the meanings of "stand": Bodily experience as motivation for polysemy. *Journal of Semantics* 11, 231-251.

Gibbs, R., Buchalter, D., Moise, J. & Farrar, W. (1993): Literal meaning and figurative language. *Discourse Processes* 16, 387-403.

Giora, R. (2003): *On our mind: Salience, context, and figurative language*. New York: Oxford.

Groesfema, M. (1995): Can, may, must, and should: A relevance theoretic account. *Journal of Linguistics* 31, 53-79.

Keysar, B., Shen, Y., Glucksberg, S. & Horton, W. (2000): Conventional language: How metaphoric is it? *Journal of Memory and Language* 43, 576-593.

Kilgarriff, A. (2001): Generative lexicon meets corpus data: The case of nonstandard Uses. In: Bouillon, P. & Busa, F. (eds.): *The language of word meaning*. New York: Cambridge University Press, 312-330.

Lakoff, G. (1987): *Women, fire, and dangerous things: What categories reveal about the mind*. Chicago: University of Chicago Press.

Lakoff, G. & Johnson, M. (1980): *Metaphors we live by*. Chicago: University of Chicago Press.

Matlock, T. (2005): Fictive motion as cognitive simulation. *Memory & Cognition* 32, 1389-1440.

McRae, K., Spivey-Knowlton, M. & Tannenhaus, M. (1998): Modeling the influence of thematic fit (and other constraints) in online sentence comprehension. *Journal of Memory and Language* 38, 283-312.

Miller, G. & Charles, W. (1991): Contextual correlates of semantic similarity. *Language and Cognitive Processes* 6, 1-28.

Moon, R. (2004): On specifying metaphor: an idea and its implementation. *International Journal of Lexicography* 17 195-222.

Nunberg, G. (1979): The non-uniqueness of semantic solutions: Polysemy. *Linguistics & Philosophy* 2, 143-184.

Potter, M., Kroll, J., Yachzel, B., Carpenter, E., & Sherman, J. (1986): Pictures in sentences: Understanding without words. *Journal of Experimental Psychology: General* 115, 281-294.

Rakova, M. (2003): *The extent of the literal: Metaphor, polysemy, and theories of concepts.* New York: Palgrave.

Ruhl, C. (1989): *Monosemy: A study in linguistic semantics*. Stony Brook, NY: SUNY Press.

Sandra, D. & Rice, S. (1995): Network analyses of prepositional meaning: Mirroring whose mind- the linguist's or the language user's. *Cognitive Linguistics* 6, 89-130.

Semino, E., Heywood, J. & Short, M. (2004): Methodological problems in the analysis of metaphor in a corpus of conversations about cancer. *Journal of Pragmatics* 36, 1271-1294.

Steen, G. (2002): Metaphor identification: A cognitive approach. *Style* 36, 286-41.

Sweetser, E. (1986): Polysemy vs. abstraction: Mutually exclusive or complementary. *Proceedings of the Twelve Annual Meeting of the Berkeley Linguistics Society.* Berkeley: Berkeley Linguistic Society, 528-538.

Swinney, D. (1979): Lexical access during sentence comprehension: (Re)consideration of context effects. *Journal of Verbal Learning and Verbal Behavior* 18, 645-659.

Taylor, J. (1995): *Linguistic categorization*. Oxford: Clarendon Press.

Vallee-Tourangeau, F., Anthony, S. & Austin, N. (1998): Strategies for generating multiple instances of common and ad hoc categories. *Memory* 6, 555-592.

Vu, H., Kellas, G., Metcalf, K. & Herman, R. (1999): The influence of global discourse on lexical ambiguity resolution. *Memory & Cognition* 28, 236-252.

Williams, J. (1992): Processing polysemous words in context: Evidence for interrelated meanings. *Journal of Psycholinguistic Research* 21, 193-218.

Winograd, T. (1983): *Language as a cognitive process*. Malden, MA: Addison-Wesley.

PART II

THE NATURE OF POLYSEMY

The Phenomenon of Polysemy and Ways to Describe It*

Anna A. Zalizniak

The Institute of Linguistics at the Russian Academy of Science, Typology Section
1/12 Bolshoj Kislovskij pereulok, 125009 Moscow
E-mail: anna-zalizniak@mtu-net.ru

1. Preliminary Remarks

One of the main constituents in the paradigm change that we have been witnessing in linguistics over the last twenty years is the gravitation of the semantic theory away from **synonymy**, which in the 1960-70s was the basic category of semantics, towards **polysemy**. Let us note that what is crucial here is the change in the methodological attitude and the general outlook on the phenomenon of linguistic meaning – one may recall the once popular understanding of **meaning** as an **invariant of synonymic transformations** relying, in particular, on the ideas of Jakobson.[1] The point is that the boundary between synonymy and polysemy is largely a matter of conceptualisation: thus, among the "synonymic resources of language" (cf. the subtitle of Apresjan's 1974 book) we find, for example, various transformations relating to diathetic change, – and these kinds of transformation as variable realisations of a word's potential are among the main concerns of the contemporary theory of polysemy. Besides, to the present time Apresjan's *Lexical Semantics* (1974) remains one of the foundational works in the study of **polysemy**, including **regular polysemy**, which is still of central interest to today's semantics.

Linguistics has at its disposal a number of basic oppositions which concern the organisation of language as a whole and against whose background one's attitude towards polysemy may be formed. These are primarily:

1. Discreteness (discontinuity) vs. gradualness (continuity). This opposition is the most global as it is essential to all levels and aspects of language functioning. With regard to the structure of polysemy it concerns the status of a particular word meaning:

---

* Publication of the present paper was supported by the Research Group for Theoretical Linguistics of the Hungarian Academy of Sciences at the Universities of Debrecen, Pécs and Szeged. An earlier version of this article appeared in *Voprosy Jazykoznanija* 2004/2: 20-45. The choice of article for inclusion in this volume was the author's own. Translated by Marina Rakova. The author would like to thank Ju.D. Apresjan, A.A. Kibrik, S.A. Krylov, I.L. Mikaeljan, E.V. Paducheva, N.V. Percov, E.Ju. Protasova and A.D. Shmelev, whose comments on earlier drafts of this paper influenced its final shape. The translator thanks Professor James Miller for comments on the English text.

1 See, for instance, Jakobson (1955), Paducheva (1974: 10-33), Mel'chuk (1999: 10).

do different meanings of a word form a multitude of discrete units or an uninterrupted continuum in which one meaning gradually merges with another?

2. Humboldt's contrast between *ergon* and *energeia* (1836: 150), for instance, do people in the process of speaking **construct** grammatical forms, phrases and sentences according to some formulae or models, – or do they **memorise** them "ready-made" (and later insert in their own speech)?

3. Is language a system of "pure significations" where the meaning of each sign is determined by its place in the system of oppositions (cf. Saussure 1973/1916), or does every word in each instance of its use express the unique sense given to it by the speaker, the sense which is a resultant of an infinite number of factors (in particular as it draws on the unique personal experience of the speaker)? In this connection: can the hearer grasp the sense which the speaker wishes to convey? Is the identification of senses generally possible?

It seems that no single answer should be sought for any of these questions, no single answer that would be the same for all linguistic units in the full complexity of their functions. Language, obviously, houses the discrete and the gradual, the reproduced and the generated, the objectively systematic and the subjectively unique. One should also remember that different styles of language acquisition and use may characterise different speakers of a language depending on their type of mentality (cf. the notion of "cognitive learning style" used in developmental psychology). Indeed, along with an unconscious identification of the structure of one's native language with the structure of language in general (which has been remarked on before) another rather common methodological aberration among linguists is the identification of one's own mastery of language with the uniquely possible. In particular, the debate about whether the language learner acquires **rules** or **chunks of language** and the opposition between theories supporting one or the other postulate seem to rest on the false premise that there is a unique way in which language is acquired and used by all people.

Plungian and Rakhilina (Plungian & Rakhilina 1996, 2000; Plungian 2001) develop an approach to the description of strongly polysemous linguistic units (prepositions and prefixes) which combines the advantages of the atomistic lexicographic approach and the holistic cognitive one. These authors begin from the premise that the central problem in the description of polysemy is finding the boundary which separates the **reproduced** from the **generated**, – that which is "remembered" from that which is "construed" (Plungian & Rakhilina 1996: 5f.). If we follow their line of thought, the description of polysemy must comprise two parts. To that which lies to the one side of the boundary there corresponds something like a list of a word's submeanings (which the speaker is supposed to know, if he/she has mastered the meaning of a given polysemous word – or must learn, if he/she wishes to master it). To that which is situated on the other side of the boundary there corresponds something like a list of "instructions", i.e. rules of meaning transformation which the speaker of a language is supposed to apply when using polysemous words. This way of formulating the problem seems entirely correct. One should, however, keep in mind that along with all the other difficulties that one will encounter when trying to separate the "reproduced" from the "generated" one may have to admit the possibility that the boundary in question will most probably have to be mapped differently not only for words of different semantic and grammatical classes but also for different speakers.

On the whole, today it seems indisputable that polysemy is an essential property of language serving its three major functions: the cognitive, the communicative and the poetic.

2. Polysemy and Ambiguity

In Russian linguistic terminology there are two terms corresponding to the English 'polysemy': *polisemija* and *mnogoznachnost'* (lit. 'many-meaningness'). They are virtually synonymous, although there are some slight differences in their use. *Polisemija* is understood as a purely paradigmatic relation: the fact that a word has more than one meaning (i.e. the term *polisemija* is reserved for **lexical** polysemy), whereas *mnogoznachnost'* may also be syntagmatic: the term may apply to the possibility of **simultaneous** realisation of two (or more) meanings for a given linguistic unit. Thus, it also encompasses *neodnoznachnost'* ('ambiguity', lit. 'not-single-meaningness').

Phrases or texts are said to be **ambiguous** (*mnogoznachnyj*) if they simultaneously have several distinct senses. Depending on the kind of senses involved one distinguishes between **lexical** ambiguity (e.g., *proexat' ostanovku*: 'cover a certain distance [between two bus stops]' and 'go past a point [a bus stop]'; *pereizbrat' Petrova*: 'elect Petrov for a further term' and 'elect somebody else to occupy Petrov's post') and **syntactic** ambiguity (e.g., Lat. *amor patris* ['love of/for the father]; *mat' ljubit doch'*: 'the mother loves the daughter' and 'the daughter loves the mother'; *flying planes can be dangerous*, etc.). Apresjan distinguishes between **language** ambiguity (lexical and syntactic) and **speech** ambiguity, which arises in an utterance because of the underdetermined character of some parameters (1974: 176ff.). He illustrates the latter type of ambiguity with examples like *John prostrelil sebe ruku* ('John shot through his (own) hand') or *Gusar zazvenel shporami* ('The hussar clanked his spurs'), where the verbs can designate both intentional and unintentional actions. However, it seems that here the distinction must be drawn in a slightly different way. With respect to the type of ambiguity involved, the use of questions like *When was Pushkin born?* in an exam context is on a par with other shifts in the illocutionary function of a question (*Can you pass me the salt?*, *Do you know what time it is?*, *How much longer do I have to wait?*, *Where are you going?*, etc.). In cases like these one and the same sentence may be used with different illocutionary functions, and therefore mean something different. The possibility to express two different meanings is guaranteed here, as in the case of syntactic or lexical ambiguity, by language structure; two different meanings cannot be "intended" simultaneously, and the hearer is usually capable of selecting the right interpretation (Percova 1988 calls this kind of ambiguity **disjunctive**). But if the hearer resolves the ambiguity incorrectly (for example, responding *Yes, I do* to the question *Do you know what time it is?*), there is a **communication failure**. The same happens when somebody takes an exam question for an ordinary one (cf. the joke in which to the teacher's question *When was Pushkin born?* the pupil responds *I wish I had your worries, Sir!*).

A different kind of ambiguity is presumably involved in sentences like *The hussar clanked his spurs*. Whereas in the examples above different meanings exclude each other, here both readings – intentional and unintentional – are quite compatible in the sense that in order to understand sentences like this one the hearer does not have to **choose** between the two interpretations. Some aspects of the situation may simply remain unknown to us (namely, whether the person did the action in question intentionally or not, just as we may not know why, with what purpose, how, etc. he did it). That is, we are dealing here not with ambiguity but rather with the **indefiniteness** of some parameters, and thus an incomplete understanding of the situation (put differently, it is not **ambiguity** that is the case here but **vagueness**). Likewise, insufficient context may not let us choose, for example, between the resultative and the non-resultative interpretation of the general-factual use of the imperfective aspect in sentences like *Kto stroil etot dom?* ([Who build$_{\text{PAST-IMPF}}$ this house?] – the construction of the house may be finished or not; cf. Paducheva 1996: 33).

Thus, while **language ambiguity** is the capacity of a word, phrase or construction to have distinct senses, i.e. it is a property of linguistic units, **speech ambiguity** is the realisation of this property in an utterance. Speech ambiguity may be unintentional (in which case either it will be resolved in the course of further communication or there will be a communication failure), but it may also be intentional, i.e. it may be used as a special device (see below).

Ambiguity as coexistence of a multitude of different interpretations a **literary text** may have is recognised by some researchers to be an inherent property of such texts: the simultaneous presence of two or more distinct understandings available for a word, phrase or whole text creates a new meaning (see Jakobson 1960; Eco 1962; Empson 1966). For this reason the meaning of a poetic text goes beyond not only its literal but also its **conveyed** meaning (according to Grice 1975): what the author of a poetic text **wanted to say** results from the interaction of its explicit and implicit meanings. From the legion of examples that could be cited here let us reproduce only one: – *Parizh? – I ja s toboj parju* (addressing a lady who is in Paris; from oral discourse), literally meaning: 'Paris?' – 'And I'm soaring with you.' Here a fusion between the idea of Paris and that of soaring, which, on the phonetic level, results from the coincidence of sound shapes of the forms *Parizh* ('Paris', pronounced as [par'ish]) and *parish'* (the 2nd person singular form of the verb *parit'*, 'to soar', also pronounced as [par'ish]) on the semantic level gives a new expression to the Russian cultural myth of Paris[2]; the three ideas together constitute the meaning of this text.

The ambiguity of a poetic text may have different origins: it may be generated both by the ambiguity of words or word forms used and the ambiguity of a text as a whole, which includes allegory, allusion, different intertextual elements, the simultaneous presence of two different planes of description (two different story lines or situations with which one and the same text correlates), etc. The latter type of ambiguity is a constitutive property of such genres as proverb, adage and riddle, for example: *Tishe edesh' – dal'she budesh'* (lit. 'The slower you go the further you get'; cf. *The lesser the more*), *Na vore shapka gorit* (lit. 'The thief's hat burns on him'; cf. *The thief gives his game away*), *What goes on four legs in the morning, on two legs at noon, and on three*

2 The idea of Paris as the capital of the world and the centre of light, carefree existence.

legs in the evening? (the riddle of the Sphinx), etc. One of the major sources of poetic ambiguity is **metaphor**, which is based on the simultaneous presence of two denotationally distinct but conceptually identical levels of representation.

Another important source of poetic ambiguity is the animation of the "inner form"[3] of a word (as a result of which a word acquires an extra sense, to a greater or smaller extent different from its literal meaning, and this leads to a peculiar stereoscopic effect). What frequently happens here is that the primary, usually spatial image or physical phenomenon which served as the basis for the creation of an abstract concept becomes reconstructed, as in:[4]

(1) *I vot eshche pochemu vsjakaja bol'shaja ljubov' s tochki zrenija ustroennogo byta* ***pre-stupna***.[5]

'And here is another reason why any big love, from the point of view of well-arranged domestic life, is **criminal**.' (lit. **trans-gressive**).

A more complex interplay of meanings is also possible, as in:

(2) [...] *a ponizhe skvozil, kak v glubokoj vode, rasplyvchato-temnyj prislon stula, stavimogo tak vvidu* ***popolznovenija*** *dverej medlenno, s* ***sodroganijami***, *raz"ezzhat'sja.*[6]

'[...] while lower down there showed through, as if in deep water, the fuzzy dark back of a chair placed in that position to foil the **propensity** of the door-leaves to crawl apart in a series of **jerks** [lit. 'in view of the door-leaves **crawling** towards sliding apart slowly, with **shudders**']'.

The expressions in bold originally denoted physical phenomena, but in today's standard Russian they have only their derived meanings which belong to the sphere of a human person's internal states. In the examples above they are used in the occasional derived meanings returning them to the sphere of physical objects; however, the standard meanings, relating them to the realm of a person's internal states, are also present.

"Poetic" ambiguity may arise from the non-obviousness of the author's position, the availability of different "interpretation levels"; genre indefiniteness (cf. Gugel 1967 on the genre of Catullus's poem LI); referential indeterminacy for personal pronouns (in particular, in lyric poetry), and many other factors. Still, even a brief examination of this fascinating field would be beyond the scope of the present article. Poetic ambiguity falls within the province of linguistics only insofar as it is based on language ambiguity (see, for instance, Jakobson 1960; Lotman 1970; Nikolaeva 1997; Uspensky 1994; Percov 2000; Zalizniak 2006: 347-391).

---

3 Meaning reconstructed from the etymology of a word or from the primary meaning of its constituent morphemes (the term of Potebnja 1976: 175).

4 My emphasis in the examples below and thereafter – A.Z.

5 Prishvin: *Dnevniki* [Journals].

6 Nabokov: *Tjazhelyj dym* [Torpid smoke]. In: *A Russian Beauty and Other Stories*. New York: McGraw-Hill International, Inc., 1973: 28.

The main difference between "colloquial" and "poetic" ambiguity is that in everyday communication only one of two possible understandings of an expression is correct with respect to the intentions of the speaker, and a broader context (linguistic or situational) should let the hearer choose the correct understanding. Otherwise there is a communication failure: 'Avoid ambiguity' is one of Grice's (1975) conversational maxims. Thus, with regard to the communicative function of language an utterance's ambiguity is speech "waste", an obstacle which leads to the speech act's failure and must be eliminated as far as possible. Ambiguity of this kind may arise if the hearer incorrectly establishes the referents of names used by the speaker, lacks the necessary presuppositions and knowledge of the world, or **infers** something that was not **implied** by the speaker (cf. Bybee et al. 1994: 285; Paducheva 2004: 101). However, in this case one cannot categorise utterances into ambiguous and unambiguous: for a non-co-operative hearer any utterance may acquire a "parasitic" interpretation. Indeed, the number of logically conceivable (but in the context of a real speech act inappropriate and therefore immediately cancelled) interpretations available for virtually any utterance is simply striking. Besides, often it is the literal meaning that is the most absurd (and is automatically rejected by "normal" speakers). This property of linguistic communication is brought to the fore in the texts of Lewis Carroll (cf. Paducheva 1982), as well as in the legend about the Golem of Prague, a creature made of clay and given life by a rabbi from Prague, who could not speak and whose ability to understand language was confined to literal meaning. That is why when the rabbi's wife told him to *bring water to the house* he began to bring buckets of water from the well and pour the water out onto the floor, and later had the following encounter with an apple stall keeper:

(3) *– Look at him! – the stall keeper was outraged – **he wants me to give him my whole stall for his groszy** [= pennies]!*[7]
*Having thought a little, Golem decided that the woman was right. **That was exactly what he wanted**. He lifted the stall with all the apples and the keeper thrown into the bargain, put it on his shoulder and headed home.*

The resolution of potential ambiguity at all levels (first of all, morphological and syntactic) is one of the main problems for automated text analysis, which remains current to the present day. Apparently,

> that which people do easily when understanding a text, relying in their choice of interpretation for ambiguous elements on common sense, world knowledge and broad communicative context, is still inaccessible to any computational system (Boguslavsky et al. 2003: 40).

With respect to lexical meaning the term **ambiguity** is often used in this field as a synonym for the term **homonymy**: when ambiguity is seen as an obstacle to the tasks of analysis, the difference between polysemy and homonymy becomes inessential.

---

7 From *Kuvshin s medom. Evrejskie legendy i skazki* [A Jug of Honey: Jewish Legends and Folk Tales]. Moscow, 1991: 75. See also Gershon Winkler (1980): *The Golem of Prague: A New Adaptation of the Documented Stories of the Golem of Prague*. Judaica Press.

3. Ambiguity and Language Games

Exploiting language ambiguity is a favourite trick of advertisers. It is a kind of **language game**, and the effect achieved by it is based on the pleasure derived from playing the game successfully: the "success" of an advert's addressee as a partner in the game is constituted by their discovery of two senses simultaneously present in the text of an advert. Note that this pleasure is of purely semiotic nature. Indeed, the secondary sense is often to some extent sexually suggestive,[8] although this is not necessary, as in:

(4) (a) *Kakaja **svjaz'** mezhdu Moskvoj i Podmoskov'em? – Moskovskaja sotovaja.*
'What is the **link** between Moscow and the Moscow Region? – Moscow CellLink.'

(b) ***S nashej obuv'ju** vy ne rasstanetes' nikogda*
'**With our shoes** you will never part.' (Caption under a picture where a man and a woman are tied to each other with the laces of their shoes.)

(c) *Gde voznikaet atmosfera **blizosti** i dushevnogo **tepla**? Konechno, na divane.*
'Where do you find the atmosphere of **closeness** and soul-**warming** concord? Of course, on a sofa.' (The picture shows a small sofa with two people sitting on it close to each other.)

(d) *Ne ostavljajte veshchi **bez vnimanija**. Novyj bol'shoj katalog IKEA.*
'Don't leave things **unattended** (lit. 'without attention'). The new big IKEA catalogue.'

Thus, functionally, advertising is closer to the poetic text than to practical communication, in which ambiguity is always negatively appraised and avoided whenever possible. The effect of a certain class of jokes also bases on language ambiguity, as in:

(5) (a) *Pis'mo iz Centra **ne doshlo** do Shtirlica. On prochital eshche raz: opjat' **ne doshlo**.*

'Shtirliz **did not get** the letter from the Centre. He reread it and still **did not get** it.'

(b) *Vstrechajutsja Brezhnev i Andropov na tom svete. Brezhnev sprashivaet:*
– Nu i kto zhe tam v Kremle sejchas glavnyj?
– A Misha Gorbachev.
*– Nu i kto ego **podderzhivaet**?*
*– A nikto ne **podderzhivaet**, on sam xodit.*

'Brezhnev and Andropov meet in the other world. Brezhnev asks:
– And who is now the boss in the Kremlin?
– Mike Gorbachev.

[8] This is reflected in the meaning of the Russian word *dvusmyslennyj* (lit. 'two-sense', cf. the English *double entendre*) as in *dvusmyslennaja shutka* (lit. 'a two-sense joke'), that is 'a joke with an obscene second sense', or *govorit' dvusmyslennosti* (lit. 'say two-sensinesses', cf. *indulge in double entendres*), etc.

– And who **supports** him?
– Nobody **supports** him, he walks by himself.'

The effect of a joke may also be obtained when one uses the same words alternating between their literal and figurative meanings, as in:

(6) *Nu chto eto za* ***cirk****? Eto* ***bordel'*** *kakoj-to, a ne* ***cirk****. Vot u moego djadi v Zhmerinke byl* ***bordel'****, tak eto byl* ***cirk****!*

'And what kind of **circus** is that? It's some **brothel**, not a **circus**. My uncle in Zhmerinka had a **brothel**, and that was a real **circus**! (*cirk* = (1) circus as a show of various performers, (2) a scene of entertaining action; *bordel'* = (1) brothel, (2) complete chaos)'

The fact that a linguistic unit can be used **ambiguously** (first of all, in puns) is the clearest evidence of its "many-meaningness" (cf. Apresjan, 1974: 180ff.). That is, if the use of a word in a given context creates the effect of **zeugma** (punning), contrasting two different understandings, it follows that these two understandings correspond to two distinct meanings of the word in question. Thus, from the sentence *Shel dozhd' i dva studenta, odin byl v shljape, a drugoj – v xoroshem nastroenii* ('There was rain and two students [lit. There was walking rain and two students], one was in a hat, and the other – in a good mood.'), which involves punning, one can conclude to the existence in the Russian language of at least two meanings for the verb *idti* ('to go, walk' and 'to fall' as of rain, etc.) as well as for the construction *byt' v* ('to be in'). However, the fact that two meanings may be contrasted in some context does not eliminate the possibility of neutralising this contrast in another context (see below).

Of course, the zeugma effect is neither a necessary nor a sufficient condition for polysemy: it is not sufficient because punning (zeugma) is neutral with respect to the difference between polysemy and homonymy (cf. *Xoroshuju veshch'* ***brakom*** *ne nazovut.* – 'A good thing won't be called *brak* [(1) marriage, (2) production waste].'), and it is not necessary for the simple reason that it is not always possible to bring together different meanings of a polysemous word in a pun. However, when one has to distinguish between **close** senses, the zeugma effect may undoubtedly be considered as showing the presence of an opposition, and therefore two **distinct** meanings.

4. Types of Non-Zeugmatic Meaning Superposition

Let us first of all consider the notion of **meaning superposition** (*sovmeshchenie znachenij*) itself.[9] Unfortunately, the term is not used unequivocally, and this may lead to some rather vexing misunderstanding, as is the case with the polemic that Sannikov (1999: 181ff.) engages in. Indeed, it would be difficult not to agree with Sannikov's view that "punning (including punning with polysemous words) has no bearing on the question about the unity of a word, the availability of an invariant, etc." (op. cit., 183).

[9] Different kinds of meaning superposition are analysed in much detail in Percova (1988). See also Percov (2000, 2001: 31f.); Empson (1966: ch. I-II).

But this does not in any way undermine Percov's view that the possibility of meaning superposition is evidence of permeable boundaries between individual meanings of a word, an argument in favour of the existence of an invariant (Percov 1996: 27ff.), for zeugmatic and non-zeugmatic meaning superposition are two different phenomena. Whereas punning contrasts and **opposes** – be it meanings of a word, homonyms or any other superficially similar entities (homophones, homographs, accidentally converging forms, etc.) – non-zeugmatic meaning superposition, on the contrary, **unifies** different meanings of a word (note that it is possible for polysemes, but not for homonyms).

Below we will concern ourselves with non-zeugmatic meaning superposition only. At least the following four types may be distinguished.

1. "Gluing" – the unification (within one utterance) of two clearly distinct but not incompatible meanings of a word which does not create any special effect: this "ambiguity" is discovered only by the linguist seeking to identify the dictionary meaning(s) of a word. Instances of "gluing" together two identical signifiers with different signifieds usually go unnoticed by both the speaker and the hearer, but when these are discovered their "de-gluing" causes no difficulty and is absolutely harmless for the meaning of the sentence as a whole. This type of meaning superposition can be illustrated with the following examples, which have been discussed in the literature before:

(7) *Pustoe* ***serdce*** *b'etsja rovno, / V ruke ne drognul pistolet.*[10]
'The empty **heart** beats steadily, / In the hand the pistol did not tremble.'

(8) *Cherez kraj polnaja* ***auditorija*** *byla nespokojna i izdavala gluxoj, sdavlennyj gul.*[11]
'Filled beyond capacity, the **lecture room** was restless and emitted an indistinct, muffled hum.'

In (7) the word *serdce* ('heart') "glues" together the meanings 'the central organ maintaining blood circulation' and 'that organ regarded as the symbol of feeling and emotion'; in (8) the word *auditorija* ('lecture room') simultaneously designates the room and the many people inside it. Percova (1988: 65) correctly characterises (7) as an instance of "conjunctive ambiguity" (i.e. ambiguity presupposing the simultaneous presence of two readings), which is not intentional on the part of the speaker.

In this connection it is interesting to consider the following example, which is discussed in detail in Percov (2000, 2001):

---

[10] Lermontov: *Na smert' poeta* [Death of the Poet]. Uryson (1997: 113) uses this example to illustrate the claim that a word may figure "in an intermediate meaning, which unites components of different (dictionary) definitions". However, it seems that what we find here is precisely a superposition (simultaneous expression) of two different meanings at the level of the given utterance; the word *serdce* ('heart') does not acquire any "intermediate" meaning. Generally speaking, the term "intermediate meaning" seems somewhat infelicitous: to characterise uses that simultaneously have features of two different meanings (which is especially characteristic of prepositions, see Zalizniak 1995) the metaphor of enveloping space would be more appropriate.

[11] Herzen: *Byloe i Dumy* [My Past and Thoughts].

(9) *Figurno il' bukval'no: vsej sem'jej,*
Ot jamshchika do pervogo poeta,
My vse ***poem*** *unylo* [...].[12]
'Figuratively or literally: the whole family,
From the coachman to the first poet,
We all **sing** gloomily [...].'

Percov sees here a non-zeugmatic unification of meanings on the basis of a semantic invariant which includes the features 'aesthetic', 'pleasant', 'rhythmicity' and 'human voice' (2001: 36).

Percov's analysis provokes a number of objections. First of all, the polysemy structure of the verb *pet'* ('to sing') has significantly changed since Pushkin's times: in contemporary Russian 'to utter musical sounds with the voice' is the main and virtually the only meaning the verb has; the meaning 'to read/compose poetry' is completely obsolete; and 'to sing, praise (in verse)' – literary and archaic. Thus, today the character of meaning superposition for this verb is different from what it was in the language of Pushkin, which greatly complicates its analysis.

On the other hand, although there is indeed no zeugma effect in this example, it is impossible to agree that here the superposition of meanings "despite the warning in the first line, is unnoticed by the majority of the readers" (Percov 2000: 58). In these lines Pushkin undoubtedly plays with the possibility of unifying clearly **distinct** senses, and only a very inattentive reader will give the fact no notice. Here the unification of meanings is a device whose aim is to create an **illusion of unity**. As for the invariant, one of the two superposed meanings of the verb *pet'* ('to sing') is 'to compose poetry', i.e. the semantic component 'human voice' is either absent or optional, and thus cannot form part of the invariant (whereas completely excluding this component from the supposed invariant would contradict the main meaning of the verb). It would seem that in this case the possibility for non-zeugmatic meaning superposition is based not on an invariant, but on a stable European cliché "poet – singer", which goes back to the actual superposition of these functions (cf. the realisation of this cliché in Pushkin's 'The poet and the crowd').

2. Fusion.[13] This type of meaning superposition is especially characteristic of poetry. Here two clearly distinct meanings are presented **as if** they were one; however, the perception of their **distinctness** is also preserved, which creates the effect of different things appearing as one, and a new, third sense emerges from their fusion. Let us give two examples for illustration:

(10) *Eshche Mandel'shtam pytalsja mne ob'jasnit', chto takoe uznavanie. [...] On dumal ne tol'ko o processe, t.e. o tom, kak protekaet uznavanie togo, chto my uzhe videli i znali, no i o vspyshke, kotoraja soprovozhdaet uznavanie do six por skrytogo ot nas, eshche neizvestnogo, no voznikajushchego v edinstvenno*

---

12 Pushkin: *Domik v Kolomne* [The little house in Kolomna].

13 Cf. the notion of conceptual blending developed by Fauconnier & Turner (2002).

nuzhnuju minutu, kak sud'ba. Tak uznaetsja slovo, neobxodimoe v stixax, kak by prednaznachennoe dlja nix, tak vxodit v zhizn' chelovek, kotorogo ran'she ne videl, no slovno predchuvstvoval, chto s nim perepletjotsja sud'ba.[14]

'Mandelstam also tried to explain to me what *uznavanie* (learning-recognition) is. [...] He thought not only of a process, i.e. the way in which we recognise something that we have already seen and learnt, but of a flash which accompanies the recognition of something that was hidden from us before, still unknown, but emerging just at the only right minute, like fate. Thus is recognised a word needed in verses, as if destined for them, thus enters our life a person whom we have not seen before but almost felt that fate would bring us together.'

According to dictionaries (for example, *MAS*), the word *uznavanie* (1.'learning'; 2.'recognition'; lit. morph. 'coming-to-knowledge') denotes the intellectual acquisition either of something **new** or of something **old** (identification with an image stored in memory). The use in (10), evidently, does not fall under either of these definitions: here (roughly speaking) we are dealing with the *uznavanie* (learning-recognition) of something new which is subjectively perceived as the acquisition of something that one has known before. However, it is clear that the reader has no difficulty understanding the intended meaning; on the other hand, it is also clear that we do not need to revise the dictionary entry for the word *uznavanie*. Here is the second example:

(11) *Vsjo stalo tjazhelee i gromadnee, potomu i chelovek dolzhen byt'* ***tverzhe*** *vsego na zemle i otnosit'sja k nei, kak almaz k steklu.*[15]

'Everything has become heavier and bigger, that is why a human person too must be **harder** than anything else on earth, and relate to it as an uncut diamond to glass.'

Here the word *tverzhe* expresses a meaning which results from a synthesis of its dictionary meanings. It is precisely synthesis rather than oscillation (see below): the property of **hardness** for a human person referred to in the text is a fusion of the word's literal and figurative meaning.

3. Oscillation. Another type of "poetic" meaning superposition is what is known in linguistics as "oscillating" meanings (see, in particular, Apresjan 1974: 179 who refers to Stern 1931): these are uses in which two or more different meanings are present in a word simultaneously thus creating the effect of oscillation (i.e. different meanings reveal themselves, as it were, in turns). Such use of the verb *videt'* ('to see') can be illustrated with the help of the following example (discussed in Apresjan 1995a):

14 Nadezhda Mandelstam (2001): *Vtoraja kniga* [Second book (*Hope Abandoned*)]. Moscow, 13.

15 Osip Mandelstam: *O prirode slova* [On the Nature of the Word].

(12) *Vot my i vstali v krestax i nashivkax, / V snezhnom dymu, / Smotrim i* ***vidim****, chto vyshla oshibka – / I my – ni k chemu!*[16]

'And thus we stood (decorated) with crosses and stripes, / In snowy smoke, / We look and **see** that a mistake has been made – / And we are not needed!'

Here the verb *videt'* ('to see') simultaneously has two different meanings (which is indicated by different contextual elements): that of visual perception and that of knowledge-understanding ('seeing in the mind's eye').

4. A special case of poetic non-zeugmatic meaning superposition can be found in the phenomenon which Nikolaeva calls "**the principle of ternary semantics**". The principle says that one and the same lexical item has meaning *X* in case 1, meaning *Y* in case 2, and in case 3 – meanings *X* and *Y*, as it were, simultaneously. Thus, in *The Lay of Igor's Campaign* the word *galki* ('jackdaws') sometimes simply denotes jackdaws, sometimes – the Polovians, and in the third case it remains unclear whether it denotes the jackdaws or the Polovians (Nikolaeva 1997: 41).

One can probably further diversify the types of poetic meaning superposition (see examples in Percova 1988), but this would be beyond the scope of the present discussion. Here we will only note that poetic meaning superposition (at least our types 2 and 3), while being quite a self-evident argument in favour of "the unity of a word", is not in any way an argument against the principle of discontinuous representation for polysemy in the dictionary (usually it is not difficult to establish **which** dictionary meanings are superposed; it may be more difficult to describe the effect of their superposition, but this, presumably, goes beyond the set task of lexicography). Moreover, poetic meaning superposition is not an argument against the principle that "normally" each concrete use of a word realises only one of its meanings (see below): it is this "norm" that is violated by poetic language, which is how it achieves its effect.

If we want to enumerate all instances when the same word within an utterance conceals a number of different senses, to one end of our list we should add punning, i.e. the use of language that creates a comical effect through unifying (usually intentionally) two clearly distinct senses neither of which is "meant" (because intentional punning has only one objective: to make others laugh).[17] From the other end, the list can be supplemented with "vagueness": the unification of two senses whose separation is impossible within a given utterance (i.e. the two senses may be separated only on the basis of some further contextual clues). An example of the latter kind may be found in the phrase *borot'sja s eretikami* ('to fight with heretics'; from Apresjan 1974: 181) which simultaneously realises two different meanings (*borot'sja s kem-to za chto-to* – 'to fight with someone for something' and *borot'sja s chem-to* – 'to fight with something'). It would be incorrect to apply the notion of **meaning superposition** to these cases; more commonly they are labelled as instances of **syncretism** or **indifferentiation** (although there is no consistency in the use of these terms). However, it would

---

16 Galich: *Oshibka* [A mistake].

17 Cf. "An utterance admitting of two or several interpretations, all of which are 'meant' [...], must be considered semantically anomalous: the purpose of such an utterance is not to express one of its meanings, but to call the hearer's attention to their interplay." (Paducheva 1982: 85)

be even more precise to say that in such cases a word has only **one** meaning, but this meaning is of a higher order, where the feature distinguishing between the meanings of a lower order is not relevant.

Thus, for example, the verb *bojat'sja* ('to be afraid of') clearly has two contrasting meanings: the "emotional" one which foregrounds the feeling of fear based on the idea of the negative character of some event and the "mental" meaning of probabilistic evaluation (see Zalizniak 1992: 86). The two meanings interact with negation differently. Thus, sentence

(13) *Ja ne* ***bojus'*** *s"ezzhat's etoj gory.*
'I'm not **afraid** to go down this mountain.'

realises the first, "emotional" meaning (= 'have no fear'), whereas sentence

(14) *Veroj v budushchee ne* ***bojus'*** */ Pokazat'sja tebe krasnobaem.*[18]
'With faith in the future I'm not **afraid** / To appear to you as a phrasemonger.'

presents the "mental" meaning: *ne bojus' pokazat'sja* ('[I]'m not afraid to appear') means 'do not think it probable that this will happen'.

The existence of contrast between these two meanings of the verb *bojat'sja* ('to be afraid of') is confirmed by the fact that it lends itself to punning, which can be illustrated with the following episode related by Shklovsky (1940; see Sarnov 2002: 11):

(15) *Majakovskomu peredali, chto Brjusov jakoby skazal o nem '****Bojus'****, chto iz Majakovskogo nichego ne vyjdet'.*
Vladimir Vladimirovich ochen' zabavno pokazyval, kak Brjusov spit i prosypaetsja noch'ju s voplem:
– ***Bojus', bojus'****!*
– Ty chego ***boish'sja****?*
– ***Boyus'****, chto iz Majakovskogo nichego ne vyidet.*
'Mayakovsky was told that Brusov had allegedly said about him: 'I'm **afraid** that Mayakovsky will be no good'.
Vladimir Vladimirovich [Mayakovsky] very amusingly showed how Brusov sleeps and wakes up in the night shouting:
– I'm **afraid**, I'm **afraid**!
– What are you **afraid** of?
– I'm **afraid** that Mayakovsky will be no good.'

Yet in other cases, including those under negation, the choice between the two meanings proves impossible – and not because the context is insufficient, but rather because the opposition is absent from what the speaker wanted to say. For example, uttering

[18] Pasternak: *Ne volnujsja, ne plach', ne trudi …* [Don't worry, don't cry, don't strain…].

(16) *Ja ne **bojus'** ostat'sja odna.*
'I'm not **afraid** of being left alone.'

the speaker may have in mind **either** that this will not happen **or** that it will not be a bad thing – but this explicit disjunctiveness is present only in our interpretation; the speaker most probably is not aware of it.[19]

To put it differently, in some context the feature which distinguishes between two meanings of word in other contexts (and justifies the lexicographer's effort to distinguish between them in dictionary definitions) may be inessential. In this connection it is appropriate to quote the following passage from D. N. Shmelev:

> The semantic structure of a whole range of words is characterised by the fact that individual meanings, clearly separable one from another in certain positions, in other positions prove compatible and are indivisible. (1973: 77)

And further:

> We have in mind not the special poetic (often, simply punning) mode of using words in context, which reveals their polysemy, but rather that in everyday speech communication the isolated meanings are not completely and fully separated from one another [...] This '**diffuseness**' of individual meanings does not pose any difficulty in speech communication, does not make utterances ambiguous, because the opposition of meanings of a polysemous word in certain contexts is compatible with the possibility (also positionally determined) of their 'superposition' (*sovmeshchenie*) in other contexts. (op. cit., 80)

That "meaning superposition" is not peripheral but, in some sense, constitutive for the semantic system follows from the nature of semantic evolution: during a period of time two meanings are superposed without differing, but later they diverge, incorporating into their semantic structure an element of contextual meaning, as a result the difference between them changes from positional to inherent – cf. the famous example from Benveniste: *le faucon vole la perdrix* ('the falcon *chases* and *in the air catches* the partridge', Benveniste 1954). It is obvious to us today that 'to fly' and 'to steal' are

---

19 Another illustration of this can be found in the following dialogue from a film by Eduard Rjazanov *Predskazanie* [The prophecy]. Having rescued his beloved from the persecutions of her villainous ex-husband, and finally finding himself safe and alone with her, the hero says:

> – *Ja **bojus'**, chto posle vsego, chto bylo, ja okazhus' ne na vysote.*
> – *Vot uzh chego ja ne **bojus'**.*
> '– I'm **afraid** that after all that happened I will not live up to the situation.
> – This is something I'm not **afraid** of at all.'

Semantic analysis produces two possible interpretations of her response: either she is certain that he will 'live up to the situation' or she does not think that it matters (does not think that it will be bad if he won't). However, it seems that, in accordance with the author's intention, we are dealing here with vagueness rather than ambiguity: the heroine simply wants to say that everything will be fine; thus, the disjunction discussed above, or the contrast between the two meanings of the verb *bojat'sja* ('to be afraid of'), is not realised in this example.

two different senses (corresponding to the two homonyms with the word form *voler* in modern French), but there was a time when they were expressed as a single whole.

With this reservation in mind (i.e. if instances of non-poetic syncretism may be considered as **one** meaning), we can agree that "normally every polysemous word is used in an utterance in one of its meanings" (Apresjan 2000a: xxvii-xxviii).

5. Ways to Represent Polysemy

Among ways of representing polysemy that are used today by different authors we can distinguish the following six:

1. a hierarchically ordered (= many-level) list of individual meanings (traditional dictionaries; Mel'chuk & Zholkovskij 1984; Apresjan 1974);

2. a list of individual meanings specifying the route of semantic derivation which links them to the primary meaning, i.e. the scheme of Kurylowicz 1960: Paducheva 2004; Mel'chuk's "semantic bridges" (Mel'chuk et al. 1995); Turovsky's (1985) operations on interpretation;

3. an invariant (≈ general meaning) and variants (= individual meanings) which can be derived from it and which are realised in different contexts, i.e. the scheme of Jakobson (1971a); Percov (2001);

4. the meaning of a word as a set of semantic, or interpretational, components which have the form of propositions expressed in a semantic metalanguage (Wierzbicka 1996). Comparison of such sets reveals similarities and differences in the meaning of synonyms within a language, translational equivalents in different languages, and also different meanings of a word (each meaning is assigned its own set);[20]

5. an image-schema: a picture which supposedly allows one to represent in a cognitively adequate way both the meaning of a word and the structure of its polysemy: different meanings "select" (profile, foreground) different parts of the schema as central, leaving its other parts beyond the scope of attention or on its periphery, which reflects the organisation of vision and other cognitive processes (Johnson 1987; Lakoff 1987; Talmy 2000; Langacker 2002; Janda 1986);

6. an abstract schema (schema-scenario) and a range of formal operations for its logical transformation whose application results in individual meanings (Kiseleva & Paillard 1998).

Without intending to review these conceptions in detail, we will pause only on some crucial points. Among the main principles of the cognitive approach to polysemy we can name the following:

1. All linguistic units are polysemous.

2. There is no single core (invariant) meaning corresponding to a polysemous linguistic unit such that all its other meanings are variants of this core.

---

20 See her description of different meanings of the word *soul* (Wierzbicka 1992: 36ff.), verbs like *ask* and *tell* (Wierzbicka 1987), and the Russian words *pravda* ('truth') and *nepravda* ('falsehood') (Wierzbicka 2002).

3. The meaning of an expression can be represented as its image-schema.

4. Meanings of an expression form a radial structure category in which the central element is linked with all the other elements via image-schema transformations (i.e. mental operations which let the speaker link conceptually close configurations as variants of the same basic image-schema) and metaphor.

5. Derived meanings cannot be predicted from the central meaning, but are motivated by the central meaning, image-schema transformations and metaphoric transfers.

6. There is no fundamental difference in the polysemy structure of words, grammatical words and morphemes.

Of all this an especially important point is the contrast between **deducibility** vs. **motivatedness**. Indeed, a derived meaning is called **deduced** if there exists for it a **deduction rule** (of the kind "**whenever** there is a set of conditions *A*, it triggers a process leading to result *B*"). One can find rules of this kind in semantics, but there are very few of them. A derived meaning is called **motivated** if there is some transparent content relation between states *A* and *B*. Presumably one should agree that in the most general case semantic derivation has the property of motivatedness, but not that of deducibility. Semantic derivation is determined by the interaction of so many factors that it cannot be generally predicted. On the other hand, when we know that some semantic change **has already taken place** within a word, then knowledge of the mechanisms of motivation (semantic derivation) can let us explain why this change took place within that word, but not, for example, a semantically close but different word (cf. Dirven 1985: 27). Thus, for example, Rozina (2005) quite convincingly explains why the verb *podogret'* ('to warm up') acquires a jargon meaning transferring the verb to the realm of social relations (= 'to bribe'), whereas a cognate verb with a different prefix *sogret'* ('to warm') – does not have any similar meaning. In other words, knowledge of the mechanisms of semantic derivation can let us uncover **possible** routes of semantic evolution which are admissible from the point of view of a language's internal logic; but whether the language will indeed follow these routes cannot be predicted.

On the whole, one cannot deny the achievements of cognitive linguistics in the study of polysemy. The idea of figure-background or profile-base interaction as the generative principle behind polysemy undoubtedly advances our understanding of it. Cognitive linguistics' conceptual apparatus is especially potent in the analysis of strongly polysemous grammatical words and morphemes – first of all, prepositions and prefixes (see, for instance, Filipenko 2000 on prepositions and Janda 1986 on prefixes). Some doubts, however, arise as to whether it can be productively used in the study of those words of abstract semantics whose abstract meaning is primary (rather than derived) – for example, words like *znat'* ('to know') or *zhdat'* ('to wait'), *zhalko* (adv.: 'it is a pity') or *naprasno* (adv.: 'in vain'). Besides, even with respect to words like *neobxodimyj* ('necessary', lit. morph. 'non-go-round-able') or *neizbezhnyj* ('unavoidable', lit. morph. 'non-runnable-out-from') one cannot be certain that the description of their meaning must appeal to the words *obojti* ('to go round') or *izbezhat'* ('avoid', lit. morph. 'to run out') in their primary, spatial meaning (see below on differences in linguistic competence of native language speakers, including those that concern a word's "inner form"). Of course, the cognitive approach may be extended to cover cases like these; however, it seems that beyond the spatial metaphor (i.e. the description of the meaning of prefixes, prepositions, verbs of physical action and some other word classes) it is not exactly ineffective, but rather effective only in so far as it loses its specific character which distinguishes it from more traditional methods of semantic analysis.

On the other hand, the principles of cognitive linguistics have always been widely employed in different branches of Russian semantics. These are the theses regarding the influence of social, psychological, cultural and other "external" factors on language; the dependence of language structure on the conceptualisation of the world and, vice versa, the existence of language-specific conceptual structures which are reflected in the meaning of words from different languages; the absence of a boundary between linguistic and encyclopaedic knowledge; the interpenetration of different linguistic levels – syntax, morphology and lexis (cf. the list of cognitive linguistic principles in Rudzka-Ostyn 1993: 1f.). In particular, these principles find their expression in the study of linguistic conceptualisation and the semantics of language-specific words (cf. Shmelev 2002). Research in the area of metaphorical collocations or "material connotations" (*veshchnye konnotacii*) for abstract words (whose principles were formulated in Uspensky 1979) as well as conceptual analyses, including modelling the meaning of such words through locating their analogues in the world of physical phenomena (Arutjunova 1976), in fact realise the central principle of cognitive linguistics (cf. Turovsky 1991 and later publications in the series 'The Logical Analysis of Language'). Quite close to cognitive linguistics is also the idea of constructing a **conceptual schema** (see below) which unifies not only different meanings of a polysemous word, but also different words, as, for example, the sets *sozhalet'* ('to regret') – *zhalet'* ('to feel pity, be sorry') – *zhal'* (pred. 'it is a pity') – *zhalko* (pred. 'to feel sorry'), and *obidet'* ('to offend, hurt') – *obidno* (pred. 'to feel hurt, resent') – *obida* ('offence, resentment') described in Zalizniak 2006 (cf. the analysis of the words *go*, *gone*, *away* in Langacker 2002: 6). It is also appropriate to mention here Paducheva's (2004) investigations in which she categorises conversives together with other types of diathetic shift occurring within a word. These investigations belong to the traditional problem area of analysing the prototypical situation and different ways of its **lexicalisation** (cf. Fillmore 1968, 1977; Apresjan 1974; Kibrik 1980). Like cognitive linguistic studies, these investigations centre on the idea of different "focussing of attention" as the generative principle of polysemy, i.e. different "foregrounding" of one participant or another in a situation and/or of a semantic component, – cf. the term "profiling" used by Langacker (2002: 5) or the term "windowing of attention" (Ungerer & Schmid 1996: 218; Talmy 2000: 76f.), etc.

The idea that polysemy is generated because distinct aspects (semantic components) of the meaning of a word realise themselves in distinct circumstances is developed in the work of Paducheva (see, for example, Paducheva 2004). Similar ideas were expressed by other researchers as well (see, for instance, Gurevich 1988: 27; Gak 1998: 30, 238; Zalizniak 1992). One of the first attempts to describe, by means of a formal metalanguage, standard relations of semantic derivation linking one meaning of a polysemous word, which is taken to be primary, with all its other meanings can be found in Turovsky (1985). Models of semantic derivation for a broad range of basic

Russian words are described in Kustova (2004) and Rozina (2005). The closeness between the notions of **regular polysemy** (**semantic derivation**) and **image-schema transformation** was noted by Filipenko (2000: 33) and Rakhilina (2000a: 5). Finally, the idea of schematic images being building blocks in the construction of linguistic meaning (cf. Goddard 1998: 79f.) is very close to the idea of semantic primitives.

Indeed, it seems highly plausible that basic elements of experience, out of which linguistic concepts are built, exist on a non-verbal level, and for this reason any attempt to translate this information into verbal form is bound to fail. However, translation into visual form cannot be done without a loss either. This is especially doubtful in the case of kinaesthetic (i.e. directly reflecting our sensorimotor experience) schemata,[21] – cf. the analysis of the English prepositions *in* and *out* on the basis of the perception of the body as a container in Lindner (1983). Thus, "pictures" manifest their obvious advantage only in those cases when the coded fragment of experience is originally of a visual nature; this may be true for spatial adverbs and prepositions (cf. a rather convincing analysis of the English preposition *over* in Dewell 1994). On the other hand, the "cognitive adequacy" of any such model is hard to verify. Another argument against any kind of "pictures" is the well-known fact that, in linguistics, graphic representations of authors' ideas, with rare exceptions, are comprehensible only to the authors themselves – in any case they do not clarify anything by comparison with their verbal versions. For example, discussing the advantages of graphic representation for spatial information, in particular when one has to establish the localisation of some object, Rakhilina (2000b) does not offer any "picture" to her readers. Similarly, a very sketchy graphic image found in Plungian and Rakhilina (2000: 118f.) merely accompanies its verbal analogue (with which the authors work in the rest of the article).

6. The Meaning of a Lexical Item as a Realisation of Its Conceptual Schema

6.1. The Notion of Conceptual Schema

There are, to our knowledge, two ways to represent polysemy which are directed towards preserving the "unity of a word": on the one hand, it is the Jakobsonian idea of **general meaning** (Jakobson 1971a; cf. also the notion of **invariant** in Jakobson 1971b), on the other hand, it is the idea of **core (basic) meaning** (Kurylowicz 1960). In both cases the unity of a word is guaranteed by derivational links connecting all its individual meanings; the main difference between them is that Kurylowicz's schema presupposes operation with "real" meanings, which reveal themselves in concrete uses, whereas adopting Jakobson's schema means turning towards some unobservable semantic essence, which is situated on a different level of abstraction and requires a different metalanguage than that used in lexicographic description. Each of them has its advantages and shortcomings, which have been much discussed in the literature (see, for example, Wierzbicka 1980, 1996; Percov 2001; Paducheva 2000), and we do not need to reproduce these arguments here.

Our main thesis is that **different** mechanisms ensuring the unity of the meaning of a lexical item coexist in language; hence, there are **many** correct ways of represent-

21 See Johnson (1987), Lakoff (1987), Deane (1988).

ing polysemy. This means that in some cases it is preferable (i.e. more adequate with regard to the object of study) to use a description that distinguishes between primary and derived meanings considered as entities of the same order (Kurylowicz's schema); in other cases the advantages of a description that distinguishes between two levels – hidden and explicit (Jakobson's schema) – become evident. The same is true with respect to the long-debated opposition between "classical" and "prototype" approaches to categorisation (cf. Wierzbicka 1996).

In this article the way of representing polysemy which ensures the semantic unity of a word is called **conceptual schema**. The use of this term allows a functional unification of several different specific metalinguistic methods, both well-established in linguistics and new: all these methods aim to represent the meaning of a polysemous word as a single whole. We can thus think of invariants, general meanings, prototypical scenarios (see Wierzbicka 1999), and so on as instances of conceptual schemata – namely, when it proves possible to find a formula which would be sufficiently rich in content and operational, but at the same time would not contain fixed values of those parameters that must remain indeterminate at this level.

6.2. Some Examples of Conceptual Schemata

6.2.1. *Naprasno*

The adverb *naprasno* ('in vain'/'mistakenly') has three particular meanings: that of the ineffectiveness of an action (*naprasno s"ezdil* 'went (somewhere) in vain' = 'without result'); that of a wrong opinion (*naprasno tak dumaesh'*, lit. 'in vain so (you) think' = 'you're wrong'); and evaluative (*naprasno otkazalsja*, lit. 'in vain refused' = 'it would have been better to accept'). For all these meanings of the word *naprasno* we can formulate the following semantic **invariant**, which is also its **conceptual schema**:

> Using the phrase *naprasno P* ('in vain'/'mistakenly *P*') the speaker asserts that *Q* which constitutes *P*'s raison d'être does not exist.[22]

Each of the particular meanings of *naprasno* ('in vain'/'mistakenly') listed above is a **realisation** of this schema: for the first, *Q* is an objective which the agent of action *P* wants to achieve via doing *P* (but fails); for the second, *Q* is the actual (from the point of view of the speaker) state of affairs: it provides foundation for or justification of the corresponding opinion (*P*); for the third, *Q* is a state of affairs (usually, some positive consequence of *P*), which serves as a foundation for a positive evaluation of *P*.

Representing polysemy with the help of conceptual schemata is in a sense complementary to the approach where semantic derivation links one of the real meanings of a word, taken to be primary, with its other, derived meanings. The model generating derived meanings is more effective for representing relatively regular polysemy (certain kinds of metaphoric and diathetic shifts, changes in arguments' taxonomic class, etc., – cf. Paducheva 2004). Conceptual schemata are more effective for representing

---

22 Note that this formulation is close to the diachronically primary but presently lost meaning of this word ('having no apparent reason or foundation', cf. *naprasnaja smert'* – lit. 'vain death').

those words whose polysemy for some reason cannot be described within the framework of the "derivational model", but whose semantic unity is nonetheless significant and calls for explication. To reveal this unity it may be necessary to use a metalanguage different from the natural language in that it leaves unexpressed certain oppositions built into the meaning of words of that natural language and uses communicatively undissociated assertions. Another important feature of conceptual schemata which distinguishes them, for example, from general meanings is that the same schema may underlie a number of different words.

6.2.2. *Sozhalet'*

Let us consider the semantics of *sozhalenie* ('regret'). The development of its conceptual schema is necessary to clarify how one and the same word can unify uses where the propositional object is given opposite valuations. Thus, on the one hand, one can *sozhalet' o sovershennoj oshibke* ('to regret a mistake made'): it is a feeling directed at something **bad** ('sozhalet'$_1$'). On the other hand, one can *sozhalet' o schastlivoj molodosti*, lit. 'to regret (one's) happy youth' (≈ 'to regret that the happy days of one's youth are gone'), and it is a feeling directed at something **good** ('sozhalet'$_2$'). Hence a sentence like *On sozhalel o godax, provedennyx vo Francii* ('He [*sozhalel*] the years spent in France') is ambiguous: either he thought that living in France was a waste of time or that it was wonderful.[23]

We can reconstruct the semantic unity of the word *sozhalet'* ('to regret') if we pay close attention to the specific functioning of the evaluative component within this verb. What is constant here is the value relation: "that which does not exist (in the actual world) is better than that which does". Different valuations of the propositional object in the two submeanings of the verb *sozhalet'*, which we noted above, are determined by the fact that in the first case the verb selects as its argument the first term of the comparison (a mistake one made is something that "exists"), and in the second case – the second term (one's happy youth is something that "does not exist"). Thus:

> Some state of affairs which **does not exist** in the actual world, but could exist in it, is thought of as BETTER than that which **does exist**.

This formula, however, is not fully adequate as it employs the linguistic operator of preference 'better', which, for the purposes of representation in terms of conceptual schemata, lacks some necessary, and, on the contrary, contains some superfluous components; the words *good* or *bad* are even less appropriate as neither of them allows us to unify the absolute and the comparative valuations without fixing a perspective at the same time (i.e. to unify the senses '*P* is bad', 'not-*P* is good', 'not-*P* is better than *P*', '*P* is worse than not-*P*). For this reason a more adequate way to represent the evalu-

[23] The polysemy in question also characterises, for example, the French verb *regretter* as in *regretter ses fautes* ('to regret one's mistakes') vs. *regretter sa jeunesse* '(lit. 'to regret one's youth', 'to regret that the happy days of one's youth are gone'), whereas the English verb *to regret* does not have the second meaning. For more details see Zalizniak (1991, 1992, 2006).

ative component is to use a **scale**, which is component (c) in the conceptual schema of *sozhalenie* ('regret'):

(a) Something is absent from the actual world
(b) This something could be present in the actual world
(c) bad good

```
                 bad                                              good
.................x.....................................x.........................
           that which                              that which
           is present                              is absent
```

Component (a) introduces a situation which has no place in the actual world (a situation from the past or from a possible world different from the actual world). Component (b) reflects one's idea of the alternative, which is constitutive of regret, – unlike other internal states which carry a negative valuation of the actual state of affairs.

The three components which constitute the conceptual schema are put into different conceptual configurations (schema realisations) in the particular meanings of a word (like the Russian *sozhalet'*, 'to regret', *sozhalenie*, 'regret', *zhalet'*, 'to be sorry', the French *regretter*, etc.): each of them becomes more articulated and acquires a definite communicative status. When the schema's realisation corresponds to the meaning '*sozhalet'*$_1$' the object position is occupied by the name of a situation which has taken place and which is *bad* or *worse* than some alternative situation which could have taken place but did not. Thus, in uses like

(17) *Ja* ***sozhaleju****, chto sjuda prishel.*
'I **regret** coming here.'

component (a) refers to the situation 'I did not come here' (that this situation does not exist follows from the factive presupposition of (17)); component (b) corresponds to the felicity conditions of the utterance (one can say *I regret coming here* only if one could choose between coming and not coming); component (c) is realised in the form 'not-*P* is better than *P*' ('did not come' is better than 'came') and constitutes assertion.

When the schema is realised with the meaning 'sozhalet'$_2$' the object position is occupied by the name of a situation which is not present and which is good (possibly better than the one which is present, although this is not stated directly). Component (a) becomes the felicity condition; (b) is shadowed; and the evaluative component (c) is realised in the form of an absolute evaluation '*P* is good'.

One advantage of conceptual schemata is that they allow us to describe even those uses of a word which do not clearly fall under one of its particular meanings.

On the whole, we can say that the smaller the distance between meanings of a lexical item is, the less different the conceptual schema is from the real definition. For this reason, for example, the conceptual schema of *raskajanie* ('repentance') virtually coincides with its lexicographic definition.

The conceptual schema for a polysemous abstract word is an informal description of the prototypical situation that contains a number of elements each of which may become central, relegating other elements to the background. The elements of the prototypical situation correspond to the constituents of a word's semantic structure, which have different communicative status in different meanings. This structure of polysemy is inherent in verbs like *bojat'sja* ('to be afraid of'), *govorit'* ('to speak'), *sochuvstovovat'* ('to sympathise'), *zhdat'* ('to wait'), *podozrevat'* ('to suspect'), etc. (see Zalizniak 1992; 2006).

6.2.3. *Sobirat'sja*

Let us consider another example. The following conceptual schema may be proposed for the verbs *sobirat'sja* ('to be going to', lit. 'to gather oneself') and *namerevat'sja* ('to intend') <to do something>:

> The person is in the stretch of time between making a decision and carrying it out.

The simple meaning of intention, which can be illustrated with examples like

(18) *On **sobiraetsja/namerevaetsja** zhenit'sja/pokupat' dachu.*
'He **is going/intends** to get married/buy a cottage.',

emerges when the first component, corresponding to the passing of the first point (making a decision), is asserted, and the second component (corresponding to the fact that the second point has not yet been passed, i.e. the action has not been carried out) functions as the felicity condition. In cases like these we are dealing with the subject's intention and nothing else, and here the verb *sobirat'sja* ('to be going to') is virtually synonymous with the verb *namerevat'sja* ('to intend') and its translational equivalents in European languages. In this case the verb *sobirat'sja* is also synonymous with the perfective verb *sobrat'sja* ('to be going$_{PF}$', lit. 'to have gathered oneself'): of every person who *sobiraetsja* ('is going$_{IMPF}$') to get married, buy a cottage, etc. it is also true that he *sobralsja* ('is going$_{PF}$') to do that, and the other way round. The difference here is purely aspectual: in one case it is the state (i.e. the intention) itself that is the focus of attention, in the other – transition into this state (i.e. they form a standard "perfect" aspectual pair, typical of inner state predicates; see Paducheva 1996: 152ff.).

The language-specific **process** meaning of the verb *sobirat'sja*,[24] which is absent from the verb *namerevat'sja* ('to intend') but found in uses of type (20), emerges from the same schema, but here two semantic shifts occur.

(19) *Uzhe chas lezhu i **sobirajus'** vstat'; **sobirajus'**, da vse nikak ne **soberus'** <otvetit' na pis'mo, komu-to pozvonit'>; vse utro **sobiralsja** sest' rabotat', da tak i ne **sobralsja**.*
'I've been lying down for an hour **going** (lit. 'gathering myself') to get up; I'm **going to** but can't really finally **make** (lit. 'gather') myself <answer a let-

[24] For more details on this meaning of the verb *sobirat'sja* see Zalizniak and Levontina (1996).

ter, phone someone>; I was **going to** get down to work the whole morning, but did not **manage** (lit. 'gather myself') to do it.'

The first shift consists in the component '*X* has not yet carried out *P*' raising its status: from the felicity condition it turns into a full-fledged semantic component, which may become the main assertive one.[25] The second shift, which occurs simultaneously with it, consists in the fact that the very idea of **making a decision** becomes blurred, as if it were decomposed into two stages like (i) 'it should be done; I will do it at some point' and (ii) 'I will do it now'. In this derived meaning *sobirat'sja* describes not the state between making a decision and carrying it out (as in the original meaning of intention), but the state between the first and the second stages of decision-making. In this case *sobirat'sja* turns into a quasi-process of mobilising one's internal resources, "gathering" them in one place (the way a person gathers and piles together things they will need in their travels). The process is terminative, and the point of termination is the event of *sobrat'sja* ('to be going to$_{\text{PF}}$', lit. 'to have gathered oneself'), i.e. having gathered sufficient internal resources to proceed to the stage 'I will do it'. Upon reaching this point *sobirat'sja*$_{\text{IMPF}}$ and *sobrat'sja*$_{\text{PF}}$ are no longer interchangeable but enter the "process – result of this process" relation. The pair *sobirat'sja – sobrat'sja* ('to be going to$_{\text{IMPF}}$ –'to be going to$_{\text{PF}}$') is assimilated with terminative aspectual pairs of the conative type, cf. *reshat'* <zadachu> ('solve$_{\text{IMPF}}$'<a problem>) – *reshit'* ('solve$_{\text{PF}}$'), with the semantic correlation "to try to achieve something – to achieve something". It is for this reason that is possible to use the formula *sobiralsja, no ne sobralsja* (≅ 'was going to but did not manage', lit. 'was gathering myself but did not gather'), which is prima facie paradoxical (and can hardly be translated into foreign languages) – by analogy with *reshal, no ne reshil* ('was trying to solve but did not solve').[26]

6.2.4. *Mimo*

Conceptual schemata of polysemous words with spatial meaning (spatial prepositions and adverbs, verbs of motion, and also verbal prefixes) include spatial images on which a certain conceptual structure is imposed, making possible the foregrounding of only some of the image's fragments and in this way giving rise to real particular meanings. Thus, depending on intonation, sentence

(20) *My proedem* ***mimo*** *Gamburga.*
'We will go **past** Hamburg.'

may express either the hope of meeting (someone who is in Hamburg) [the word *mimo* ('past') is unstressed: meaning 'mimo$_1$'] or the regret that such a meeting will not take place [*mimo* ('past') carries phrasal stress: meaning 'mimo$_2$']. To analyse the word

---

[25] A similar rise in status affects the component 'without getting into contact' in the meaning of the word *mimo* ('past') – see below.

[26] However, it seems that this assimilation remains incomplete and retains an element of language game.

mimo ('past') we can propose the following **conceptual schema** admitting of different realisations (this explains the possibility of two divergent meanings coexisting within one and the same word):

> There are three entities: a moving object (*X*), an immobile object (*Y*) and the vicinity of object *Y*. Object *X* moves in such a way that at some point in time it passes through the vicinity of *Y*.

'Mimo$_1$' and 'mimo$_2$' split this picture differently: for 'mimo$_1$' the difference between *Y* and its vicinity is unimportant: the situation is conceptualised in terms of *X* passing through the vicinity of *Y* or, possibly, *Y* itself. In contrast, for 'mimo$_2$' the difference between *Y* and its vicinity is essential: here it is important that *X*'s trajectory does not take it through *Y* itself.

Each element of the conceptual schema 'mimo' may be correlated with a semantic component of this word. Taking one of its meanings to be primary (namely the one that is realised with neutral phrasal stress) we can describe the same relation in the following way: the meaning 'mimo$_2$' emerges from the meaning 'mimo$_1$' through reorganising the latter's semantic structure. Namely, the component ('*X* does not come into contact with *Y*'), which is "weak" in 'mimo$_1$', in 'mimo$_2$' is foregrounded, becoming the main assertive component (for more details see Zalizniak 1994). The type of shift described above is one of the major mechanisms of semantic derivation.

Let us note that the notion of conceptual schema is different from that of primary meaning first of all because it does not contain any information about the constituents' relative communicative significance. Hence, in those cases when the communicative hierarchy of the components is inessential or if there is only one component, a word's conceptual schema simply coincides with its primary meaning.

7. Concluding Remarks

It seems that the solution to the task of describing polysemy should be sought in the attitude which distinguishes between questions about the **real functioning** of polysemy (i.e. how speakers use it in speech comprehension and production: which individual meanings are "memorised"? which are generated in accordance with certain schemata or patterns? which are not perceived as distinct at all?) and the **correct description** of it in the dictionary (the dictionary as a reference book whose users are not professional linguists, as opposed to the lexicon as a recently popular genre of linguistic investigation). We believe that dictionary representation of the meaning of a polysemous word should not strive to reflect the way information about polysemy is stored in the mind of the speaker, nor the way the speaker uses it. There are several reasons for this.

First, we do not know in what format information about polysemy is stored in the mind of the speaker.

There are reasons to believe that, ontologically, the development of polysemy proceeds not from the "concrete" to the "abstract", but rather from the most **general** representation, in which metaphorically or metonymically motivated transfers are simply not perceived as generating distinct entities, to gradual **differentiation** and opposition between particular meanings. This is evidenced by both phylogenetic and ontogenetic data: cf., on the one hand, studies in the semantics of classical languages (see, in particular, Ivanov 1999: 550 on the syncretism of the ancient Greek *frénes* and Swadesh 1972: 183ff.), and, on the other hand, studies in the area of first language acquisition (cf. Barrett 1995 and references therein). Thus, three- or four-year old children reject adults' use of words in their transferred meaning (cf. *Moloko ne mozhet ubezhat', u nego zhe net nog*, 'Milk cannot run off [boil over], it doesn't have legs', Cejtlin 2000: 199). On the other hand, in children's speech, for example, an acorn and an object resembling an acorn are one and the same thing (cf. words like *shar* ('ball') or *krug* ('circle') which can mean 'an object with the form of <a ball, a circle>' in everyday "adult" language). Saying that resin drops on a fir tree are *slezy, kotorymi elka plachet* ('tears with which the fir tree cries'),[27] the child does not do anything different in principle from using the same word to designate its own and a dog's ears. A two-year-old child may use the word *babah* ('bang!') to refer to a blow, the sound of a blow, the fact that it hurts, as well as a ball and generally any spherical object. In all these cases there is no metaphor or metonymy, because there is no **transfer** as such. In other words, children reject metaphor in so far as they are able to discover it; they need identity rather than similarity (a drop of resin shaped like a tear **is** a tear).

Second, as mentioned above, there are good reasons to believe that information storage and manipulation to some extent **differ** among individuals depending both on the speaker's type of mentality and other factors (social, age-related, professional).

Third, as those working with dictionaries (both bilingual and monolingual) might have noticed, a lexicographic definition often gives a less clear understanding of the meaning of a word than several examples illustrating its use in a given meaning. Presumably, the explanation for this is that the meaning of a word is not stored in the speaker's mind as a list of meanings represented by their definitions. (In particular, even if there is a **lingua mentalis**, it is even less accessible to the speaker than to the researcher.) One should also remember that many contextually motivated distinctions are not perceived by the speaker at all (in particular, distinctions concerning arguments' taxonomic class, cf. the analysis of the verb *razbit'* ('break') in Paducheva 2006). Thus, both postulated meanings and rules of their generation model the metalinguistic activity of the linguist to a greater degree than the linguistic competence of the speaker, and one cannot exclude the possibility that not only **definitions** but also **particular meanings** belong only to the metalanguage of linguistic description.

The real functioning of a lexical item's polysemy is the resultant of so many factors that the most adequate conception of this phenomenon can be formed only if we have at our disposal several different, complementary or even alternative, ways to describe it. There must be at least two such types of description:

---

27 Cf. *Prozrachnoj slezoj na stenax prostupila smola* ('Resin oozes from the walls, a transparent tear', Mandelstam, *Za to, chto ja ruki tvoi ne sumel uderzhat...* – 'Because I could not keep hold of your arms...', transl. A.S. Kline at www.tonykline.co.uk/PITBR/Russian/MoreMandelstam.htm). See also Cejtlin (2000: 195) on similarities in the mechanisms of child and poetic speech creativity.

1. the traditional dictionary description as a list of particular meanings (where most emphasis should be given to the selection of examples encompassing the relevant multitude of a word's uses);

2. an analysis of this list or a **hypothesis** about the way this system of meanings is stored in the mind of the speaker and is used by him/her (which, in principle should admit of multiple representational formats).

Representing polysemy as a multitude of particular meanings – either with or without established hierarchies between them and proposed models of semantic derivation – will always remain imperfect (in the sense of being not fully adequate to facts), and this imperfection results not from the lack of thoroughness or insight, but from the nature of polysemy itself which functions **non-discretely** in language as a system: realised in speech, this non-discreteness is significantly reduced but is not eliminated completely. This, however, does not mean that one should give up the "dictionary type" of description.

Thus, there are two different tasks. One is to organise in the most effective way the information which may be required by the language user. The other is to understand how polysemy works, which means drawing a boundary, in one way or another, between the **reproduced** and the **generated**, and discovering the mechanisms of semantic derivation used by the speaker (and, correspondingly, the hearer, who carries out the reverse operation) in the "generation zone". As for the first task, the optimal approach today is probably the one which represents the meaning of a word in the form of its "lexicographic portrait" (see Apresjan 1995b and chapter 9 of Apresjan 2000b). As for the second task, we believe that, along with the model generating derived meanings from the primary meaning, the model operating with the notions of conceptual schema and its realisations will prove effective.

The meaning that a word has in a concrete use is the resultant of twofold operations on the constituents composing its conceptual schema: on the one hand, it is the selection of the most important semantic components and their arrangement in accordance with their communicative status (presumption, assertion, implication, etc.); on the other hand, it is the reinterpretation of the selected components motivated by changes in the taxonomic class of the arguments. The interaction between these operations produces a concrete set of semantic derivation rules which generate (more or less regular) polysemy.

Bibliography

Apresjan, Ju.D. (1974): *Leksicheskaja semantika: Sinonimicheskie sredstva jazyka*. Moskva: Nauka.

Apresjan, Ju.D. (1995a): Novyj ob'jasnitel'nyj slovar' sinonimov: Koncepcija i tipy informacii. In: Apresjan, Ju.D. (ed.): *Novyj ob''jasnitel'nyj slovar' sinonimov. Prospekt*. Moskva: Jazyki russkoj kul'tury, 7-118.

Apresjan, Ju.D. (1995b): Leksikograficheskij portret glagola *vyjti*. In: Apresjan, Ju.D.: *Izbrannye trudy*. Vol. II. Moskva: Jazyki russkoj kul'tury, 485-502.

Apresjan, Ju.D. (2000a): Struktura slovarnoj stat'i slovarja. In: Apresjan, Ju.D. (ed.): *Novyj ob''jasnitel'nyj slovar' sinonimov russkogo jazyka. vyp. 2*. Moskva: Jaz. rus. kul'tury, VIII-LIV.

Apresjan, Ju.D. (2000b): *Systematic Lexicography*. Transl. K. Windle. New York: Oxford University Press.

Arutjunova, N.D. (1976): *Predlozhenie i ego smysl*. Moskva: Nauka.

Barrett, M. (1995): Early lexical development. In: Fletcher, P. & MacWinney, B. (eds.): *Child Language*. Oxford: Blackwell, 362-392.

Benveniste, E. (1954): Problèmes sémantiques de la reconstruction. *Word* 10, 251-264.

Boguslavsky, I., Iomdin, L., Sizov, V. & Chardin, I. (2003): Ispol'zovanie razmechennogo korpusa tekstov pri avtomaticheskom sintaksicheskom analize. In: *Conference Proceedings*, Varna, 1-7 Sept.

Bybee, J.L., Perkins, R. & Pagliuca, W. (1994): The evolution of grammar: Tense, aspect and modality in the languages of the world. Chicago: University of Chicago Press.

Cejtlin, S.N. (2000): *Jazyk i rebjonok. Lingvistika detskoj rechi*. Moskva: Vlados.

Deane, P. (1988): Polysemy and cognition. *Lingua* 75, 325-361.

Dewell, R. (1994): Over again: Image-schematic transformations in semantic analysis. *Cognitive Linguistics* 5, 351-380.

Dirven, R. (1985): Metaphor and polysemy. In: Jongen, R. (ed.): *La polysemie: lexicogaphie et cognition*. Louvain-la-Neuve : Cabai, 9-27.

Eco, U. (1962): *Opera aperta*. Milano: Bompiani.

Empson, W. (1966): *Seven types of ambiguity*. New York: New Directions.

Fauconnier, G. & Turner, M. (2002): *The way we think: Conceptual blending and the mind's hidden complexities*. New York: Basic Books.

Filipenko, M.V. (2000): Problemy opisanija predlogov v sovremennyx lingvisticheskix teorijax (obzor). In: Paillard, D. & Seliverstova, O.N. (eds.): *Issledovanija po semantike predlogov*. Moskva: Russkie slovari, 12-54.

Fillmore, Ch. (1968): The case for case. In Bach, E. & Harms, R.T. (eds.): *Universals in linguistic theory*. New York: Holt Rinehart & Winston, 1-88.

Fillmore, Ch. (1977): The case for case reopened. In: Cole, P. & Sadok, J. (eds.): *Syntax and semantics*. Vol. 8. Grammatical relations. New York: Academic Press, 59-82.

Gak, V.G. (1998): *Jazykovye preobrazovanija*. Moskva: Jazyki russkoj kul'tury.

Goddard, C. (1998): *Semantic Analysis*. New York: Oxford University Press.

Grice, H.P. (1975): Logic and conversation. In: Cole, P. & Morgan, J.L. (eds.): *Syntax and Semantics*. Vol. 3. New York: Academic Press, 41-58.

Gugel, H. (1967): *Catull, Carmen* 8. Athenaeum. Studi periodici di Letteratura e Storia dell'Anticita. Università di Pavia. Nuova serie, vol. XLV, 278-293.

Gurevich, V.V. (1988): *Semanticheskaja proizvodnost' v grammatike*. Moskva: MGPI.

Humboldt, W. v. (1836): *Über die Verschiedenheit des Menschlichen Sprachbaues und ihren Einfluß auf die geistige Entwicklung des Menschengeschlechts*. Berlin: Druckerei der Königlichen Akademie der Wissenschaften.

Ivanov, V.V. (1999): *Structura Gomerovskix tekstov, opisyvajushchix vnutrennie sostojanija*. Iz rabot Moskovskogo semioticheskogo kruga. Moskva: Jazyki russkoj kul'tury, 547-575.

Jakobson, R. (1955): On linguistic aspects of translation. In: Brower, R.A. (ed.): *On translation*. Cambridge, Mass.: Harvard University Press, 232-239.

Jakobson, R. (1960): Linguistics and poetics. In: Sebeok, T. A. (ed.): *Style in Language*. Cambridge, Mass.: MIT Press, 130-144.

Jakobson, R. (1971a): Beitrag zur allgemeinen Kasuslehre: Gesamtbedeutungen der russischen Kasus. In: Jakobson, R.: *Selected Writings* II. Paris: The Hague, 133-175.

Jakobson, R. (1971b): Morfologicheskie nabljudenija nad slavjanskim skloneniem. In: Jakobson, R.: *Selected Writings* II, Paris: The Hague, 176-197.

Janda, L. (1986): A semantic analysis of the Russian verbal prefixes 'za-', 'pere-', 'do', and 'ot-'. *Slavistische Beiträge* B. 192. München: Sagner.

Johnson, M. (1987): *The Body in the Mind: The Bodily Basis of Meaning, Imagination, and Reason*. Chicago: University of Chicago Press.

Kibrik, A.E. (1980): Predikatno-argumentnye otnoshenija v semanticheski ergativnyx jazykax. *Izvestija AN SSSR, Literatura i jazyk series* 39, 324-335.

Kiseleva, K.L. & Paillard, D. (1998): Diskursivnye slova kak ob''ekt lingvisticheskogo opisanija. In: Kiseleva, K.L. & Paillard, D. (eds.): *Diskursivnye slova russkogo jazyka*. Moskva: Metatekst, 7-44.

Kurylowicz, J. (1960): *Esquisses linguistiques*. Wroclaw & Kraków: Ossolineum.

Kustova, G.I. (2004): *Tipy proizvodnyx znachenij i mexanizmy jazykovogo rasshirenija*. Moskva: Jazyki slavjanskoj kul'tury.

Lakoff, G. (1987): *Women, Fire, and Dangerous Things: What Categories Reveal about the Mind*. Chicago: University of Chicago Press.

Langacker, R. (2002): *Concept, Image, and Symbol*. Berlin: Mouton de Gruyter.

Lindner, S. (1983): *A lexico-semantic analysis of English verb particle constructions with OUT and UP*. Blumington, Indiana: Indiana University Linguistics Club.

Lotman, Ju.M. (1970): *Struktura xydozhestvennogo teksta*. Moskva: Iskusstvo.

MAS (Malyj Akademicheskij Slovar'): *Slovar' russkogo jazyka v 4 tomax*. Evgen'eva, A.P. (ed.) (1999). Moskva: Russkij jazyk.

Mel'chuk I.A., Clas A. & Polguère A. (1995): *Introduction a la lexicologie explicative et combinatoire*. Louvain-la Neuve: Editions Duculot.

Mel'chuk, I. (1999): *Opyt teorii lingvisticheskix modelej "Smysl⇔Tekst"*. Moskva: Jaz. rus. kul'tury.

Mel'chuk, I.A. & Zholkovskij, A.K. (1984): *Explanatory-Combinatorial Dictionary of Modern Russian*. Wien: Wiener Slavistischer Almanach.

Nikolaeva, T. M. (1997): *"Slovo o polku Igoreve" i Pushkinskie teksty*. Moskva: Indrik.

Paducheva, E.V. (1974): *O semantike sintaksisa*. Moskva: Nauka.

Paducheva, E.V. (1982): Tema jazykovoj kommunikacii v skazkax L'juisa Kerolla. *Semiotika i informatika* 18, 76-119.

Paducheva, E.V. (1996): *Semanticheskie issledovanija*. Moskva: Jazyki russkoj kul'tury.

Paducheva, E.V. (2000): O semanticheskoj derivacii: slovo kak paradigma leksem. *Russkij yazyk v nauchnom osveshchenii* 1, 87-111.

Paducheva, E.V. (2004): *Dinamicheskie modeli v semantike leksiki*. Moskva: Jaz. slavjanskoj kul'tury.

Percov, N.V. (1996): O nekotoryx problemax sovremennoj semantiki i komp'juternoj lingvistiki. *Moskovskij lingvisticheskij al'manax* 1, 9-66.

Percov, N.V. (2000): O neodnoznachnosti v poeticheskom jazyke. *Voprosy jazykoznanija* 3, 55-82.

Percov, N.V. (2001): *Invarianty v russkom slovoizmenenii*. Moskva: Jazyki russkoj kul'tury.

Percova, N.N. (1988): *Formalizacija tolkovanija slova*. Moskva: Izdatel'stvo MGU.

Plungian, V.A. (2001): Pristavka *pod-* v russkom jazyke: k opisaniju semanticheskoj seti. *Moskovskij lingvisticheskij zhurnal* 5 (1), 95-124.

Plungian, V.A. & Rakhilina, E.V. (1996): Polisemija sluzhebnyx slov: predlogi *cherez* i *skvoz'*. *Rusistika segodja* 3, 3-21.

Plungian, V.A. & Rakhilina, E.V. (2000): Po povodu 'lokalistskoj' koncepcii znachenija: predlog *pod*. In: Paillard, D. & Seliverstova, O.N. (eds.): *Issledovanija po semantike predlogov*. Moskva: Russkie slovari, 115-133.

Potebnja , A.A. (1976): Mysl' i jazyk [Thought and language]. In: Potebnja, A.A.: *Estetika i poetika*. Moskva: Iskusstvo.

Rakhilina, E.V. (2000a): O tendencijax v razvitii kognitivnoj semantiki. *Izvestija RAN, Literatura i jazyk* 59, 3-15.

Rakhilina, E.V. (2000b): 'Bez konca i bez kraja' ['Without end and without edge']. In: Paillard, D. & Seliverstova, O.N. (eds.): *Issledovanija po semantike predlogov*. Moskva: Russkie slovari, 243-262.

Rozina, R.I. (2005): *Semanticheskoe razvitie slova v russkom literaturnom jazyke i sovremennom slenge*. Moskva: Azbukovnik.

Rudzka-Ostyn, B. (1993): Introduction. In: Rudzka-Ostyn, B. & Geiger, R.A. (eds.): *Conceptualizations and Mental Processing in Language*. Berlin: Mouton de Gruyter, 1-20.

Sannikov, V.Z. (1999): *Russkij jazyk v zerkale jazykovoj igry*. Moskva: Jazyki russkoj kul'tury.

Sarnov, B. (2002): *Nash sovetskij novojaz*. Moskva: Materik.

Saussure, F. de (1973 [1916]): *Cours de linguistique générale*. Paris: Payot.

Shklovsky, V. (1940): *O Majakovskom*. Moskva: Sovetskij pisatel'.

Shmelev, D.N. (1973): *Problemy semanticheskogo analiza leksiki*. Moskva: Nauka.

Shmelev, A.D. (2002): *Russkaja jazykovaja model' mira. Opyt slovarja*. Moskva: Jaz. slav. kul'tury.

Stern, G. (1931): *Meaning and Change of Meaning*. Göteborg: Elanders.

Swadesh, M. (1972): *The Origin and Diversification of Language*. London: Routledge.

Talmy, L. (2000): *Toward a Cognitive Semantics*. Cambrigde, Mass.: MIT Press.

Turovsky, V.V. (1985): O sootnoshenii znachenij mnogoznachnogo slova. In: *Semiotika i informatika*. Vol. 26, Moscow: VINITI. 83-104.

Turovsky, V.V. (1991): Pamjat' v naivnoj kartine mira: *zabyt', vspomnit', pomnit'*. In: Arutjunova, N.D. (ed.): *Logicheskij analiz jazyka. Kul'turnye koncepty*. Moskva: Nauka.

Ungerer, F. & Schmid, H.-J. (1996): *An Introduction to Cognitive Linguistics*. London: Longman.

Uryson, E.V. (1997): Nesostojavshajasja polisemija. (Tipy tolkovanij s sojuzom *ili*). In: Krysin, L.P. (ed.): *Oblik slova: sbornik statej v pamjat' Dmitrija Nikolaevicha Shmeleva*. Moskva: Russkie slovari, 113-121.

Uspensky, V.A. (1979): O veshchnyx konnotacijax abstraktnyx sushchestvitel'nyx. In: *Semiotika i informatika*. Volume 11. Moscow: VINITI, 142-147.

Uspensky, B.A. (1994): Anatomija metafory u Mandel'shtama. In Uspensky, B.A.: *Izbrannye trudy*. Vol. II. Moskva: Jazyki russkoj kul'tury, 246-274.

Wierzbicka, A. (1980): *The Case for Surface Case*. Ann Arbor: Karoma.

Wierzbicka, A. (1987): *English Speech Act Verbs. A Semantic Dictionary*. Sydney: Academic Press.

Wierzbicka, A. (1992): *Semantics, Culture, and Cognition. Universal Human Concepts in Culture-Specific Configurations*. Oxford: Oxford University Press.

Wierzbicka, A. (1996): *Semantics: Primes and Universals*. Oxford: Oxford University Press.

Wierzbicka, A. (1999): *Emotions across Languages and Cultures*. Cambridge: Cambridge University Press.

Wierzbicka, A. (2002): Russkie kul'turnye skripty i ih otrazhenie v jazyke. *Russkij jazyk v nauchnom osveshchenii* 2, 6-34.

Zalizniak, A.A. (1991): De la nature du regret. *Bulletin de la Société de linguistique générale et appliquée* 17, 67-78.

Zalizniak, A.A. (1992): Investigations in the Semantics of Inner State Predicates. *Slavistische Beiträge* 298. München: Otto Sagner Verlag.

Zalizniak, A.A. (1994): Prazdnik zhizni proxodit mimo (Zametki o neodnoznachnosti nekotoryx russkix slov). *Wiener Slavistischer Almanach* 34, 261-278.

Zalizniak, A.A. (1995): Opyt modelirovanija semantiki pristavochnyx glagolov v russkom jazyke. *Russian linguistics* 19, 143-185.

Zalizniak, A.A. (2006): *Mnogoznachnost' v jazyke i sposoby ejo predstavlenija*. Moscow: Jaz. slav. kul'tur.

Zalizniak, A.A. & Levontina, I.B. (1996): Otrazhenie nacional'nogo xaraktera v leksike russkogo jazyka (razmyshlenija po povodu knigi Anna Wierzbicka, Semantics, Culture, and Cognition. Universal Human Concepts in Culture-Specific Configurations. New York: Oxford University Press, 1992). *Russian Linguistics* 20, 237-264.

On Irregular Polysemy[*]

Gergely Pethő

Department of German Linguistics, University of Debrecen
H-4010 Debrecen, Pf. 47.
E-mail: pethog@inf.unideb.hu

Most research on polysemy has so far concentrated (for understandable reasons) primarily on data which show meaning variation that is in some sense systematic (regular). According to common wisdom, these are the only phenomena in connection with which there is a reasonable chance for meaning variation to be explained and predicted (namely, by revealing its underlying regularities). A general definition of systematic polysemy is commonplace: systematic polysemy involves at least two lexical items (lexemes) which have different readings (or interpretations; these two terms will be used interchangeably throughout this paper), and among these one can distinguish at least two types of reading which occur with each of these lexemes. In other words, the lexemes have several different parallel readings. Let us introduce the term 'polysemy type' to designate a particular pattern of (polysemic) meaning variation. There are several different systematic polysemy types in each language – for example, Pethő (2004) presents about sixty (more or less productive ones) in Hungarian nouns. Let us see two examples for such types from English and German, respectively.[1]

(1) 'legal relation' – 'document which proves that this obtains'
Some examples: *insurance*, *permission*, *agreement*, *commission*, *contract*

(a) 'legal relation'
All employees have the permission to park their vehicles in the parking lot of the company.

(b) 'document'
Show me your permission!

---

[*] Publication of the present paper was supported by the Research Group for Theoretical Linguistics of the Hungarian Academy of Sciences at the Universities of Debrecen, Pécs and Szeged. The author would like to thank Marina Rakova, Csilla Rákosi, Piroska Kocsány, Mária Ladányi, András Kertész, Péter Csatár and Péter Pelyvás for their helpful comments on different versions of this paper. This research was supported by Grant F42664 of the Hungarian Scientific Research Fund.

[1] In the numbering P indicates a proposition, Q a question, D a definition and plain numbers everything else.

(2) 'figure (number)' – 'coin or bank note with this value'
Some examples: German *Zehner*, *Zwanziger*, *Tausender;* cf. also Hungarian *tízes*, *húszas*, *ezres*, meaning: '10', '20', '1000', respectively

By looking at the literature we can conclude that research during the past approximately twenty years has led us significantly closer to understanding the nature of systematic lexical meaning variation. But whereas our knowledge of systematic polysemy has grown considerably, research has barely taken up non-systematic polysemy. The topic of this paper will be this latter group of phenomena, which should be examined even though interpretations varying in a non-systematic way cannot be predicted.

In the following I will try to show that non-systematic polysemy phenomena do not form a homogeneous set. They can be subclassified, and the examination of each class can lead to important conclusions in connection with theories of polysemy and other linguistic phenomena (especially metaphor). The main point of my argument will be that the identification of metonymically motivated polysemy with systematic polysemy and that of metaphorically motivated polysemy with non-systematic polysemy (which is wide-spread in the literature) is in fact not correct. On the one hand, systematicity in some sense can also be observed in connection with metaphorically motivated polysemy, as is quite well-known thanks to research in the framework of the theory of conceptual metaphors. Nevertheless, the nature of this systematicity is quite different from the one that can be attributed to metonymic polysemy. On the other hand, metonymically motivated polysemy is not necessarily systematic: its predictability is restricted by factors (independent of the basis for meaning variation) such as the aspect of communicative needs or arbitrary lexicalisation.

The subject of this study will be nouns which show non-systematic polysemy phenomena. The material will consist of examples from English, German and Hungarian. The choice of languages is arbitrary and essentially unimportant, as the argumentation of this text should be adequate for nominal polysemy in any other language as well, although the choice of examples would obviously have to be partly different. The restriction to nouns, however, is relevant from a theoretical perspective: the concepts that are required for the explanation of the polysemy of nouns are different from those that are needed to explain polysemy of adjectives and verbs. Verb polysemy, for example, is closely connected to the notion of argument structure alternations, cf. e.g. Levin (1993) and Ladányi (this volume). From this it follows that it makes sense to restrict the study to a specific part of speech, in order to be able to present a relatively coherent and self-contained account.

The theoretical background and the general approach are akin to the versions of two-level semantics modified by Dölling (2001). This approach is cognitive in the (relatively wide) sense that it follows the principles codified by Chomsky's transformational and generative grammar for approaches to linguistics, e.g.: The ultimate goal is not the description of individual phenomena, but rather the explanation of how the language faculty that is contained in the minds of the speakers works. Language is treated as a mental property (instead of a social construct), and interrelation between language and other systems of knowledge is not ruled out as such (i.e. language is not pictured as a closed system which is independent of everything else, as in classic structuralism).

The structure of the paper is as follows: In chapter 1, I will present a brief overview of some attempts to explain systematic polysemy, and I will also discuss the notion of metonymical and metaphorical motivation. Chapter 2 contains five case studies, which indicate that the relationship between the systematicity of polysemy and its metaphoric/metonymic motivation is not as straightforward as is generally taken for granted. On the basis of the case studies, a theoretically founded classification of non-systematic polysemy phenomena is also developed. Finally I will summarize the conclusions of the paper in chapter 3.

1. The Notions of Systematicity and Motivation of Polysemy

The goal of this chapter will be to introduce the main concepts which will be employed in later parts of the paper (this will include references to important contemporary work on the topic). First, I will delimit the notion of systematic polysemy more precisely, namely, by explicating it as polysemy that can be described by rules. Then I will introduce two types of rule (so-called focussing and shifting rules), which are required according to the more recent literature to explain systematic polysemy phenomena. Finally I will outline, on the one hand, the notion of the metonymic motivation of polysemy, which appears as a collateral consequence of the rules presented earlier, and on the other hand the notion of metaphoric motivation, which is generally regarded as the counterpart of the former in the literature.

In the introduction I gave a rather imprecise characterisation of what systematic polysemy is. There I did not mention an important complex property that is generally associated with systematic polysemy: the possibility to be described by rules. Systematic polysemy is considered a more interesting phenomenon than non-systematic polysemy exactly because meaning variation of a certain type occurring with several words can be potentially described by rules. For such rules, similar considerations apply as to rules in morphology (e.g. word formation). There is a reason to assume that a linguistic phenomenon is based not merely on the learning of individual forms and meanings, but also, and to a greater extent, on the application of rules, if the following conditions are satisfied (for a more detailed discussion cf. e.g. Haspelmath 2002).[2]

(P1) A phenomenon can be described by a rule if and only if it is equally true that

(a) The distribution of the phenomenon can be exactly described (in other words, the conditions of the rule's application can be specified) and the relation of the elements involved in the phenomenon can be exactly characterised (i.e. the input and the output of the rule can be specified). If on the basis of the element to which the rule is applied (the input) and of the assumed rule the form and meaning of the derived element (the output) cannot be predicted, or no

---

[2] Note that these conditions only apply to rules which derive a structure from another one, i.e. relate two structures to each other. They do not tell us anything about rules which, for example, regulate whether a given structure is well-formed on its own, like the principles of generative grammar, e.g. principles A, B and C of Binding Theory. Rules of the latter type are not usually discussed in the literature in connection with the phenomena in question, so I will ignore them in what follows.

conditions of application can be found which correctly characterise the distribution of the phenomenon, it is not correct to talk about a rule.

(b) The phenomenon is productive. Conditions of the use of a rule always have to be put in such a form that they characterise, in an abstract manner, the circumstances under which the rule can be applied. In other words, if the conditions of the application of the rule could only be formulated in a way that eligible input elements are exhaustively enumerated (not characterized by their properties, but rather identified by their names), it is not correct to talk about rule application. If the conditions are given in the form of abstract properties, the rule can be applied potentially to input elements to which it has not been applied earlier, for example because the input element has been newly created, did not exist in the language previously, or because there has been no communicative need earlier to derive the output element.[3]

If either of the conditions in (a) and (b) does not hold for a phenomenon (note that (b) cannot hold if (a) is not fulfilled), then it can only be attributed to learning, but not to rule application. In practice, a condition stronger than (b) is employed when deciding whether something should be described by a rule: the number of elements exhibiting the phenomenon should not be just potentially unbounded, but it should be in fact observable in connection with a large number of elements. In section 2, I will argue that this further condition does not hold for certain polysemy phenomena which can be described by rules according to (P1).

It is mostly explicitly stated in the literature – or sometimes presupposed tacitly – that systematic polysemy conforms to rules according to principle (P1). For example, the above conditions hold of the polysemy type 'figure'[4] – 'money' mentioned above: The conditions of application can be exactly determined language-specifically (any numeral with the suffix *-er*), as well as its input element (refers to a figure) and its output element (refers to a coin or bank note). The type is productive, i.e. if there is a communicative need to name money of a denomination that has not existed before (Germ. *Sechser* '6', *Dreitausender* '3000' etc.), then the numeral can be used for this purpose. Because the type is productive, its extension is not just a small finite number of elements, but a potentially unbounded number of them.

---

[3] The applicability of these two principles is limited by the phenomenon of analogy. If we notice that a specific pattern that could only be used in a bounded (not extendable) number of cases earlier (i.e. it was either not productive or it only appeared in connection with a single element, so the question did not even arise that it could be a case of rule application) is now used sporadically in further cases as well, it is still not justified to talk about rule application, but rather about analogy. According to some researchers (e.g. Pinker 1999) there is a qualitative difference between analogy and rule application in terms of mental representations and processes. However, it does not seem possible in theory to draw a strict distinction between the two on the level of the data. In other words, it is not possible to provide either clear quantitative or qualitative criteria for when a given phenomenon should be regarded as a result of an analogy or a rule. The decision therefore depends on the linguist's discretion in practice.

[4] For lack of a better simple designation, I will use "figure" to refer to the graphic representation of a number, even if it is not a single digit, i.e. both 5 and 555 will be called a figure.

There are two main types of rule suggested in the literature for the description of systematic polysemy phenomena, which I will refer to as focussing and shifting rules in the following. This terminology is based on the one introduced in Pethő (2001a), since there are no generally accepted terms for the processes in question (nor is there any clear consensus with respect to the question whether these two kinds of rule are sufficient). I will not present a detailed survey of the literature from this field here, but refer to my more detailed discussion of earlier literature (which ignores most work on generative lexicon theory, unfortunately) in Pethő (2001b).

1.1. Focussing Rules

Before we can define the notion of focussing rule, some preliminary assumptions are required. Let L be a lexeme (lexical item) and M the concept that is assigned to it in the dictionary (i.e. L's meaning, assuming we take meanings to be concepts). The concept M is complex in the sense that it identifies distinct but interrelated entities (parts of reality, events etc.). The concept BOOK, for example, is complex in this sense: the essence of a book is that there is a given closed form (mostly an object made of paper), and this form carries a certain content (mostly a text that is formulated in some language). We also know that the content usually deals with a more or less defined topic, it has one or more authors, the book has a publisher etc. Let us assume that concepts can be approximately described by specifying the entities (x, y, z etc.) that the concept refers to (in a non-technical sense of referring), properties assigned to those entities (P, Q etc.), and relations that hold between those entities (R_1, R_2 etc.): $M = [x, y, z, \ldots P(x), Q(y), \ldots R_1 (x, y), R_2 (y, z), \ldots]$. To connect to the previous example: Let x be the variable denoting the object made of paper, y denoting the content, z the author, P the property of being a physical object, Q the property of being information, R_1 the containment relation that holds between an object that can be called a book and its content, and R_2 the relation that holds between a content and its author. Let us set a terminological convention that the entities, properties and relations pertaining to these entities which are connected to M can be called parts of the concept M.

Against the background of these assumptions, the function of a focussing rule can be defined as follows:

(D1) A focussing rule is a rule that makes it possible, on the basis of the complex concept M connected to the lexeme L, for a speaker to refer to an entity x, which is a part of concept M, using lexeme L in a given context.

To use the previous example, we can use the word *book* to refer to (i.e. denote) a book as a physical object, which is entity x (*the book is on the shelf*), or in a different context to a book as content, which is entity y (*the book is interesting*). According to a widespread assumption, the meaning of the lexeme *book* itself is underspecified, i.e. it is not defined whether it denotes a physical object or content, but it is rather assigned a complex concept as outlined above. The word can be used in a way that is unspecific in this respect. For example, whereas the word *book* clearly refers to books as physical objects in the compound *bookshelf*, it cannot be definitely said that it would exclusively refer to either aspect of books in the compound *book-printing.* (Rather it refers to the process when some content is combined with a physical object, i.e. both aspects at the same time.) However, if the word is used in one of these specific senses, it is a focussing rule that derives the intended interpretation.

Focussing rules are present in the works of several authors in different forms. For example, in his relatively early writings on this topic (Bierwisch 1983; Bierwisch & Lang 1987), Bierwisch proposed that systematic polysemy phenomena can always be described by such rules, which he called (somewhat confusingly) "conceptual shift" or "konzeptuelle Verschiebung". Later, Dölling in several of his publications (2001) and Pustejovsky in his Generative Lexicon theory (1995) suggested similar underspecified semantic representations and rules. Dölling (2001: 88) lists the word *newspaper* in the lexicon as an item that is not assigned to a single semantic sort, i.e. either physical object, mental object (content) or institution (the newspaper's publisher) specifically, but rather to the union of these three sorts. Pustejovsky introduces the "dot" operator for this same purpose, which generates complex semantic types (types play essentially the same role in his ontology as sorts in more traditional formal semantics). Both authors use a focussing rule (which Dölling calls 'sort specification rule' and Pustejovsky 'type pumping rule') to select a more specific interpretation. For essentially the same reason, Pethő (2001a) introduced – in a more traditional semantic decomposition framework – the rule of conceptual focussing, according to which the operation of focussing can be described according to the following schema, where the double arrow signifies the application of a focussing rule to *M*:

(3)
$$M = P(x)\ \&\ Q(y)\ \&\ O(z)\ \&\ \ldots\ \&\ R_1(x, y)\ \&\ R_2(y, z)$$
$$\Rightarrow M_x = \lambda x\ \exists y\ \exists z\ [P(x)\ \&\ Q(y)\ \&\ O(z)\ \&\ \ldots\ \&\ R_1(x, y)\ \&\ R_2(y, z)]$$
$$\Rightarrow M_y = \lambda y\ \exists x\ \exists z\ [P(x)\ \&\ Q(y)\ \&\ O(z)\ \&\ \ldots\ \&\ R_1(x, y)\ \&\ R_2(y, z)]$$
$$\Rightarrow M_z = \lambda z\ \exists x\ \exists y\ [P(x)\ \&\ Q(y)\ \&\ O(z)\ \&\ \ldots\ \&\ R_1(x, y)\ \&\ R_2(y, z)]$$
...

A free variable in the conceptual representation *M* (assigned to lexeme *L*) is bound by a lambda operator, whereas the remaining free variables are bound by an existential quantifier each. In this way, we obtain a representation (M_x, M_y, M_z etc.) by which the lexeme can be used to refer to that particular aspect of the concept which is represented by the given variable. Here and in the following, I will provide the formal representations of concepts (like *M*) in a way as if they were propositions.

One of the most interesting questions of polysemy research, for which there is as yet no definite answer to be found in the literature, is the following:

(Q1) Which parts of a concept *M* may be focussed upon by a focussing rule?

For example the words *book* and *newspaper* can both be used to refer to an object or some content. However, with the word *newspaper* we can refer to the institution which publishes the newspaper as well (*the newspaper employs 20 editors*), i.e. a further part of $M_{\text{NEWSPAPER}}$, whereas the word *book* cannot be used to refer to the author in general, for example (*#the book has long brown hair*), but only to the author via the thoughts and opinions expressed in the text (*A new book claims William Shakespeare wrote none of his plays [...]* – example taken from the British National Corpus, BNC).

We can find two kinds of answer for (Q1) in the literature: Some authors (most clearly Bierwisch 1983) claim that it is the concepts in question – i.e. elements of categorisation, of thought (which are essentially extralinguistic) – that determine what focussed readings are possible. Along this line, the explanation for the difference noted above may be that the status of the publishing institution within the concept NEWSPAPER is different (e.g. more important) than that of the author within the concept BOOK. On the basis of the works of other authors, it can be assumed (although this is not explicitly stated usually) that the mental lexical entry of the lexeme (i.e. a genuinely linguistic factor) determines the availability of focusable interpretations. For example, as has been mentioned above, Dölling specifies in the lexicon what aspects of the concept the word *newspaper* can be used to refer to.

Since Bierwisch's solution would obviously have greater explanatory power, this approach would seem preferable. It has a fundamental problem, however: it is not obvious, how the status of the author in the concept M_{BOOK} differs from the status of the publishing institution in the concept of $M_{\text{NEWSPAPER}}$. Unless this and similar questions can be answered, this explanation will be at least incomplete.

After having outlined the notion of focussing rule, let us address the question of what this rule type has to do with systematic polysemy. The literature mentions several types of polysemy where the systematically recurring readings can be derived by a focussing rule from an underspecified representation. We have already seen one such example in connection with the nouns *book* and *newspaper:* there are several nouns that exhibit the meaning variation 'information carrier' – 'content'. Further examples of this are *novel*, *letter*, *cassette*, *recording*, *CD*, *DVD* etc. This meaning variation seems to be systematic and can be reasonably described by a rule: the two interpretations in question can be characterised relatively well, the conditions of the use of an alternation rule can be specified, and the phenomenon is productive (as proven by nonce words like *CD* and *DVD*). Another well-known meaning variation that can be described by focussing rule is the alternation 'building' – 'institution' which is exemplified by the words *school*, *university*, *police*, *shop* etc.

It should be noted, however, that this systematicity is not necessarily due to a focussing rule that functions according to schema (3). For there are two possibilities:

1. The focussing rule is an extremely general rule that only says that, on the basis of any underspecified conceptual representation which has several distinct entities as its parts, we can refer by the word connected to this concept to any of these entities.[5] In other words, there is a single common focussing rule underlying all specific meaning variations like 'information-carrier' – 'content', 'building' – 'institution',

---

[5] For exactly this reason Dölling (2001 [1997]) does not introduce a focussing rule at all, but attributes the derivations that follow schema (3) to a general mechanism of abduction which works on the basis of context. I will not explore this possibility any further here, because I believe that it is the assumption of underspecified conceptual representations rather than of an actual focussing rule that is essential in connection with the polysemy phenomena in question. Dölling's (2001 [1997]) model is fully compatible with what is said here in connection with focussing rules.

'plant' – 'relevant part of that plant that is used for eating etc.', 'event' – 'object that is a result of that event', 'event' – 'people connected to that event', and many more. The general rule states the overall conditions for all these latter specific focussing operations and their effects. Dölling's sort specification and Pustejovsky's type pumping rules are formulated in this way.

If we take this approach, the focussing rule itself does not directly say anything about the variations 'information-carrier' – 'content' and 'building' – 'institution' at all. Consequently, the focussing rule itself is not enough to explain their systematicity. This systematicity can only arise if the inputs for the focussing rule for each relevant lexeme are similar in the respect that they have entities of the same kind as parts and these are equally accessible to the focussing rules.

Let us consider the following: if there are several lexemes associated with conceptual representations which have an entity x characterised by a certain property P as a part, and which also have an entity y as a part that is characterised by a certain property Q, and both x and y are accessible for the focussing rule, then there will be several lexemes that exhibit the meaning variation $P – Q$. If there is only a single lexeme like this, then only that single lexeme will exhibit it. The fact that several concepts are structured in a similar way (and we can therefore observe the same kind of meaning variation in the case of their associated words, e.g. 'information-carrier' – 'content') does not follow from the schema of the focussing rule as such, but has to be explained by other rules, which are presumably not linguistic rules, but rather regularities of concept formation.

This observation also provides an indirect argument for Bierwisch's answer to question (Q1), namely, that the reason for the meaning variations is to be found in the structure of the concepts. Because if we go with the other alternative, the solution chosen by Dölling to state the possible focusable readings for each word individually in the lexicon, we should expect that the readings available for each word are essentially idiosyncratic and cannot be predicted. However, this does not seem to be the case, as the productivity of the polysemy patterns in question suggests.[6]

2. The second possibility is that a separate focussing rule has to be formulated for each group exhibiting a certain meaning variation pattern. If we assume such rules, then the productivity of the meaning variations according to given patterns can be regarded as a consequence of the focussing rule itself. I do not know of a theory in the literature that claims this, and the phenomena to be discussed in section 2.1 below do not seem to be compatible with such an interpretation of focussing rules, so I will ignore this possibility in what follows. I will assume that the focussing rule is not formu-

---

6 Although according to Pustejovsky (1995) the focusable entities are also specified in the lexicon for each word, in his case the problem stated above arises in a different form. In his ontology, individual words, e.g. *school*, inherit their focusable interpretations from a superordinate word, e.g. *institution*. So words belonging to a common superordinate category are expected to show consequently the same meaning variation. Nevertheless, there are some problems in this framework as well that have to be taken care of. On the one hand, the non-trivial rules that guide this inheritance between categories have to be stated (for not all subordinate categories inherit their possible readings from a superordinate category necessarily, cf. the examples in Pustejovsky (1991) like *novel* and *dictionary*). On the other hand, this ontology does not explain differences like the one stated between *newspaper* and *book*, either, but can at best state them.

lated for specific meaning variations individually, but that it is rather a more general mechanism.

1.2. Shifting Rules

Whereas focussing rules relate to some inherently given part of a concept, and foreground such a part, there is a relatively clear consensus within polysemy research that further kinds of meaning derivation rules are also required if we want to account for the whole range of systematic polysemy phenomena. The reason for this is that in certain cases it is not obviously justified to claim that several systematically related interpretations can be identified with different aspects of one and the same complex concept.

Let us take as an example the polysemy 'figure' – 'money' that has been mentioned earlier. A possible solution to describe this would be to assign a conceptual representation of the form (3) to German words of the form *N-er* (*Fünfer*, *Zwanziger*, *Hunderter* etc.), where x is the variable referring to the figure, y refers to the coin or bank note, and both interpretations can be derived by focussing rules. But the problem with this solution is that it contradicts the intuition that the interpretation 'money' is secondary to the interpretation 'figure', which is relatively independent of the former. Let us see how this problem appears in connection with this group of examples.

Firstly we can plausibly assume that there are two distinct concepts (for each number relevant at this point) represented in our minds. One is the concept of the number itself (e.g. FIVE), which can itself be taken to be complex: it refers to the number as an abstract mathematical entity, the appropriate amount, the figure representing it in writing etc. The other is the concept of the money of the appropriate value (e.g. FIVE-EURO NOTE), which includes the information whether the money of that denomination is a coin or a bank note, what it looks like, what real value it represents etc. Whereas it is a fundamental property of the latter concept that it refers to the concept of the number FIVE (as we necessarily know of five-euro notes that their value is equal to five units), it is not a fundamental property of the concept of the number FIVE (as opposed to SIX, for example) that there is a coin or bank note that has this value. We can easily count, add, multiply etc. using the number five without even knowing anything about five-euro notes. Thus the relation of the two concepts to each other is not symmetric: we do not need FIVE-EURO NOTE in order to define FIVE, but we do need FIVE in order to define FIVE-EURO NOTE.

Assuming that we try to describe the meaning variation in connection with the word *Fünfer* according to schema (3), i.e. by a focussing rule operating on an underspecified semantic representation, we have to assign the concept FIVE-EURO NOTE or FIVE-CENT COIN as the underspecified representation to this word. The reason for this is that according to what was said above, both the concept FIVE (the number) and reference to the money are parts of these concepts. On the other hand, the M assigned to the word *Fünfer* cannot be the concept FIVE itself, as the money with the value of five units is not part of this concept, so the reading 'bank note' cannot be derived from it by focussing.

Firstly we encounter the complication that FIVE-EURO NOTE or FIVE-CENT COIN are clearly two quite different concepts, so the word should be regarded as essentially homonymous if these should be its primary meanings instead of FIVE. Whereas the assumption of homonymy here seems rather implausible in itself, there are further problems as well. In order not to make the discussion more complicated than necessary, I will ignore in the following the fact that *Fünfer* can refer to all manners of things beside the figure (in principle anything that can be identified with the help of the number 5, e.g. a bus line, a shoe or a screwdriver of this size etc.) and concentrate on the relation between the 'bank note' and the 'figure' interpretations.

As stated above, the assumption that would have to be made in order to account for this meaning variation by a focussing rule is that the word *Fünfer* is primarily assigned the concept of the bank note, and reference to the figure 5 only arises indirectly through this. Therefore, we should expect that speakers should feel that the primary meaning of this word is 'bank note', or 'bank note' and 'figure' should at least be felt to be equally basic. However, in fact it is felt that the interpretation 'number' or 'figure' is basic and 'bank note' is derived in some sense, even though the latter is probably somewhat more frequent in actual language use. Thus a prediction which can be plausibly derived from the focussing account does not agree with the intuitions of the language users.

Let us further assume that the interpretation 'figure' would be derived from the concept FIVE-EURO NOTE by focussing, in approximately the following way:

(4) $M_{\text{FIVE-EURO\_NOTE}} = \text{BANK NOTE}(x) \,\&\, \text{FIGURE}(y) \,\&\, \text{FIVE}(z) \,\&\, \text{VALUE}(x, z) \,\&\, \text{REPRESENT}(y, z) \,\&\, ...$

$\Rightarrow M_{\text{FIVE-EURO\_NOTE}, y} = \lambda y\, \exists x\, \exists z\, [\text{BANK NOTE}(x) \,\&\, \text{FIGURE}(y) \,\&\, \text{FIVE}(z) \,\&\, \text{VALUE}(x, z) \,\&\, \text{REPRESENT}(y, z) \,\&\, ...]$

where the representation in the second row is gained by applying a focussing rule according to schema (3), and it is the interpretation through which the figure 5 can be referred to by the word *Fünfer*.

According to representation (4), in a context where the actual interpretation of this word is the figure (e.g. *auf dem Blatt steht ein Fünfer* 'there is a figure five on the sheet of paper'), the interpretation of that word should be something like 'a figure that corresponds to the value of the five-euro note/that is written on the five-euro note etc.', which sounds rather bizarre and counterintuitive. An interpretation like this would result because focussing does not delete all the information that belongs to the complex concept but is not in focus, e.g. the component BANK NOTE (x). This information is still available in the background, as signalled by the existential quantifiers. This approach seems to be justified and compatible with our intuitions for groups of examples like those mentioned in 1.1, but not for this example or further ones to be mentioned shortly.

It should be added that in the works of authors who employ semantic processes analogous to focussing (type-pumping, sort specification), the fact that focussing rules are unsuited for the description of the phenomenon in question does not reveal itself so transparently, because of notational differences. Apparently, however, the reason why they introduce shifting rules in addition to focussing rules is a similar one.

Above I tried to argue (by reductio ad absurdum) for the claim that focussing rules are not suited to describing certain systematic polysemy phenomena. It follows that we need different rules to be able to account for these. The shifting rules are supposed to fulfil exactly this function.

Shifting rules can be defined in the following way:

(D2) A shifting rule is a rule that makes it possible to refer by a lexeme L to an entity x which is not part of the concept M assigned to L, but stands in a relation R specified by the rule to some entity y which is part of the concept M.

In connection with the example above we can assume that the word *Fünfer* is assigned primarily the complex concept of the number 5, which includes reference to the figure but does not include reference to money. Therefore, on the basis of the underlying concept M by itself, the word *Fünfer* is unable to refer to an entity x which is some money. It is a shifting rule deriving the interpretation 'coin' or 'bank note' on the basis of M that enables us to use this word to refer to these entities x. The fact that x stands in a certain relation R ("value of") to an entity that forms part of M, namely, to the amount "five" (y), satisfies the condition mentioned in the definition.

According to (D2) the schema of shifting rules can be given as follows:

(5) $M = P(y)\ \&\ \ldots$
$\Rightarrow M_O = \lambda x\ \exists y\ [O(x)\ \&\ P(y)\ \&\ R\ (x, y)\ \&\ \ldots]$

where the double arrow signals the application of the shifting rule that introduces the entity x and the relation R, and M_O is the representation on the basis of which lexeme L can refer to an entity x that has property O. In the case of the example above, O is the property BANK NOTE, P is the property FIVE, R is the relation VALUE, and there is a further property Q (FIGURE) with an entity it is assigned to.

Apart from this example, several further polysemy types are known that can presumably be described adequately by shifting rules. A particularly well-documented example is so-called "grinding", by which a mass noun is derived from a count noun without any morphological change, and the mass noun refers to the material that constitutes the thing denoted by the count noun. The most common cases of grinding are to be found in connection with the names of animals or plants, e.g. *I ate chicken for lunch, there is too much onion in the salad* etc., where we do not refer to individual animals or onion bulbs by the noun, but rather chicken meat or the "meat" of onions as a material. Another similar operation is "packaging", which is the reverse of grinding, i.e. it derives a count noun from a mass noun, e.g. *I drank a beer.* Yet a further example is the polysemy 'colour' – 'person characterised by the colour', which has at least three more specific versions: 1) 'colour' – 'person having hair of this colour', e.g. German *ein Blonder* 'a blonde', 2) 'colour' – 'person having skin of this colour', e.g. *ein Schwarzer* 'a black person', and 3) 'colour' – 'person who belongs to a political party or movement symbolised by this colour', e.g. *ein Grüner* 'a person belonging to the Green Party'. Further shifting rules can be used to describe metonymic uses of proper names when the proper name does not represent the individual normally denoted by the name, but rather another entity (a person, a thing etc.) that is connected to this individual. For example, ***Newcastle** called* 'someone who is in Newcastle', ***London** denied the news* 'the British government' and *the museum has bought a **Picasso*** 'a work of art by Picasso' etc.

There are several authors who employ shifting rules in their theories of polysemy, e.g. Dölling (2001) who calls them shift rules, or Copestake & Briscoe (1996) who talk about sense extension rules. The type coercion rules introduced in Pustejovsky (1995) also conform to definition (D2) above.

Among the shifting rules we can distinguish two subtypes. On the one hand there are shifting rules deriving interpretations of a lexeme *L* which are relatively independent of specific contexts, often usual interpretations which are presumably listed in the lexicon (the above examples, with the possible exception of the proper names, belong to this group). On the other hand there are some which are triggered by specific contexts and are determined specifically by the properties of such contexts. Type coercion rules mostly belong to this latter group. For example, we can reasonably assume that the verb *hear* demands as its object an expression that denotes a sound phenomenon, e.g. *she can hear the music.* However, this verb can also be used with direct objects which do not primarily denote a sound phenomenon, but rather a person or a thing, e.g. *I can hear the piano/the announcer.* In such cases the selection restriction that applies to the direct object of the verb *hear* triggers a shifting (type coercion) rule, the result of which is that a noun (that primarily denotes a thing or object) can be used to refer to the sound emitted by that thing or person.

Although it is mostly accepted now that both rule types outlined above are needed to describe the whole range of systematic polysemy phenomena, this was not the case earlier. Interestingly, for example Bierwisch (1983) only assumed rules which are, according to the terminology used here, focussing rules (to describe phenomena which are relevant for us), whereas Nunberg (1979) in turn only assumed shifting rules, cf. Pethő (2001b). The more recent literature (e.g. Nunberg 1996) usually uses focussing rules to describe metonymically motivated polysemy that is symmetric, in the sense that none of the readings in question seems either primary or derived in relation to the others. On the other hand, shifting rules are employed to describe asymmetric metonymically motivated polysemy, i.e. one where one reading is felt to be primary in relation to another derived one.

To conclude the discussion of the two rule types, it makes sense to briefly mention the issue of the psychological reality of these rules. Murphy (this volume) convincingly argues against the common practice that polysemy phenomena are described by rules for the sole reason that the use of rules makes the description more economical. He notes, referring to the results of experimental psycholinguistic research on this topic, that speakers apparently do not use rules to derive different readings of systematically polysemous words, but retrieve these readings from the mental lexicon instead. Since the capacity of the lexicon is very large, there is ample space in it for the explicit representation of many different readings for each systematically polysemous word. In other words, the mental lexicon of speakers is not organised in an economical way. Therefore, if one chooses the principle of economy as the guiding methodological principle and suggests, merely on the basis of this principle, rules to describe systematic polysemy, this description will not be psychologically plausible.

Nevertheless, contrary to Murphy's position, I believe that it is in fact justified to use rules to describe the phenomena in question, because this practice is not only motivated by a methodological principle of parsimony, but more importantly by the productivity of the phenomena in question, cf. (P1)(b) above. As e.g. Pustejovsky (1995) stresses very emphatically, systematic polysemy phenomena can be employed in rather creative and productive ways, so if one chooses a lexicon that simply enumerates the meanings for each word to describe these phenomena, then even the fundamental requirement of observational adequacy is not met. There is an analogous situation in inflectional morphology as well. As Pinker (1999) explains in detail, there are good reasons to believe that not only irregular past tense forms of English verbs are stored in the mental lexicons of the speakers, but a large number of regular past tense forms as well, which could also be derived by the speakers using rules. Still, according to Pinker, we have to assume that the speakers do in fact have a rule for deriving regular past tense forms as well, exactly because of the productivity of regular past tense morphology, and some facts point to the possibility that during language processing the derivation of regular forms by rule in fact competes against the process of looking them up in the lexicon. Thus it does not necessarily follow from Murphy's (this volume) arguments that we should deny the psychological reality of the rules discussed in 1.1 and 1.2.

1.3. Metonymic and Metaphoric Motivation

At least since Apresjan (1973), the idea that systematic polysemy is in most cases metonymically motivated, whereas non-systematic polysemy is metaphorically motivated, has been generally accepted. One of the main aims of the case studies in section 2 will be to refine this claim. In order to be able to do this, it will be useful to clarify how metonymic and metaphoric motivation are to be understood. This is made rather difficult by the fact that we do not have a good definition of either metaphor or metonymy at our disposal. Theories of metaphor and metonymy usually only characterise their respective object phenomena and take it for granted that we can decide whether an expression is e.g. a metaphor. In other words, they do not define the object of their inquiry, and it is not possible to reconstruct an operationalisable definition of metaphor or metonymy even on the basis of their characterisations (cf. Pethő & Csatár 2006). For lack of a better alternative, I will use the classic, but unfortunately very vague "definitions" in attempting to explain why we speak about metonymic and metaphoric motivation in connection with polysemy phenomena.

1.3.1. Metonymic Motivation

Metonymy is the phenomenon when we use a lexeme *L* to refer to some object *y* that is different from the thing *x* that *L* would name if we used this lexeme in its normal, literal sense. This other object *y* stands in the relation of "contiguity" to some *x* that could be literally denoted by *L*. "Contiguity" is not to be understood as the spatial closeness of *x* and *y*, but rather as a superordinate abstract concept that subsumes an unspecified number of relations of many different kinds, from spatial or temporal location proper through the part-whole relation to the cause-effect relation, with the significant exception of the relation of similarity. To put it another way, *x* can be said to be "contiguous" to *y* if *x* has something to do with *y*, except if they are similar to each other.

Therefore, the relations that are described by the shifting and focussing rules above can be basically said to be metonymic, cf. schemas (3) and (5). In both cases there are at least two distinct entities which can be referred to by a lexeme *L*, and these entities are connected by some relation *R* to each other. In the case of focussing rules, this relation *R* is an inherent part of the concept assigned to *L*, whereas the shifting rules introduce the relation *R* themselves. It is also clear that in the examples mentioned above it is never a relation of similarity which relates the two entities to each other, but rather relations like "value of", "material of", "product of" etc. Still there is an important difference between shifting and focussing rules on the one hand and true metonymy on the other: in the case of the latter, reference to the entity *y* is extraordinary, non-literal, whereas in connection with the former, this is not the case, or at least not always. The literature generally agrees that readings derivable by focussing rules are without doubt fully literal, and even have the same status, i.e. one does not get the impression that one reading is derived from or "less primary" than the other. For the shifting rules this is not completely obvious, but still it is usually (e.g. in examples like *I ate* ***chicken*** *for lunch*, *I hear the* ***announcer*** etc.) true that the word that is subjected to a shifting rule is not felt to be less literally used than in examples that are not affected by such rules, e.g. *there are* ***chickens*** *in the yard*, *I see the* ***announcer***. Therefore systematic polysemy phenomena are usually not regarded as true metonymies, but rather as metonymically motivated meaning variations (assuming that none of the meanings is clearly felt to be non-literal).

1.3.2. Metaphoric Motivation

Let us now turn to metaphorically motivated polysemy phenomena. We have not seen any examples of these above, because according to the generally accepted opinion they cannot be described by the kinds of rule that apply to the metonymically motivated ones, and they do not exhibit systematicity either.

Metaphor is the phenomenon when a lexeme *L* is used to characterise a thing *x* for which the property that is expressed by *L* in its unmarked, literal use is not in fact true, but some properties of *x* are similar to the properties that are literally expressed by *L*. This definition is somewhat different from that of metonymy, because metonymy can in general be described as a kind of reference, whereas this is not always the case for metaphor. Specifically, in complete metaphors – e.g. *John is a hippopotamus* – the non-literally used word is not employed to refer to John (this has already been done by the name *John*), but rather to characterise John, namely, that he has some property that is similar to the property of being a hippopotamus. In the case of short (simple) metaphors, however, this "related" property is in fact used to refer to some entity, namely, one that has a property that is similar to the property expressed literally by *L* (but is not identical to it), e.g. *the hippopotamus has arrived* 'John has arrived'.

The similarity between the literally expressed property and the property that in fact holds for the topic of the metaphor is not (or at least not necessarily) objectively given. Metaphor as a stylistic tool presumably owes its effect exactly to the fact that it can point out similarities that are not obvious, and can therefore open up new perspectives for the recipient, cf. e.g. Loewenberg (1975), Glucksberg (2001).

Metaphorically motivated polysemy always follows the pattern of a short metaphor, i.e. a lexeme *L* is used to refer to an entity *y* to which we could not refer by some primary meaning of *L*, but the entity *y* is in some respect similar to some entity or entities *x* which can be referred to on the basis of this primary meaning of *L*.

To illustrate this with an example: Let *L* be the lexeme *horn*, its relevant primary meaning L_1 being 'hard, pointed thing growing on the head of an animal, for example a cow'. This property clearly does not hold of either musical instruments made of metal that resemble a trumpet, nor of things in vehicles that make loud sounds as a signal, yet the word *horn* can be normally used to refer to such objects. This is made possible ultimately by the fact that horns of animals can be used as instruments to create a loud sound. When horns are used in this way, they are similar to the musical instrument (both in their function and the way they are used, i.e. by blowing) and the car part as well (the sound of which is similar to that of an animal horn, and similarly serves as a signal tool).

Metaphorically motivated polysemy is usually not regarded as true metaphor either, for a reason similar to the one we have seen in connection with metonymically motivated polysemy: the non-primary meanings (in this case 'musical instrument' and 'car part') are not felt to be less literal than the primary one. Historically it can probably be shown, and it is at least intuitively quite transparent that the uses of *horn* in question are based on a metaphoric extension similar to what was described above. It also must have been a creative operation originally, its non-literal nature probably being very apparent to the speakers. In the current state of the English language, however, *horn* is a dead metaphor with respect to the meanings in question. It is a completely normal, everyday name for the respective items. Because the metaphorically motivated meanings of *horn* and its ilk are stored in the mental lexicon, most theories of metaphor do not regard these as true metaphors and consider them uninteresting (e.g. Loewenberg 1975). An exception is the theory of conceptual metaphors (Lakoff & Johnson 1980; Lakoff 1987), in which many dead metaphors play an especially important part (although these are not nouns, mostly).

In this section I have outlined the notion of the systematicity of polysemy, I have introduced the two types of rule which are usually employed to describe systematic polysemy phenomena in the current literature, and introduced the notions of metaphoric and metonymic motivation. These will be necessary at several points for the understanding of the case studies in section 2.

2. Case Studies

This part of the paper consists of several case studies discussing different kinds of non-systematic polysemy phenomena. I will try to show that specific assumptions concerning systematic polysemy that have been alluded to above are incorrect or incomplete. Additionally, in case study 2.4 the systematicity that is characteristic of metonymically motivated polysemy will be compared to the systematicity that can be observed in connection with some examples of metaphorically motivated polysemy. On the one hand, the case studies will lead to conclusions which are relevant to the theory of polysemy, and on the other hand a typology of non-systematic polysemy phenomena based on considerations relating to the theory of polysemy will emerge.

As I indicated in section 1, the following two propositions are mostly assumed in the current literature on polysemy:

(P2) Systematic polysemy (i.e. polysemy that occurs with several lexemes, follows a certain pattern and is productive) can always be derived by (focussing, shifting and possibly other) rules.

(P3) Non-systematic polysemy (i.e. polysemy that is restricted to single specific lexemes) can never be explained by the application of rules as in (P2).

Let us note that the conditions of systematicity outlined in (P2) and used in (P3) as well, which are usually followed by the literature at least in practice, are not completely identical to the explication of systematicity introduced in section 1, according to which phenomena that can be explained by rules of the form (P1) can be called systematic. This is because (P2) includes the further condition mentioned above in connection with (P1), that a phenomenon has to be observable in a large number of elements. This latter notion of systematicity will be referred to as "systematicity in a quantitative sense" in what follows. If I do not make explicit whether I am talking about systematicity in this sense or in the sense explicated in section 1, I assume that in the given context the conditions for systematicity in both senses are satisfied and equally relevant.

A further three propositions are also generally taken to be true, which are consistent with (P2) and (P3):

(P4) Polysemy phenomena which can be explained by the application of a focussing rule are always systematic in a quantitative sense.

(P5) Polysemy phenomena which can be explained by the application of a shifting rule are always systematic in a quantitative sense.

(P6) Polysemy phenomena which can be explained neither by the application of focussing, nor of shifting (or possibly further) rules are never systematic in a quantitative sense.

The case studies will examine the question whether the propositions (P2) to (P6) are correct.

It should be added that (P2) to (P6) are usually not stated as explicit theses in the literature, but can rather be read out of (or into) it as background assumptions. I cannot provide specific passages that directly say something similar to these propositions, because the aim of this paper is not a detailed overview of the literature. I can only refer to Pethő (2001b) here which contains bibliographic references of especially Deane, Kilgarriff, some proponents of two-level semantics and of generative lexicon theory. They tend to accept one or more of (P2) to (P6) at least as idealisations.

It is also important, however, that when it comes to experimentally verifying the psychological plausibility of theories of polysemy, researchers do this on the basis of assumptions like (P2) to (P6), cf. especially Klepousniotou (2002) and in part Klein & Murphy (2001, 2002), Murphy (this volume). So it is reasonable to ask the question what the relation is between, on the one hand, motivation and the possibility of description by rules, and, on the other hand, quantitative systematicity and the possibility of description by rules, independently of the question how unanimous the consensus actually is with regard to these assumptions.

2.1. Individual, Metonymically Motivated Polysemy

The first case study will investigate the question whether proposition (P4) is true. I will argue with the help of examples that there are cases when polysemy can be straightforwardly described by the application of a focussing rule, but is nevertheless not systematic in a quantitative sense. To put it another way, their non-systematicity is contingent, not necessary.

Let us first look at the Hungarian examples *posta* 'post, mail' and *telefon* 'telephone', which can be used to form the following sentences: *A **posta** egy hét alatt kézbesíti a belföldi leveleket.* 'The post delivers domestic letters within a week.' (institution) – ***Postád** érkezett.* 'Some post has arrived for you.' (thing sent); *A **telefon** meghibásodott.* 'The telephone is broken.' (appliance) – ***Telefonod** van.* 'You've got a call. (lit: You've got a telephone.)' (call). Both sentences contain the lexemes *posta* and *telefon*, respectively, in the second sentences affixed with the 2nd person singular possessive morpheme *-d* (literally meaning 'your mail', 'your phone'), which combines with the stem of the nouns, i.e. *telefono-* and *postá-*, instead of their nominative case forms.

It is plausible to say that metonymic relations hold between the 'institution' – 'thing sent' and 'appliance' – 'call' interpretations in the sense outlined in 1.3. Similarly to the examples discussed in section 1.1, it seems that the meaning variation can be derived on the basis of the complex inner structure of the concepts in question, the relevant details of which may be characterised by the following decomposition structures:

(6) M_{POST} = INSTITUTION (x) & THING SENT (y) & POSTMAN (z) & EMPLOY (x, z) & DELIVER (z, y) & ...

(7) $M_{\text{TELEPHONE}}$ = EQUIPMENT (x) & PHONE CALL (e) & TOOL (x, e) & ...

From these initial representations, the readings in question can be derived according to schema (3). However, the meaning variation that is observable here is not systematic in a quantitative sense: there are no other Hungarian words that show the readings 'institution' – 'thing sent' and 'appliance' – 'call', although the readings 'appliance' – 'thing sent' of the word *fax* 'fax' (and possibly further words) are at least quite similar to the latter (and it could possibly be argued that at some level of abstraction this is the same meaning variation). A similarly unique metonymically motivated polysemy is observable in the case of the word *mouth*, which can refer to at least the mouth cavity and the lips.

It should be noted that it is not completely clear in the case of *posta* and *telefon* whether the intuition holds that the individual readings of a polysemous word are equal in status (i.e. do not seem to be primary or derived with respect to each other). This was mentioned earlier as a widely accepted condition for the assumption of focussing rules in individual cases. There does in fact seem to be an intuition that for *posta*, the 'institution' interpretation is more basic, more salient, and for *telefon*, it's the interpretation 'equipment'. In the case of *fax*, there does not seem to be a clear difference in salience. It is not completely clear what these intuitions mean, but there is another property that these words and other purported examples of focussing have in common: the relevant interpretations are not independent of each other, but are rather interdefinable. For example, there is no phone call without telephone equipment, and the primary function of the telephone equipment is to make phone calls. Therefore it is plausible to describe these examples as instances of focussing rather than shifting.

Assuming that this is the case, we can conclude that the metonymically motivated polysemy phenomena that can be described by a focussing rule are not always systematic in the quantitative sense: the meaning variation pattern that we experience with these words does not occur among other lexemes. How is this possible? The answer to this question is relatively simple: As discussed already in section 1.1, it does not follow from the schema of focussing rules in (3) that the described meaning variation has to be present in several lexemes. This only depends on whether there are several lexemes in the given language to which concepts of a similar structure are assigned. More exactly:

(P7) The polysemy derived by a focussing rule is systematic in a quantitative sense if and only if there are several lexemes L_1, L_2, ... to which conceptual representations M_1, M_2, ... are assigned (in a way that M_n is assigned to L_n), and there are properties P, Q, ... such that each representation M_n has at least two entities x_n, y_n, ... as its parts to which a focussing rule can be applied, and for which it is true that $M_n \vdash P(x_n) \& Q(y_n) \& ...$

Remarks: the representations M_k, M_m that are assigned to two different lexemes L_k, L_m can be identical, in case L_k, L_m are true synonyms. The properties P and Q characterise the two distinct interpretations that recur systematically among the lexemes L_1, L_2, ... In case there are not just two, but more systematically observable readings, there have to be additional focusable entities as parts of each M_n, for which a further respective property follows from every M_n.

Let us apply (P7) to a specific example for the sake of illustration. Let L_1 be the lexeme *school*, L_2 the lexeme *university*, M_1 the concept SCHOOL (M_{SCHOOL}), M_2 the concept UNIVERSITY ($M_{\text{UNIVERSITY}}$), x_1 the school as an institution, y_1 the school building(s), x_2 the university as an institution, y_2 the university building(s), P the property INSTITUTION, and Q the property BUILDING. Furthermore,

(8) $M_{\text{SCHOOL}} = \text{INSTITUTION}(x)\ \&\ \text{BUILDING}(y)\ \&\ \text{PLACE}(y, x)\ \&\ \ldots$
$\Rightarrow M_{\text{SCHOOL}, x} = \lambda x\, \exists y\, [\text{INSTITUTION}(x)\ \&\ \text{BUILDING}(y)\ \&\ \text{PLACE}(y, x)\ \&\ \ldots]$
$\Rightarrow M_{\text{SCHOOL}, y} = \lambda y\, \exists x\, [\text{INSTITUTION}(x)\ \&\ \text{BUILDING}(y)\ \&\ \text{PLACE}(y, x)\ \&\ \ldots]$

(9) $M_{\text{UNIVERSITY}} = \text{INSTITUTION}(x)\ \&\ \text{BUILDING}(y)\ \&\ \text{PLACE}(y, x)\ \&\ \ldots$
$\Rightarrow M_{\text{UNIVERSITY}, x} = \lambda x\, \exists y\, [\text{INSTITUTION}(x)\ \&\ \text{BUILDING}(y)\ \&\ \text{PLACE}(y, x)\ \&\ \ldots]$
$\Rightarrow M_{\text{UNIVERSITY}, y} = \lambda y\, \exists x\, [\text{INSTITUTION}(x)\ \&\ \text{BUILDING}(y)\ \&\ \text{PLACE}(y, x)\ \&\ \ldots]$

Clearly (8) and (9) are consistent with (P7), therefore the polysemy 'intitution' – 'building' qualifies as systematic.

The following also seems to be true:

(P8) A meaning variation that can be described by focussing rule is always productive in the sense that any lexeme L_i that enters the language will show the same meaning variation as an already available lexeme L_j, if it is the case that the conceptual representation M_i of L_i is similar to M_j of L_j in the following way: both M_i and M_j have entities x_i, y_i, and x_j, y_j as parts respectively, which are equally accessible for the application of a focussing rule, and there are properties P, Q for which it is true that $M_n \vdash P(x_n)\ \&\ Q(y_n)$, $n = \{i, j\}$.

When a lexeme that newly enters a language is a true synonym of an already existing lexeme, or if the new lexeme is a hyponym or co-hyponym of a certain kind of an already existing lexeme, then the conditions given in (P8) are satisfied, and we can indeed observe that the already given and the newly created word allow the same focussed interpretations.

An example of the first case is when a new synonym for the word *school* appears in the language, e.g. a slang term. According to (P8), this will be expected to allow the same focussed interpretations as *school* itself. For the second case, let us look at a further group of examples. The use of words meaning electronic communication (German and Hungarian *SMS*, *e-mail* etc.) is somewhat similar to the meaning variation mentioned in connection with the word *posta* above, with the difference that here it is not an 'institution' reading that can be observed alongside the 'thing sent', but rather a reading that can be paraphrased as 'service/technology'. If a new technology appears which allows its users to communicate electronically, the lexeme that denotes this technology is expected to be usable with both the 'communication (thing sent)' and 'service/technology' readings (if the conditions demanded in (P8) are satisfied).

On the basis of these examples, we can state that it is completely irrelevant from the perspective of the properties of focussing rules whether a meaning variation describable by a focussing rule is systematic in the sense that it is observable in connection with several different words, or whether it only occurs in a single word. For as long as there was a single technology that transported electronic communication, e.g. e-mail, only a single word like this was needed. The word *e-mail* was therefore unique, and its characteristic meaning variation was not systematic in a quantitative sense. It only became systematic in this sense when other words with a similar meaning appeared as well: on the one hand, words that name other, more recent technologies that transport electronic communication, and, on the other hand, words that are synonyms of these (like *text* for 'SMS message'). The appearance of new technologies and the necessity of naming them is trivially an extralinguistic change that has to do with the cultural and technological environment, whereas the demand for synonyms is often a social phenomenon (e.g. the introduction of native synonyms for foreign words like *e-mail* in Hungarian). Both of these factors are completely contingent with respect to the theory of focussing rules. Because quantitative systematicity is therefore a consequence of factors that are partially irrelevant for the explanation of meaning variation, quantitative systematicity or non-systematicity itself should not be relevant either.

To summarize the conclusions of this case study: Proposition (P4) turned out not to be true (and neither is proposition (P3), consequently): not all polysemy phenomena that can be explained by the application of a focussing rule are systematic in a quantitative sense. Nevertheless, they are always potentially systematic, i.e. they become systematic by the appearance of new synonyms and (co-)hyponyms in the lexicon. Whether a polysemy phenomenon of this kind is actually systematic or non-systematic in a qualitative sense is not relevant from the perspective of whether it can be described by a rule. So we may conclude that it is more useful to employ the notion of systematicity explicated in section 1, i.e. systematicity in the sense of productive rule application, instead of the more usual quantitative notion.

2.2. Pseudo-Systematic, Metonymically Motivated Polysemy

The second case study examines the question whether proposition (P5) is true. I will argue with the help of examples that it is not true: we find cases when polysemy can be straightforwardly explained by shifting rules, but is not systematic.

The non-systematic polysemy phenomena to be discussed in this subsection can arguably be regarded as having started out as cases of systematic, metonymically motivated polysemy. However, single words which had originally exhibited systematic meaning variation can "fall out of" the given polysemy type in the sense that a meaning is lexicalised for the word which is more specific than what would be derived by the shifting rule, and which is in this sense independent of the rule. It is also possible that a word still retains its original interpretation derived by a shifting rule, and therefore continues to show a systematic meaning variation alongside this more specific lexicalised meaning. This will be illustrated with two examples below.

2.2.1. First Example: Packaging

Let us start with the word *glass*, which is primarily a mass noun. As with other mass nouns, we can apply to *glass* a shifting rule that is most commonly known in the literature as "packaging" (cf. section 1.2), which derives a count noun from a mass noun. By this latter use we can refer with any count noun to individualised entities that consist of the material in question, e.g. *a beer* 'a portion of beer', *a rubber* 'a piece of rubber to remove pencil marks etc.'. The general rule of packaging can be specified in roughly the following way:

(10) $M_{\text{GLASS}} = \text{MATERIAL}(x) \,\&\, \ldots$
$\Rightarrow M_{\text{GLASS, OBJECT}} = \lambda x \exists y\, [\text{OBJECT}(x) \,\&\, \text{MATERIAL}(y) \,\&\, \text{CONSIST OF}(y, x) \,\&\, \ldots]$

The double arrow signifies the application of the shifting rule "packaging". I will not elaborate on specific parts of the analysis here, e.g. properties of the relation CONSIST OF or the ontological status of the entities x and y. Such questions are addressed in more detail e.g. in several chapters of Dölling (2001), and what is said there can be applied here as well.

If we apply the shifting rule of packaging to the mass noun *glass*, we can use this word to refer to objects that consist of (or are made of) *glass*. It should be noted, however, that the actual use of this version of the word is constrained by a more general cognitive principle that appears in different forms on all levels of human language (in phonology, morphology, syntax and semantics) and is usually called the "elsewhere condition" in the linguistics literature: If two different rules could be applied to the same input element, a more specific and a more general one, then the more specific one will be applied, and this blocks the application of the more general rule. In this particular case, if there is a word with a more specific meaning that usually denotes objects of a certain kind made of glass, then the packaged version of the word *glass* will normally not be an adequate expression to name such an object. In Hungarian, for example, objects like mirrors, spectacles, drinking glasses etc. are not called *üveg* 'glass'. Instead words are used that name specifically these kinds of object, e.g. *tükör* 'mirror', *pohár* 'drinking glass' etc.

The example *glass* is relevant for our discussion because, as indicated above, there are lexicalised uses of this word that can not be derived by the rule application (10), because they are on the one hand more specific and on the other hand broader. Let us concentrate on the meaning 'drinking glass' of *glass*. This is more specific than what would be derived by the rule in that it can be specified relatively well what form and function a container has that can be called a glass in English, and it is broader in the sense that the object does not have to be made necessarily of glass, at least in everyday language use (but can be made of plastic, for example). This kind of specific lexicalisation of mass nouns is widespread in other languages as well. The Hungarian word for glass, *üveg* cannot be used to refer to drinking glasses, for example, but instead is used in the sense 'bottle'. In German, there is also a meaning 'drinking glass' available for the lexical equivalent *Glas*. At the same time, English *glass* can refer to mirrors as well (as an archaic form) and in its plural form to spectacles, neither of which is possible in either Hungarian or German.

This example shows that there are polysemy phenomena for which the use of a shifting rule has to be assumed at one point in the history of the word, but which are not systematic, because in addition to the shifting rule a further factor has also contributed to their current use: the idiosyncratic lexicalisation of a specific interpretation.

2.2.2. Second Example: The Polysemy 'Body Part' – 'Part of Clothing that Covers It'

Our second example will illustrate that a previously presumably productive polysemy type that could be derived by a shifting rule can "fall apart" because several words belonging to it are lexicalised for a more specific, non-predictable use. This may have happened with the polysemy 'body part' – 'part of clothing that covers it' in Hungarian, which may have been productive.

Words that belong to this polysemy type behave in a way that can be derived by an appropriate shifting rule that conforms to the following schema:

(11) $M_{\text{BACK}} = \text{BODY PART}\ (x)\ \&\ \ldots$
$\Rightarrow M_{\text{BACK, PART OF CLOTHING}} = \lambda y\ \exists x\ \exists z\ [\text{CLOTHING}\ (x)\ \&\ \text{PART}\ (y, x)\ \&\ \text{COVER}\ (y, z)\ \&\ \text{BODY PART}\ (z)\ \&\ \ldots]$

The following examples behave accordingly: *shoulder of a coat/a shirt* 'part covering a shoulder', *fingers of a glove* 'parts covering the fingers', *back of a dress* 'part covering the back', *leg of trousers* 'part covering a leg' etc.

In Hungarian, the exact equivalents of many of these expressions also exist. But in case we try to describe this by a rule like (11) and assume that the condition of its use is that it can apply to body part terms if the appropriate body part is covered by some part of clothing, we find that the variation does not strictly work this way. The sleeve of a shirt/coat etc. is called *kabát/ing ujja*, literally 'finger of a coat/shirt', and there are several body part terms that are used metaphorically instead of metonymically, e.g. *cipő orra* 'tip of a shoe', literally 'nose of a shoe', *cipő nyelve* 'tongue of a shoe'. On the other hand, and more importantly, it is somewhat arbitrary what body part terms can be used to name which parts of clothes. The expression *zokni ujja* 'finger of a sock' is not possible, and although *nadrág dereka* 'waist of trousers' can be used, *nadrág csípője* 'hip of trousers' or *nadrág térde* 'knee of trousers' is less possible (although there are differences among speakers as to which of these forms they would accept). Also, *kabát feje* 'head of a coat' with the meaning 'hood' is impossible, although this can arguably be explained by the existence of the lexical item *kapucni* 'hood' and the elsewhere condition. The problem is not just that the general condition for the use of (11) mentioned above is incorrect, but it does not seem to be possible to provide such conditions that would correctly describe the data but not simply enumerate the lexemes to which it can apply. Because therefore condition b) of (P1) is violated, it is not justified to talk about rule application in this case.

There seem to be two ways to explain how it is possible that polysemy phenomena that seem to be straightforwardly describable by shifting rules are nevertheless not productive and not systematic. It can be useful to review these possibilities, as they can lead to interesting conclusions as to what shifting rules really are. The first possibility was mentioned at the beginning of this subsection: a given meaning variation that seems to be systematic at first sight was caused by an existing active shifting rule in an earlier state of the language, and the meaning variation was truly systematic and productive back then. However, this systematicity was disturbed, and as a consequence the rule disappeared from the language. Those words that exhibit this at least superficially systematic polysemy in the current language state are really only "fossils" of a previously systematic polysemy type. If we accept this hypothesis, the question arises what the reason could be for the disintegration of a previously systematic polysemy phenomenon.

A plausible answer to this question seems to be the following: As we have seen in 2.2.1, if a specific version of their secondary use becomes lexicalised, individual words can leave a systematic polysemy type that can be described by a shifting rule. If there are other words in the lexicon that specifically serve to name an entity which could in principle be referred to a polysemous word as well in case we apply a shifting rule to it, this also constrains the application of the shifting rule: in such a case the entity in question often cannot be referred to by the polysemous word. As a consequence of both factors, the systematicity of the polysemy phenomenon is reduced on the level of the data. If such disruptive factors appear in large numbers in connection with a given systematic polysemy phenomenon, it is possible that a new generation of speakers will not be able to acquire the shifting rule on the basis of the linguistic stimuli they have access to. It is also conceivable that there is a sufficient number of data to learn the rule, but the number of potential inputs to the rule that behave in a way that constitutes an exception to the rule (for the two independent reasons mentioned) is very large. Such a rule that would compete with the retrieval of information from the lexicon would inhibit the speakers in looking up the exceptions in the lexicon, but would lead to a useful output only in a relatively small number of cases itself. In such a situation the language processing faculty of the speakers presumably "notices" that the application of a shifting rule would be more expensive than useful, and the rule is not employed in a steadily growing number of cases. The disintegration of systematic polysemy phenomena could therefore be in this sense similar to the process when regular inflection classes of verbs become irregular.

Another possibility of explaining the non-systematicity of such polysemy phenomena is the following: These specific variations are in fact not based on shifting rules as outlined in 1.2 at all, but are rather lexicalisations of individual metonymies that are not regular in this sense. These are similar to shifting rules in the sense that they are sense extension operations that function according to schema (5), but they are different in the respect that they cannot be formulated as specific rules, i.e. by providing the relevant properties of the inputs and outputs and conditions of application. A metonymic sense extension can in general be applied to any input (i.e. the conditions of application are empty), and the relationship between the input and the output can only be characterised in an extremely general way (cf. for this Deane 1987).

If, in a given language, individual metonymic extensions are lexicalised for a large number of similar lexemes, these lexemes will show meaning variations that can be similar in that both the inputs and the outputs have a certain common property. If a given meaning variation appears in connection with a sufficiently large number of lexemes and there are not many exceptions that would reduce the systematicity (in a loose sense) of a given meaning variation, it is possible that a following generation of speakers does not only learn the relevant readings of the lexemes that exhibit a certain meaning variation, but also develop a shifting rule by induction. As a result, a truly systematic, productive polysemy phenomenon that follows a shifting rule could arise instead of the earlier individual metonymies that were lexicalised sporadically.

Note that these sketched explanations of the non-systematicity of these phenomena may be plausible, but are in fact completely speculative, because no diachronic studies have been carried out, to the best of my knowledge, to confirm the actual historical development of these or other systematic meaning variations.

On the basis of the phenomena that we have examined in this case study, we can conclude that (P5) is not true: there are polysemy phenomena that can be explained by a shifting rule but are not in fact systematic.

Thus this case study affirmed what has been concluded in 2.1 as well, i.e. that the apparent quantitative systematicity of a polysemy phenomenon is not as relevant from a theoretical point of view as one would believe at first sight: neither does it follow from the absence of quantitative systematicity that the phenomenon cannot be explained by a rule (cf. 2.1), nor does the observation of such a systematicity entail that all relevant examples can be adequately described by a rule (2.2).

2.3. Pseudo-Systematic, Metaphorically Motivated Polysemy

The largest group of non-systematic polysemy phenomena is probably that of metaphorically polysemous words. Although the literature usually regards these as homogenous, I will distinguish three groups in what follows, which possess different theoretically relevant properties: pseudo-systematic, quasi-systematic and non-systematic metaphorically motivated polysemy.

This case study examines the question whether (P6) is correct. For this we will examine the properties of polysemy phenomena that are not metonymically, but metaphorically motivated, and nevertheless appear to be systematic. I will argue that the systematicity of the examples examined is indeed only apparent, and therefore they do not contradict the proposition (P6).

Literature relating to cognitive linguistics often notes that metaphorically motivated polysemy frequently shows a systematicity of certain kind, i.e. words that have a similar primary meaning can get similar secondary meanings. For example, several body part terms can refer metaphorically to parts of certain objects which have a similar form, function, relative position etc. to that human (or animal) body part. We have already encountered the examples *cipő orra* 'nose of a shoe' and *tongue of a shoe*. *Sole of a shoe* is a further possible example (although this could be regarded as metonymically motivated as well). Similar cases are *mouth* for the open part of containers, *leg of a chair/table*, *nose of a plane*, *spine of a book*, *bill of a cap* etc.

On the basis of what has been said in section 1.3., we could conclude that metaphorically motivated polysemy phenomena that seem to be systematic in this way could be derived by a sense extension rule, one that has a schema similar to the shifting rules, except for the difference that the characteristic relation in the background of the rule is similarity. Thus we can try to describe metaphorically motivated polysemy phenomena with a rule that has the following form:

(12) $M = P(y)\ \&\ \ldots$
$\Rightarrow M_O = \lambda x\ \exists y\ [O(x)\ \&\ P(y)\ \&\ \text{RESEMBLE}\ (Q, x, y)\ \&\ \ldots]$

where the relation RESEMBLE (Q, x, y) expresses that entity x is similar to y by the property Q (i.e. in this respect). This relation is not symmetric with respect to x and y, cf. Glucksberg (2001).

We can devise a rule on the basis of schema (12) that would work in a way similar to (11), apart from the fact that it derives a reading 'part of an object' instead of 'part of clothing', and its characteristic relation is RESEMBLE rather than COVER.

(13) $M_{\text{BACK}} = \text{BODY PART}\ (x)\ \&\ \ldots$
$\Rightarrow M_{\text{BACK, PART OF OBJECT}} = \lambda y\ \exists x\ \exists z\ [\text{OBJECT}\ (x)\ \&\ \text{PART}\ (y, x)\ \&\ \text{RESEMBLE}\ (P, y, z)$
$\&\ \text{BODY PART}\ (z)\ \&\ \ldots]$

It can be easily argued, however, that such a rule is not adequate to account for the phenomenon in question, just as (11) did not turn out to be adequate in connection with the meaning variation in 2.2.2.

Let us first examine with the help of further examples what resemblance relations can be involved in this kind of polysemy. One such relation that is relatively frequently observable is the following: In its metaphorically motivated use, the body part term names a part of an object, the relative position of which in relation to the whole of the object is analogous to how the body part in question relates to the whole of the human or animal body. This relation seems to motivate expressions like the following: *sole of a shoe*, *leg of a table*, *chair*, *bridge etc.*, *foot of a mountain*, *ladder*, *trunk of a tree*, *wing of a plane*, *fin of a plane*, *arm of a machine*, *neck of a bottle*, *a violin* etc. Furthermore, the resemblance that underlies the metaphoric sense transfer can also be based on just functional similarity, e.g. *mouth of a bag*, just formal similarity, e.g. *elbow of a pipe*, *tooth of a comb*, *a head of lettuce*, *eye of a potato*, *a storm* etc. In other cases, the relation cannot be easily characterised, but is felt to be metaphorical (e.g. *head of a department*). In yet further cases we find a combination of more than one type of similarity: *tooth of a saw:* function + similar form.

Whether we approach the problem of describing these examples in the way that we try to provide a specific metaphorical extension rule for each of these more specific types of similarity, or by trying to account for all examples by a general rule resembling (13), we necessarily encounter the problem that the phenomena in question do not have a well-defined distribution. Therefore, no general conditions for the application of a rule like (13) or a more specific version of this can be provided. For example, it is not possible to characterise in general the range of body parts or the parts of objects for which an extension rule that is based on functional resemblance could be stated. The only possible solution seems to be that we allow a rule to apply to the name of any body part to derive a name for any part of any object that has an appropriate function etc. However, this is not strict enough. By examining actual language use and native speaker intuitions, we find that the variation at hand cannot be used in a productive way to name any part of an object by any term that refers to a similar body part. This use of body part terms follows restrictions that are unpredictable and idiosyncratic.

For example, in Hungarian the noun *láb* 'leg, foot' can be used to refer to a part of something that is close to the ground, e.g. *hegy lába* 'foot of a mountain', *töltés lába* 'foot of a dyke', or to parts that have more specific properties, e.g. *asztal*, *szék lába* 'leg of a table, chair' can only refer to parts of these objects that are similar to a pole and support the object, and not a lower part of any form. It seems quite arbitrary that in some cases such a metaphorically motivated use of a word is possible, e.g. *hegy*, *??torony lába* 'foot of a mountain, a tower', but not in others, e.g. **fa lába* 'foot of a tree', **lépcső lába* 'foot of stairs', etc. Similar observations can be made about the metaphorical use of body part terms in other languages as well.

Thus it neither seems possible to provide specific conditions for the use of the metaphorical extension rules that would be needed to account for these polysemy phenomena, nor can we just state a very general condition, because in this case our rule would predict that the meaning variation is productive in an unrestricted way. That this is not (or at least not always) true can be seen from the examples above, and in similar examples in other languages. The only solution seems to be to state specifically for each body part term in the lexicon what parts of what objects that term can apply to, either by enumerating the objects or by describing the properties of the parts that can be referred to by the word (which would presumably work in the specific case of *foot* or *back* in English for most of these words' uses).

It can also be shown that the productivity of the metaphorical extension in question is not just restricted by independent principles, in particular the elsewhere condition or a lack of communicative need, as has been suggested in connection with the shifting rules in the previous section. If one assumes a sense extension rule that is similar to (13), this would mistakenly predict for example that the expression *skin of the wall* should be an adequate way to refer to the surface of a wall, since this would be a case of both functional and positional similarity. There can often be a need to refer to the surface of a wall specifically, and there is no lexicalised expression for this in the dictionary that should block this metaphorically motivated use, as this information can only be expressed by non-lexicalised descriptions like *surface of the wall.*

Such examples suggest that the metaphorically motivated polysemy in question is not in fact productive in the sense that metonymically motivated polysemy phenomena that can be derived by shifting rules are productive. But neither is it productive in the same sense as the polysemy that can be described by focussing rules turned out to be productive. For the latter, we have stated that true synonyms exhibit the same meaning variation because of the way the rule works. In case a body part term that is used metaphorically in the relevant way to refer to a part of an object is replaced by one of its true synonyms, e.g. an informal expression for the same body part, the resulting metaphorical use is unacceptable and will sound rather bizarre, e.g. *mouth of the bottle – *gob of the bottle*. In the case of focussing rules, this is not the case. For example, true synonyms of Hungarian *iskola* 'school' like *suli* 'school' (informal), show the meaning variation 'institution' – 'building' as naturally as *iskola* itself.

Thus the metaphorically motivated polysemy 'body part' – 'part of an object' indeed only seems to be superficially systematic. It is not productive, and therefore speakers probably do not have a rule like (13) or a more specific rule that could account for the phenomenon in question. If this is correct, the observed meaning variations must be due to individually learned lexical properties, and the fact that the variation is observable for several body part terms can be either a fossil of a rule that was available in an earlier stage of English or a convergent series of individual metaphorical transfers. Thus it does not follow from the results of this case study so far that the proposition (P6) should be incorrect.

Note that it is not trivial whether it is appropriate to call the relevant uses of body part terms cases of polysemy at all. The 'part of an object' reading can in most cases only appear in possessive constructions or compounds with a similar semantic structure (e.g. *table leg*), but not on its own. Therefore, the examples mentioned above both in English and Hungarian can be considered not to be semantically complex expressions formed with a polysemous body part term, but rather idiomatic possessive constructions that receive a metaphorically motivated interpretation as a whole in the lexicon. I will not discuss this possibility further here.

Let us briefly examine a further example of pseudo-systematic, metaphorically motivated polysemy as well. Names of animals can be used to refer to humans, by which one highlights a certain property of the person and also expresses some kind of (mostly negative) estimation of that person. People can be called *pig*, *chicken*, *goose*, *shark*, *donkey*, *ass*, *dog*, *viper*, *snake*, *hyena*, *gorilla*, *cow*, *toad*, *worm*, *rat* etc. The property that is expressed by the word may be a psychological or intellectual property, e.g. *pig* 'unpleasant', *goose* 'silly', *shark* 'ruthless', or an external one (relating to the body), e.g. *gorilla* 'big, muscular'.

Similarly to the polysemous body part terms above, the polysemy involving names of animals is not truly systematic: **1.** The meaning of the name of the animal (the structure of the concept assigned to it) does not allow us to predict what kinds of object (persons with what properties) can be referred to with the word in question metaphorically, and what information will be conveyed about these objects. **2.** It is not possible either to provide the conditions for the use of such a rule, i.e. to specify the set of animal names and properties for which this phenomenon appears. The variation is not productive, i.e. the list of animal names cannot be extended at will. E.g. the sentence *John is a real beaver* cannot be simply used to convey that 'John swims well/is diligent/has big front teeth'. By contrast, *John is a hyena* has a rather straightforward interpretation. This can again only be explained by assuming that the words in question each have a secondary (metaphoric) meaning lexicalised, which is only rather indirectly motivated by our knowledge of the animal, and often even such an indirect motivation is not apparent (for example, it is unclear why *dog* should have the interpretation 'unattractive woman' or *fox* 'sexually attractive person').

In both the body part term and animal name cases, it seems more reasonable to talk about motivation in the sense that the existence of these meaning variations is most probably no coincidence, especially because they are present in many languages (and may even be universal). Therefore, we can assume that there is a tendency in our thinking to view things in the world in an anthropomorphic way (body parts) or to deny accepting the human status of persons we do not appreciate (animal names). I do not want to discuss here whether such mechanisms of thought are present in the everyday thinking of all of us, but I refer to Lakoff (1987) and Lakoff & Johnson (1999) where several speculations of this nature can be found.

2.4. Quasi-Systematic, Metaphorically Motivated Polysemy

Cognitive research on metaphors (Lakoff & Johnson 1980) has pointed out that according to data, some metaphor phenomena are not simply based on particular similarities between two things, but can rather be regarded as mappings of the concepts of one conceptual domain to elements of another conceptual domain. Such mappings are believed to underlie the use of metaphoric expressions. Thus it makes sense to ask whether polysemy motivated by such metaphoric relations satisfies the conditions of systematicity. This case study (like 2.3 above) will examine this question, i.e. whether (P6) is correct.

Let us first look at an example of the groups of expressions that will form the subject of discussion in this subsection. It seems that the following examples are motivated by a linguistic regularity that can be stated as "We talk about money as if it were a liquid."

Money itself can be referred to as ***liquid assets*** or as ***currency***, which is related to the Latin word for *flow*. The organisation etc. one gets money from can be called a ***source***, the original meaning of which is 'spring'. One can talk about ***cash flow*** or an ***outflow*** of capital. If money is made available to an organisation etc., it can be said that money is ***injected*** or ***pumped*** into it. Money can also be ***channelled*** or ***funnelled*** to some use or through some institution. Funds can ***dry up*** or be ***frozen*** to prevent their movement. If someone is very rich, they can be said to be ***swimming in money*** or even ***drowning in money***. If someone is paid small amounts of money, money can said to be ***dripping*** to them, and if they receive a lot of money, it can be said to be ***pouring*** in.

The underscored expressions all have a primary use that applies to liquids, but to which another use attaches as a parasite, as it were, which is metaphoric and refers to something in connection with money. We use metaphorically motivated expressions like the above to talk about several (typically abstract, immaterial) subjects to a significant degree, e.g. time, communication, emotions, human relations (friendship, marriage etc.), cf. Lakoff & Johnson (1980), Kövecses (2002). Polysemy that is motivated in this way possibly affects a rather large percentage of the basic vocabulary overall.

In the following, I will examine in more detail how the regularity behind the phenomenon that was informally mentioned above, i.e. "We talk about money as if it were a liquid", can be characterised more explicitly, and what the nature of such a regularity is. I will outline two conflicting ideas, the first of which I believe to be more convincing.

First we can try to formulate a rule that is able to describe adequately the metaphorically motivated, apparently systematic meaning variation that we have seen above. Let us assume that there is a lexeme L_1 which is connected (according to the intuitions of an overwhelming majority of speakers) primarily to a concept M_1, which is a part of the conceptual domain C_1. For example, *drip* 'fall in drops (of a liquid)' is a concept belonging to the conceptual domain of liquids. Its secondary, derived meaning belongs to a conceptual domain C_2 different from C_1, i.e. 'receive small amounts of money' belongs to the conceptual domain of money. The concepts M_1 and M_2 are not directly related to each other, except for the similarity that in both cases something changes place in some sense. It could be suggested that the apparently systematic metaphors in general and the metaphorically motivated polysemies in particular are based on rules of the following form:

(P9) If a lexeme L_1 is assigned in the lexicon primarily a concept M_1 that entertains the same relationship to a certain conceptual domain C_1 as a concept M_2 to a certain conceptual domain C_2, we can use lexeme L_1 in the sense M_2.

If we replace C_1 by LIQUID and C_2 by MONEY, we get the secondary sense of the word *inject* by considering what type of event is referred to by *inject* in connection with liquids and what the counterpart of this event could be in connection with money.

Let us call a rule of the form (P9) an analogy rule, because it specifies an analogical relationship between M_1 and M_2. (P9) characterises a class of specific analogy rules in which the conceptual domains of C_1 and C_2 are set.

There is a striking difference between the polysemy phenomena that can be described by rules of the form (P9) and those that are based on shifting and focussing rules. Whereas lexemes that exhibit a certain metonymically motivated polysemy type are hyponyms or co-hyponyms of each other, lexemes that exhibit a metaphorically motivated polysemy according to (P9) are not necessarily hyponyms or co-hyponyms. The only thing that they have to have in common is that they (or rather their primary meanings) belong to a common conceptual domain. For example, whereas *pour*, *channel* and *injection* all have to do with liquids, there is no superordinate concept to which they belong (i.e. of which they are hyponyms).

The question arises whether this phenomenon can indeed be described adequately by rules of the form (P9). Firstly, it seems that words that primarily belong to liquids cannot be used at will to refer to money. For example, we cannot use the verb *water* to express that someone is helping out someone else with money, a wallet that does not contain money cannot be called *dry* or one that contains money *wet*, etc. We should expect that this is possible if speakers used an analogy rule like the above to refer to concepts in the conceptual domain MONEY by the lexemes mentioned.

However, as these phenomena are not as idiosyncratic as the ones that were discussed in 2.3 and show certain features of productivity, I will refer to them as quasi-systematic polysemy phenomena. Further well-known examples are expressions about war that are used to talk about arguments and expressions about buildings that are used to talk about theories.

The theory of conceptual metaphors (Lakoff & Johnson 1980; Kövecses 2002) suggests a radically different explanation for the quasi-systematic polysemy phenomena in question from what has been said so far. I will briefly outline this approach below.

The key idea of the theory of conceptual metaphors is a psychological entity called conceptual metaphor. It is a mapping from a more concrete conceptual domain (the source domain) to a more abstract one (a target domain), by which the abstract conceptual domain becomes (more) differentiated, (more) structured, and (more) manageable. The theory of conceptual metaphors would regard the group of expressions "money as liquid" above as a linguistic symptom or reflection of a conceptual metaphor MONEY IS A LIQUID.

According to the conceptual theory of metaphors, regularities that are counterparts of (P9) are present in the minds of the speakers, although they are not stated as such, because they are simply linguistic reflections of conceptual metaphors (or, to put it in another way, epiphenomenal). In (P9), C_1 is the equivalent of a source domain and C_2 of a target domain. According to this theory, regularities belonging to the class (P9) follow from the fact that speakers think about C_2 by invoking concepts from C_1. Thus the metaphorically motivated quasi-systematic polysemy phenomena are definitely not analogical formations in the lexicon, as has been suggested in 2.4.1, but rather indispensable requisites of human concept formation. Metaphors essentially have a cognitive function rather than a linguistic one, namely, that we would not be able to think about the abstract concepts in question without them (or at least not as effectively).

Certain points of criticism ought to be mentioned in connection with this approach to quasi-systematic polysemy. Firstly, it is questionable whether expressions that could just as well be considered to have a general meaning should be regarded as metaphors. For example, intuitively it seems that expressions like *attack*, *defend*, *adversary* etc. are not primarily expressions for physical force (and even less for war, which is seldom a part of our everyday experience), but for conflicts in general. If this is correct, it is still true that we talk about arguments as if they were wars, but the reason for this is not that a conceptual metaphor ARGUMENT IS WAR makes us do this. Instead, this fact would result from the application of such banal rules as "we talk about arguments as about conflicts" and "we talk about wars as about conflicts", for the trivial reason that both are indeed conflicts. Similar observations are made in connection with adjectives by Rakova (2003).

Secondly, Murphy (1996) points out that the strongest interpretation of the theory of conceptual metaphors, according to which conceptual metaphors are indispensable for the development of abstract concepts and the reasoning with such concepts leads to too strong empirical predictions. To illustrate this by our example: There is an extremely large number of expressions that are used exclusively or mostly to talk about money (e.g. *cash*, *money*, *account*, *tax*, *wage*, *spend* etc.), which suggests that we do not need expressions related to liquids or other more "concrete" concepts to talk about money. For related reasons, conceptual metaphors can at most be reasonably attributed the cognitive function that they make our abstract concepts (that are available and can be used anyway) more differentiated in some sense (Gibbs 1996; Murphy 1997).

In this section we have outlined two possible explanations for quasi-systematic metaphorically motivated polysemy phenomena. Of course, there are other possibilities beside these two extremes. An approach that is in some sense halfway between them is Gentner's theory of metaphor, who assumes that metaphors are analogical formations, but also believes that they do play an important role in cognition and are not just lexical phenomena, e.g. Gentner & Medina (1998), Bowdle & Gentner (2005).

Like in the case study in section 2.3, we have again reached the conclusion that the apparently systematic metaphorically motivated polysemy phenomena do not necessarily contradict proposition (P6).

Finally, the above discussion begs the question why quasi-systematic, metaphorically motivated polysemy phenomena should exist at all, if the reason for this is not that they are based on conceptual interrelations that are necessary to make sense of the world (as the theory of conceptual metaphors claims). One significant reason for the creation of word groups that exhibit a meaning variation of a certain type could be the fact (which is well-known from historical linguistics and lexicology) that speakers do not like to coin completely new words to refer to concepts that cannot yet be verbalised (e.g. because they are new). Instead, speakers create compounds, borrow words from another language, or employ an already existing word, often by extending its meaning metaphorically. Thus metaphoric sense extension can plausibly be derived from the same principle of the economy of the lexicon as other examples of polysemy in general: to satisfy new communicative needs, speakers are forced to employ metaphorisation among other strategies if they want to avoid using words they have never before heard others use (which seems to be a very strong factor even though it is not well understood why this is so).

2.5. Individual, Metaphorically Motivated Polysemy

In this final section, we will take a brief look at metaphorically motivated polysemy phenomena in connection with which speakers refer to an object or other entity by a lexeme on the grounds of a particular, individual association, without following a larger pattern. For example, beside the animal, a computer part can be called *mouse; ring* can refer not only to a piece of jewellery, but also to other circular objects, e.g. onion rings, or even non-circular objects, e.g. the ring in boxing; *chalice* can refer not only to drinking cups, but also parts of a flower; and *fork* not only to a tool for eating, but also to a place where e.g. a road or a river splits into two parts.

The secondary meanings are motivated by the fact that the thing or entity to be named is similar to the thing or entity denoted in the primary use of the word. Thus we find the same motivation as in connection with the examples in section 2.3, cases of pseudo-systematic, metaphorically motivated polysemy. Like in those cases, lexicalisation seems to play a crucial role. However, it also seems that such individual, particular metaphors can be used much more freely for new, so far unnamed objects or entities than what we can observe in connection with the groups in 2.3, which are mostly closed sets of metaphorically motivated polysemous expressions. As a consequence, metaphorical uses of words are extremely common in technical and group languages.

Uses of polysemous words like *mouse* for a computer part, *blade* for pieces of grass, *basket* in basketball, *fork* as a part of bicycles and motorcycles, *stirrup* in ear anatomy, or *finger* as in *fish fingers* refer to concrete, immediately observable objects, and the metaphor that motivates these expressions is obviously based on a similarity of form between the primarily and the metaphorically denoted objects. Other types of similarity cannot be found, e.g. functional (the stirrup in the ear serves not to support something, we do not touch anything with fish fingers etc.) or relational (there is no saddle belonging to the stirrup, no palm for the finger, no spoon or knife for the fork etc.).

Thus such designations do not help at all to understand the objects in question. They are based on superficial similarities, which should be distinguished from more interesting structural resemblances (cf. e.g. Gentner & Medina 1998's distinction between mere-appearance similarities and analogies). If one tries to think about the "metaphorically" designated object in terms of the "literally" designated one, the same problem crucially appears that was noted by Murphy (1996) in connection with conceptual metaphors, i.e. that this leads to incorrect conclusions about the "metaphorically" named object. So in order not to derive false assumptions spontaneously, e.g. that the ball should stay in the basket if thrown into it or that fish fingers contain a bone, speakers have to be aware that they must not derive any conclusions from the metaphorically motivated names in question about the object named. Thus it is highly unlikely that such metaphoric transfers could play any role at all in concept formation and reasoning, but rather can only serve a communicative function, namely, the satisfaction of the communicative need of naming the objects in question by using an already available expression, cf. 2.4.

3. Summary

I believe that the case studies above confirm that the lack of interest toward non-systematic polysemy phenomena in the literature is undeserved, because they can potentially lead to similarly interesting theoretical conclusions as systematic polysemy phenomena.

We have seen that the propositions (P4) and (P5), which are mostly taken for granted in the literature, are not true without further qualifications, and thus a strong interpretation of (P2), which is also commonplace, is incorrect. In particular, polysemies that can be derived by focussing rule are potentially always systematic, but this potential is not always actually exploited, and it is therefore sometimes the case that only a single lexeme exhibits a meaning variation of a certain type. On the other hand, groups of lexemes that have lost their systematicity or have arisen from convergent processes of analogy can be mistaken for systematic polysemy phenomena that can be described by shifting rules. Note that being able to be described by rules does not imply that these meaning variations are in fact derived in the minds of the speakers instead of being simply stored in and retrieved from the lexicon (which Murphy, this volume, claims to be the case in most non-creative uses of polysemous words). However, on the other hand, the reverse is in fact true: if some variation cannot even be described by rules, because it is not systematic enough, one can safely assume that it is stored in the lexicon. One of the substantial morals of the thoughts laid out in this paper is that careful attention must be paid to whether some semantic variation is truly or just superficially systematic when one is planning experiments that aim to examine the mental representation of different types of polysemy.

In section 2.2 we have seen that from a metonymically motivated meaning variation we cannot automatically infer that the variation is based on a rule, i.e. that the meanings in question are not simply lexically stored. And in section 2.1 I argued that there is no necessary theoretical difference between a meaning variation that appears only with a single word and one that can be observed in connection with several lexemes, and therefore the former should not be excluded from the range of examples that are potentially relevant to polysemy research. As I mentioned above, both of these attitudes are widespread in the literature, regardless of whether they are just methodologically motivated or are based on theoretical considerations.

On the basis of the case studies, we can arrive at the following classification of non-systematic polysemy phenomena:

	motivation	**quantitative aspect of meaning variation**	**regularity involved**	**productivity**
1.	metonymic	individual	focussing rule	productive
2.	metonymic	several words	shifting rule	not productive
3.	metaphoric	several words	similarity-based metaphoric extension	not productive
4.	metaphoric	several words	analogy/conceptual metaphor	unclear
5.	metaphoric	individual	similarity-based metaphoric extension	not applicable

I have left several relevant issues open. For example, I have not been able to discuss creatively used figurative and quasi-idiomatic expressions, which I believe are much more relevant than their treatment in the literature would suggest (notable exceptions include Riehemann 2001). I have also not discussed sense extensions in connection with proper names. It would have to be decided whether these are to be regarded as cases of polysemy (and if so, what consequences this would entail for the definition of the object of theories of polysemy), and in what sense this meaning variation is systematic. Finally, it should be carefully examined how productive the quasi-systematic, metaphorically motivated polysemy phenomena are.

References

Apresjan, J.D. (1973): Regular polysemy. *Linguistics* 142, 5-32.

Bierwisch, M. (1983): Semantische und konzeptuelle Repräsentation lexikalischer Einheiten. In: Růžička, R. & Motsch, W. (eds.): *Untersuchungen zur Semantik* (Studia Grammatica XXII). Berlin: Akademie-Verlag, 61-99.

Bierwisch, M. & Lang, E. (eds.)(1987): *Grammatische und konzeptuelle Aspekte von Dimensionsadjektiven* (Studia Grammatica XXVI + XXVII). Berlin, Akademie-Verlag.

Bowdle, B. & Gentner, D. (2005): The career of metaphor. *Psychological Review* 112, 193-216.

Copestake, A. & Briscoe, T. (1996): Semi-productive polysemy and sense extension. In: Pustejovsky, J. & Boguraev, B. (eds.), 15-67.

Deane, P.D. (1987): *Semantic theory and the problem of polysemy.* (Ph.D. Dissertation.) Chicago: University of Chicago.

Dölling, J. (2001 [1997]): Ontological domains, semantic sorts and systematic ambiguity. In: Dölling, J. (2001), 71-92.

Dölling, J. (2001): *Systematische Bedeutungsvariationen: Semantische Form und kontextuelle Interpretation* (Linguistische Arbeitsberichte 78). Leipzig: Institut für Linguistik, Universität Leipzig.

Gentner, D., & Medina, J. (1998): Similarity and the development of rules. *Cognition* 65, 263-97.

Gibbs, R.W. Jr. (1994): *The poetics of mind: Figurative thought, language, and understanding.* Cambridge: Cambridge University Press.

Gibbs, R.W. Jr. (1996): Why many concepts are metaphorical. *Cognition* 61, 309-19.

Glucksberg, S. (2001): *Understanding figurative language: from metaphor to idioms.* Oxford: Oxford University Press.

Haspelmath, M. (2002): *Understanding Morphology.* Oxford: Arnold.

Klein, D.E. & Murphy, G.L. (2001): The representation of polysemous words. *Journal of Memory and Language* 45, 259-82.

Klein, D.E. & Murphy, G.L. (2002): Paper has been my ruin: conceptual relations between polysemous senses. *Journal of Memory and Language* 47, 548-70.

Klepousniotou, E. (2002): The processing of lexical ambiguity: Homonymy and polysemy in the mental lexicon. *Brain and Language* 81, 205-223.

Kövecses, Z. (2002): *Metaphor: a practical introduction.* Oxford: Oxford University Press.

Lakoff, G. (1987): *Women, fire, and dangerous things. What categories reveal about the mind.* Chicago: University of Chicago Press.

Lakoff, G. & Johnson, M. (1980): *Metaphors we live by.* Chicago: University of Chicago Press.

Lakoff, G. & Johnson, M. (1999): *Philosophy in the flesh. The embodied mind and its challenge to Western thought.* New York: Basic Books.

Levin, B. (1993): *English verb classes and alternations: A preliminary investigation.* Chicago: University of Chicago Press.

Loewenberg, I. (1975): Identifying metaphors. *Foundations of Language* 12, 315-338.

Murphy, G.L. (1996): On metaphoric representation. *Cognition* 60, 173-204.

Murphy, G.L. (1997): Reasons to doubt the present evidence for metaphoric representation. *Cognition* 62, 99-108.

Nunberg, G. (1979): The non-uniqueness of semantic solutions – polysemy. *Linguistics and Philosophy* 3, 143-84.

Nunberg, G. (1996 [1995]): Transfers of meaning. In: Pustejovsky, J. & Boguraev, B. (eds.), 109-32.

Pethő, G. (2001a): Konzeptuelle Fokussierung. Bemerkungen zur Behandlung der Polysemie in der Zwei-Ebenen-Semantik. In: Kocsány, P. & Molnár, A. (eds.): *Wort und (Kon)text.* Frankfurt am Main: Lang, 49-101.

Pethő, G. (2001b): What is polysemy? A survey of current research and results. In: Németh T., E. & Bibok, K. (eds.): *Pragmatics and the flexibility of word meaning.* Amsterdam: Elsevier, 175-224.

Pethő, G. (2004): *Poliszémia és kognitív nyelvészet. Rendszeres főnévi poliszémiatípusok a magyarban* [Polysemy and cognitive linguistics. Types of systematic polysemy in Hungarian nouns]. (Ph.D. dissertation). Budapest: ELTE.

Pethő, G. & Csatár, P. (2006): Recognition and processing of figurative language. Talk presented at workshop 11 (Korpusbasierte Behandlung nichtkompositioneller Phänomene) of the 28th annual conference of the DGfS in Bielefeld, Germany, on the 24th February 2006.

Pinker, S. (1999): *Words and rules.* New York: Basic Books.

Pustejovsky, J. (1991): The generative lexicon. *Computational Linguistics* 17, 409-41.

Pustejovsky, J. (1995): *The generative lexicon.* Cambridge: MIT Press.

Pustejovsky, J. & Boguraev, B. (eds.)(1996): *Lexical semantics. The problem of polysemy.* Oxford: Clarendon.

Rakova, M. (2003): *The extent of the literal: metaphor, polysemy and theories of concepts.* Basingstoke: Palgrave Macmillan.

Riehemann, S. (2001): *A constructional approach to idioms and word formation.* (Ph.D. dissertation). Stanford: Stanford University.

Polysemy, Transfers of Meaning and Integrated Metonymy*

Georges Kleiber

4 rue de Luttgerbach
F- 67 1090 Strasbourg, France
E-mail: kleiber@umb.u-strasbg.fr

1. Introduction

We will begin with a statement that has become banal: words are not always used for the "things" they seem destined for. To provide an account for these glides or shifts of reference, it seems preferable today to make use of general principles or rules of derivation that apply to the whole ensemble of lexical units or expressions, rather than opt for an uncontrolled and more or less arbitrary multiplication of the number of senses assigned to one and the same expression. Such a solution, one can say, is more elegant and far more economical, and above all it has the advantage of foregrounding the fundamental mechanisms of semantic and cognitive structuring.

However, the problem of the relevance of such general rules of interpretation certainly arises. An even more crucial problem is that there are considerable drawbacks, not only for lexical semantics, but also for referential functioning and the processes of inference involved in interpretation. Therefore, one cannot but be attentive to new proposals made in this field, and try to see how they come to regulate "the polysemous affairs" that animate the world of meaning.

Taking as the starting point the referential situation of utterances like:

(1) *Je suis (garé) sur la place.*
'I am (parked) in the square.'

we propose in this article to work in that direction in two ways. On the one hand, by examining the new approach of Nunberg (1995) in terms of **predicate transfer**, and on the other hand, in the spirit of our previous work in this field (Kleiber 1984, 1989,

* Originally published as Georges Kleiber (1995): Polysémie, transferts de sens et métonymie intégrée. *Folia Linguistica* XXIX/1-2: 105-132. Included here with the permission of the author and with support of the Research Group for Theoretical Linguistics of the Hungarian Academy of Sciences at the Universities of Debrecen, Pécs and Szeged. The choice of article for inclusion in this volume was the author's own. Translated by Marina Rakova.

1991, 1992a, 1992b, 1994; Kleiber & Riegel 1989, 1991), by further combining our analysis based on the principle of integrated metonymy with a new pragmatic principle, namely that of **meronomic integration** or **meronomisation**.

First, we will recapitulate the analysis in terms of referent change and the critique that this standard treatment provoked. Then we will present the theory of predicate change before proposing, on the basis of certain critical considerations that Nunberg's thesis may give rise to, an approach which does not involve either predicate change or referent transfer, but which, in order to obtain the desired interpretative inference, brings into play general pragmatic principles, and essentially that of integrated metonymy. The final goal envisaged here is to pave the way for an analysis, different from the ones proposed by current compositional models – such as the generative model of Pustejovsky (1991), presently much in vogue –, regulating certain cases of principal or complementary polysemy (cf. the phenomenon of **coercion**). Apart from that, it is the general problem of meaning that will be addressed here.

2. Referent Change: The Phenomenon of Indirect Reference

Everybody agrees that utterances (1) and (2):

(1) *Je suis (garé) sur la place.*
'I am (parked) in the square.'

(2) (a) *Je suis dans l'annuaire de telephone.*
'I'm in the phone book.'

(b) *Picasso est au Louvre.*
'Picasso is in the Louvre.'

(c) *George Sand est sur l'étagère de gauche.*
'George Sand is on the left shelf.'

(d) *Paul a été heurté à l'aile par un camion.*[1]
'Paul was hit in the fender by a truck.'

(e) *Alain Prost perd de l'huile.*
'Alain Prost is losing oil.'

(f) *Maman, je suis sur la liste* (des reçus au baccalauréat).
'Mum, I am on the list (of those who have passed the baccalaureate).'

(g) *Mammouth est aussi à Strasbourg.*
'Mammouth [a supermarket chain] is also in Strasbourg.'

(h) *Marie se reboutonne.*
'Mary is buttoning (herself) up.'

---

[1] Cf. the example of Jackendoff (1992: 6): *A truck hit Ringo in the fender when he was momentarily distracted by a motorcycle.*

do not have the reading that one would predict on the basis of the "normal" or "literal" sense of their subject (or object in the case of (2)(h)), but more or less correspond to interpretations (1') and (2'):

(1') *Ma voiture est (garée) sur la place.*
'My car is parked in the square.'

(2') (a) *Mon nom est dans l'annuaire du telephone.*
'My name is in the phone book.'

(b) *Des oeuvres de Picasso sont au Louvre.*
'The works of Picasso are in the Louvre.'

(c) *Des oeuvres de George Sand sont sur l'étagère de gauche.*
'The works of George Sand are on the left shelf.'

(d) *La voiture de Paul a été heurtée à l'aile par un camion.*
'Paul's car was hit in the fender by a truck.'

(e) *Le moteur de la voiture* ou *la voiture d'Alain Prost pert de l'huile.*
'The engine of Alain Prost's car *or* Alain Prost's car is losing oil.'

(f) *Maman, mon nom est sur la liste.*
'Mum, my name is on the list.'

(g) *Il y a un ou des magasin(s) de Mammouth aussi à Strasbourg.*
'There is one or there are some Mammouth shop(s) in Strasbourg.'

(h) *Marie reboutonne son corsage* (ou un autre vêtement à boutons).
'Mary is buttoning up her blouse (or another item of clothing with buttons).'

The most natural solution for this problem of interpretation consists in claiming that there is a phenomenon of indirect reference, i.e. one expression that normally corresponds to such-and-such type of referent serves the purpose of taking one to a different type of referent, realizing a relation which unites the two types of referents in question. We will further clarify that we are dealing here with indirect **metonymic** reference, as the relation is that of metonymy, like the one that unites a car with its owner or driver, or works of art (novels, paintings, etc.) with the person who created them (author, painter, etc.), a shop with an enterprise or establishment that owns it, an item of clothing with the person wearing it, etc. It does not matter much whether we talk about **metonymic polysemy** or **open polysemy** (Deane 1988). The essential point is that this type of approach postulates a change of referent on the basis of the existence of a metonymic relation: in (1) and (2) the expressions *I*, *Picasso*, *George Sand*, *Mammouth*, etc. do not refer to their usual referent, but to the referents of the subject (and object, in the case of (2')(h)) of utterances (1') and (2') by virtue of a link, or rather a **pragmatic** or **connector function** (Nunberg 1978; Fauconnier 1985). This function, which, as formulated in rule (3) of Fauconnier (1985: 3), allows one to use the name of one referent, the **trigger** referent, for the other referent, the **target** referent:

(3) If two objects (in the most general sense), *a* and *b*, are linked by a pragmatic function $\boldsymbol{F}$ $(b = F(a))$, a description of *a*, d_a, may be used to identify its counterpart *b*.

Such an analysis intuitively seems satisfactory and it draws further power from the fact that it applies to other phenomena of interpretation. It also accounts for utterances of the type *ham omelette* (**closed** polysemy in the work of Deane, **closed connector** in the work of Fauconnier), where it is similarly a relation between the target referent, the customer, and the referent normally denoted by the expression, namely the dish ordered by the customer, that allows one to use the name of the dish to refer to the customer:

(4) (a) *L'omelette au jambon est parti(e) sans payer.* (Fauconnier 1985)
'The ham omelette left without paying.'

(b) *L'hépatite du 3 ne mange toujours pas.*
'The hepatitis in 3 still eats nothing.'

(c) *Les culottes bleues ont gagné par 3 à 0.* (of a football team)
'The blue shorts won 3 to 0.'

On the other hand, it is equally well-suited to explain the restricted referential interpretation of utterances of type (5):

(5) (a) *Paul est bronzé.*(= Paul's skin)
'Paul is tanned.'

(b) *Marie est maquillée.* (= Mary's face)
'Mary is made-up.'

(c) *Paul est voûté.*(= Paul's back)
'Paul is bent.'

If, in the case of (5)(a), for example, Paul's name can indeed be used to refer to Paul's skin only, this is because a part-whole relation unites these two types of referent.[2]

This seems too good to be true, however. And it is not the case that, because this solution directly corresponds to the intuition one may have about the interpretation of utterance types (1) and (2), it is automatically the right one. In fact, the thesis of metonymic transfer too soon meets with difficulties that force us to look for a different solution.

First, it turns out to be far too powerful in that it predicts cases of transfer that are not allowed. Thus, despite the metonymic relation that exists between a car and its owner or driver, we nonetheless cannot use an utterance like (6):

2 For a more detailed analysis of this problem see Kleiber (1991, 1992a, 1994, ch. 8-9).

(6) ?*Je suis grand.*[3]
'I am big.'

to say that the speaker's car is big, not even in a favourable context which already presents such a transfer and permits one to establish a link of coherence between the utterances. Sequence (7):

(7) *Je suis (garé) dans le parking des autocars, parce que je suis trop grand.*
'I am (parked) in the parking lot because I am too big.'

cannot really be interpreted as 'I am parked or my car is parked in the parking lot because my car/it is too big'. One can envisage similar situations for the other transfers given in (2). The result is the same. Even if the conditions for a similarly metonymic understanding of the second part of the sequence were provided, it does not get "launched":

(8) (a) ?*Paul n'est pas dans l'annuaire de téléphone, parce qu'il a trop de lettres.* (*il* = son nom)
'Paul isn't in the phone book because he's got too many letters.' (he = his name)

(b) ?*Picasso est au Louvre. Il est recouvert de poussière* (*il* = les tableaux)[4]
'Picasso is in the Louvre. He is covered with dust.' (he = the paintings)

(c) ?*George Sand est sur l'étagère de gauche. Elle est reliée en cuir.* (*elle* = les livres de George Sand)
'George Sand is on the left shelf. She is bound in leather.' (she = the books of George Sand)

(d) ?*Paul a été heurté à l'aile par un camion, parce qu'il est trop large.* (*il* = la voiture)
'Paul was hit in the fender by a truck because he is too wide.' (he = the car)

(e) ?*Alain Prost perd de l'huile. Il devra être révisé.* (*il* = le moteur ou la voiture)
'Alain Prost is losing oil. He will need checking.' (he = the engine or the car)

(f) ?*Maman, je suis sur la liste* (des reçus au baccalauréat).
Je suis tout petit. (*je* = mon nom)

---

[3] See Kleiber (1989, 1991, 1992b, 1994) and Kleiber & Riegel (1989, 1991). See also Jackendoff (1992) and examples like: **Ringo repainted himself* (i.e. his car). Nunberg (1994: 113) also emphasizes this fact: even if the speaker's car was once driven by Jean Gabin, one cannot, however, say: ??*I was once driven by Jean Gabin*.

[4] One will notice an interesting fact here: the utterance is perfectly acceptable if it is about a "reproduction" of Picasso, namely his photograph or a statue representing him, which shows that the relation of representation that Jackendoff (1992) calls the **statue rule** is not to be assimilated with referential situations in force in (1) and (2).

'Mum, I am on the list (of those who have passed the baccalaureate).'
'I am very small.' (I = my name).

(g) ?*Mammouth est aussi à Strasbourg. Il est tout neuf.* (*il* = le ou les magasins)
'Mammouth is also in Strasbourg. It is brand new.' (it = the shop or shops)

(h) ?*Marie se reboutonne, car elle est ouverte.* (*elle* = le corsage de Marie)
'Mary is buttoning (herself) up, because she is undone.' (she = Mary's blouse)

All these examples clearly show that, contrary to rule (3) of Fauconnier, a metonymic connection does not suffice to ensure transfer. A predicate that may apply to the target referent would not be able to accommodate itself to the expression of the trigger referent. In other words, there are predicates which block referent change, even if the conditions of a switch between the two types of referent are satisfied. This fact, even if it noticeably weakens the thesis of referential transfer and may thus be considered as a sign of its inadequacy, would not however make it invalid all by itself. It is enough, in fact, to add to it a pragmatic constraint which explains why it does not apply in all the cases so that it could be retained in situations of type (1) and (2).

On the other hand, the arguments which question not the generality of the rule, but the very reality of referent change turn out to be decisive. They are of different kinds:

1. The anaphoric data strongly contradict the hypothesis of referent change. If in (1):

(1) *Je suis (garé) sur la place.*
'I am (parked) in the square.'

je ('I') effectively refers to a different referent, one could expect that referent, in this case the car, to be picked out by a pronoun further applied to this new referent as established by the metonymic relation. However, such transfers do not occur. One cannot have a pronoun which reflects the grammatical features of the target referent and no longer those of the trigger. Examples (9) and (10) of Fauconnier intended to illustrate that such transfer can take place, indeed seem to us unacceptable (Kleiber 1989):

(9) *George Sand est sur l'étagère de gauche.* ***Il*** *est relié en cuir.* (Fauconnier 1984: 18)
'George Sand is on the left shelf. **It** is bound in leather.'

(10) *Françoise Sagan n'est pas, en* ***lui-même****, un sujet de thèse passionnant.* (Fauconnier 1984: 20)
'Françoise Sagan is not in **itself** a fascinating dissertation topic.'

We will verify this with the help of (1) and (2)(e) which cannot be followed by a pronoun corresponding to the gender of *car*:

(11) (a) ?*Je suis (garé) sur la place.* ***Elle*** *est tout au bout.* (*elle* = la voiture)
'I am (parked) in the square. **It** is at the very back.' (it = the car)

(b) ?*Alain Prost perd de l'huile.* ***Elle*** *devra être révisée.* (*elle* = la voiture)
'Alain Prost is losing oil. **It** will need checking.' (it = the car)

nor by another anaphoric expression that would be coreferential:

(12) ?*Je suis (garé) sur la place.* ***La voiture/cette voiture*** *est tout au bout.*
'I am (parked) in the square. **The car/that car** is at the very back.'
(in the interpretation where *je* and *la voiture/cette voiture* are in the relation of coreference)

On the other hand, one finds that a pronominal continuation referring to the non-transferred initial referent is always possible, if it respects the condition of discourse coherence:

(13) (a) *Paul est garé sur la place.* ***Il*** *est venu jusqu'ici à pied.*
'Paul is parked in the square. **He** has come here on foot.'

(b) *Paul n'est pas dans l'annuaire de téléphone.* ***Il*** *n'a pas voulu donner son nom.*
'Paul is not in the phone book. **He** did not want to give his name.'

(c) *Marie est sur la liste des reçus.* ***Elle*** *l'a mérité.*
'Mary is on the list of those who have passed. **She** deserved it.'

(d) – *George Sand est sur l'étagère de gauche entre Hugo et Musset.*
Si elle revenait sur terre, cela ne ***lui*** *plairait peut-être pas.*[5]

'George Sand is on the left shelf between Hugo and Musset.
If she returned to earth, it probably would not please **her**.'

– *C'est parce qu'* ***il*** *est un écrivain populaire que Victor Hugo figure chez nous sur l'étagère de gauche.*

'It is because **he** is a popular writer that Victor Hugo is on the left shelf in our home.'

(e) *Picasso est au Louvre. Cet honneur* ***le*** *laisse indifferent.*
'Picasso is in the Louvre. This honour leaves **him** indifferent.'

(f) *Alain Prost perd de l'huile, mais* ***il*** *ne se laisse pas abattre et repart à l'attaque.*

'Alain Prost is losing oil, but **he** doesn't give up and continues the fight.'

---

5 N. Flaux (personal communication) made me notice that the sequence *George Sand est sur l'étagère de gauche. Tu verras qu'elle écrit divinement bien.* ('George Sand is on the left shelf. You will see that she writes divinely well.') (Fauconnier 1984: 18) is not natural either. This seems to be due to coherence reasons.

(g) *Mammouth est aussi à Strasbourg. **Il** compte s'installer bientôt en Allemagne.*
'Mammouth is also in Strasbourg. **It** plans to set up in Germany soon.'

It is, of course, conceivable to talk about divergent anaphora with respect to (13), explaining that the trigger can remain a possible pronominal antecedent, even if it is the target that is referred to in the first instance. Fauconnier (1984: 18), who proposes such an analysis, thus sees in examples of type (13) a situation of referential disjunction between the antecedent and the pronoun: the antecedent, for example *Paul* in (13)(a) refers to the target, that is to say the car, whereas the pronoun, in the present case *il* ('he'), continues to refer to the trigger of the metonymy, that is to say Paul in our case. Such a description is, however, only pertinent within the hypothesis where we also have the situation of co-reference: **target** referent (antecedent) – **target** referent (pronoun). Now, we have seen that such a situation does not occur: *Paul*, *George Sand*, *Picasso*, etc. cannot be the antecedents for the anaphoric expressions referring to the referents that are metonymically connected to them (the car, books, paintings, etc.). As a consequence, it is preferable to abandon the thesis of referent transfer.

2. Co-predications with predicates referring manifestly to the "non-transferred" referent are possible without the production of zeugma:

(14) (a) *Je suis (garé) sur la place depuis dix minutes et y retourne à pied dans un quart d'heure.*
'I've been (parked) in the square for about 10 minutes and will return there on foot in a quarter of an hour.'

(b) *Alain Prost perd de l'huile, mais ne se laisse pas abattre par ce coup du sort.*
'Alain Prost is losing oil, but he doesn't get give up because of this blow of fate.'

(c) *Picasso est au Louvre, mais n'en est pas heureux.*
'Picasso is in the Louvre, but is not happy about it.'

(d) *Paul a été heurté à l'aile par un camion et est décédé trois heures après.*
'Paul was hit in the fender by a truck and died three hours later.'

(e) *Mammouth est aussi à Strasbourg et prend ainsi une dimension de plus en plus européenne.*
'Mammouth is also in Strasbourg and is thus taking a more and more European dimension.'

3. As the glosses in (16) show, the thesis of referent change can only account for utterances like (15) with difficulty. There, the referent assigned to the metonymic term appears explicitly in another place:

(15) (a) *Je suis dans l'annuaire de téléphone sous le nom de Dupont.*
'I am in the phone book under the name of Dupont.'

(b) *Je suis (garé) sur la place avec la voiture de Pierre et pas avec la mienne/je suis (garé) là-bas avec mon camion.*
'I am (parked) in the square with Pierre's car and not mine/I am (parked) there with my truck.'

(c) *Mammouth est à Strasbourg avec un seul magasin.*
'Mammouth is in Strasbourg with only one shop.'

(d) *Picasso est au Louvre grâce à quatre tableaux.*
'Picasso is in the Louvre with [lit. thanks to] four paintings.'

(16) (a) (?) *Mon nom est dans l'annuaire de téléphone sous le nom de Dupont.*
'My name is in the phone book under the name of Dupont.'

(b) ?*Ma voiture est (garée) sur la place avec la voiture de Pierre et pas avec la mienne./Mon camion est (garé) là-bas avec mon camion.*
'My car is (parked) in the square with Pierre's car and not mine./My truck is (parked) there with my truck.'

(c) ?*Des/un magasin de Mammouth sont/est à Strasbourg avec un seul magasin.*
'Mammouth shops/shop are/is in Strasbourg with only one shop.'

(d) ?*Des tableaux de Picasso sont au Louvre, grâce à quatre tableaux.*
'Picasso's paintings are in the Louvre with [lit. thanks to] four paintings.'

3. Predicate Change

3.1. Nunberg's (1995) Solution of "Transfers of Meaning"

In 1978, Nunberg opted for the analysis in terms of referent change, aligning the mechanism of descriptive reference in (1) and (2) with that of indirect ostension working in utterances like (17), where the demonstrative does not have the key of the car that is being shown as its referent, but the car itself:

(17) *This is parked out back.* (showing the key of the car)[6]

In his 1995 article he abandons this assimilation, observing that whereas the properties of (17) are well linked to the indirect referent 'car', the properties of such utterances as *I am parked out back* would rather lead to the "literal" referent of *I*.[7] He concludes that

---

6 The example is not as obvious as that and it would be appropriate to question the real relevance of the mechanism of **deferred ostension** (Quine 1971). We do not think that in the case of *This is parked out back* there is first an indexical designation of the key, which is then, thanks to the relation between the key and the car, upgraded to the car.

7 He thus observes that:

- the demonstrative agrees in number and grammatical gender with the indirect referent and not with the demonstrated referent. If there are several keys and only one car, it will nevertheless be:

in the referential situations of type (1) and (2) there is no mechanism of indirect reference, and thus no change of referent for the NP.

The new hypothesis formulated is that it is the predicate that changes. It no longer expresses the property it normally does, but a new one. It is still a transfer process, but with respect to the predicate, rather than a nominal referent. As Nunberg (1995) says:

> The principle here is that the name of a property that applies to something in one domain can sometimes be used as the name of a property that applies to things in another domain, provided the two properties correspond in a certain way. (p. 111)

Just as the thesis of referent change for the NP presupposes a relation or a mechanism of transition between the trigger referent of the NP and the new intended referent (or target), for example, between the owner and the car in (1), the thesis of predicate change or transfer presupposes a relation between the original predicate and the derived predicate.

This is the first condition on predicate transfer:

> The property denoted by the derived predicate has to correspond in a certain way to the property denoted by the original predicate. (p. 112)

In the case of (1), for example, there is functional correspondence between the location of cars in a parking lot and the properties of the owners of these cars (or, more precisely, the persons they belong to): if you know the location of a car, you also know a useful property of its owner. Thus, it is necessary that two domains of properties correspond to each other in an appropriate or useful fashion, so that the denomination of one of them could be used for the other. The first condition on predicate transfer can also be expressed in terms of functions, connecting, however, not two types of referent but two domains of properties:

(18) Let $\mathcal{P}$ and $\mathcal{P}$' be sets of properties that are related by a salient transfer function gt: $\mathcal{P} \rightarrow \mathcal{P}'$. Then if F is a predicate that denotes a property $P \in \mathcal{P}$, there is also a predicate F', spelt like F, that denotes the property P', where $P' = \text{gt}(P)$. (p. 112)

The fact that (19) and (20):

This is parked out back, whereas if there are several cars and only one key, it will be: *These are parked out back*;

- the copredications occur for the demonstrative with the car, but not with the key, whereas the inverse holds in the case of utterances of type (1):

(a) *This is parked out back and may not start.*
??*This fits only the left front door and is parked out back.*
(b) *I am parked out back and have been waiting for 15 minutes.*
* *I am parked out back and may not start.*

(19) *Nous sommes à Pittsburgh.* ('tous nos magasins sont installés à Pittsburgh')
'We are in Pittsburgh.' ('all our shops are set up in Pittsburgh')

(20) *Nous sommes à présent à Singapour.* ('nous avons un ou des magasins à Singapour')
'We are in Singapore now.' ('we have one or more shops in Singapore')

do not correspond to the same quantificational interpretation scheme – the first one gives rise to a universally quantified interpretation, the second one requires only an existentially quantified interpretation – leads Nunberg to postulate two instantiations of the rule of predicate transfer, which we will call **definite** predicate transfer (a) and **indefinite** predicate transfer (b):

(21) If ft is a transfer function from a property domain $\mathcal{P}$ to $\mathcal{P}'$, then for every P belonging to $\mathcal{P}$, if $ft(P) = P'$, we can conclude either (a) or (b):

(a) $\forall y\, (P'(y) \rightarrow (\exists x(Px)\ \&\ R(x,y)))$
(b) $\forall y\, (P'(y) \rightarrow (\forall x\, R(x,y) \rightarrow (Px)))$

where R is a contextual relation that depends on the domains $\mathcal{P}$ and $\mathcal{P}'$.

The same risk of being far too powerful, which was regarded as unacceptable with respect to the rule of referent transfer (3), is involved with a rule like (21). According to (21), as Nunberg emphasizes, one should be able to say (22) or (23):

(22) *?J'ai été conduit une fois par Jean Gabin.*
'I was once driven by Jean Gabin.'

(23) *?Je suis dans une caisse dans le sous-sol.*
'I am in a crate in the basement.'

if the speaker's car was once driven by Jean Gabin or if some paintings of the speaker (who happens to be a painter, e.g. Elizabeth Murray) are in a crate in the basement.[8] It obviously doesn't work that way, and to avoid such undesirable transfers, Nunberg postulates a second constraint on the process of predicate derivation: it can only be successful if the transferred predicate reveals itself as noteworthy for its bearer. Thus one understands why (22) and (23) do not get over the threshold: they do not ascribe any sufficiently noteworthy properties to the subject. This condition of **noteworthiness** depends crucially on the context. A sufficiently restricted context is enough for the realization of a transfer which by default seems impossible. If the crates with Elizabeth

8 For examples similar to *?George Sand est par terre.* ('George Sand is on the floor.') or *?Paul est sec.* ('Paul is dry.') for 'La peau de Paul est sèche.' ('Paul's skin is dry.') see Kleiber (1989, 1990, 1991, 1992a, b, 1994).

Murray's paintings are to be shipped to the Biannual Exhibition in Venice and thus their localisation in such a place has a significance that bestows a certain distinction on the painter, it is then possible to resort to an utterance like (23).

The interpretation of this property of salience can give rise to discussion. Thus, Nunberg contradicts Jackendoff (1992) concerning the analysis of example (2)(d):

(2) (d) *Paul a été heurté à l'aile par un camion.*
'Paul was hit in the fender by a truck.'

For Jackendoff (24):

(24) **Paul a été heurté à l'aile par un camion deux jours après sa mort.*
'Paul was hit in the fender by a truck two days after he died.'

shows that (2)(d) is possible only if Paul is in the act of driving or has his car parked in a parking lot. Nunberg regards this condition as too strict. In his opinion, the decisive fact is that the property which the owner inherits from his car has interesting consequences for him. If a truck hits Paul's car on the fender, he is obviously affected by it in different ways, whereas if he is dead, it no longer has any significance for him.

The two instantiations of predicate transfer put forward in (21) correspond to two possible ways in which a property can be noteworthy. Examples of type (1) illustrate mode (b), the mode of universal quantification. The transferred predicate serves the function of assigning the bearer to the class of people who parked their cars in a such-and-such place and (1) is interpreted more or less as 'I belong to the class of people whose car or cars are parked in the square'. The "noteworthy" property does not need to have any importance or inherent interest for the one who satisfies it: its role consists in placing the subject referent in a class unambiguously determined by the context. Mode (a), that of existentially quantified interpretation, is exemplified by (2)(b)-(c) or (2)(f). The transferred predicate of (2)(b):

(2) (b) *Picasso est au Louvre.*
'Picasso is in the Louvre.'

does not aim not to identify a unique class of things which the referent satisfying the derived property would be part of, but rather to signal an intrinsic property of this referent as witnesses the gloss 'Picasso has the property that one acquires if a painting that one produced has the property of being in the Louvre'.

3.2. Corollaries

3.2.1. Lexical Polysemy

According to Nunberg, the thesis of predicate transfer paves the way for a unitary treatment of lexical polysemy. It applies equally to **lexical** transfers and seems pertinent to describe transfers concerning nouns, adjectives and other lexical categories. The transition is mediated by situational metonymy[9] of type (25) in predicative use:

(25) *Qui est l'omelette au jambon?* (prononcé par un garçon de restaurant)
'Who is the ham omelette?' (said by a restaurant waiter),

where the mechanism of predicate transfer seems clear, as there is a relation between the domain of properties of dishes ordered and that of customers who ordered them: the customers acquire the identifying properties of the distinctive properties of the dishes they ordered. Thus it is reasonable to claim that if the same expression is used referentially as in (4)(a), instead of predicatively, it is justified to extend the analysis to such cases and regard them as phenomena of predicate transfer:

(4) (a) *L'omelette au jambon est parti sans payer.*
'The ham omelette left without paying.'

There is no longer a reason not to make this move, because the classic cases of lexical metonymy known under the names of **regular polysemy**, **systematic polysemy**, **logical metonymy**, etc. are also approached in terms of predicate change:

(26) **examples of systematic polysemy** (Nunberg 1995: 117)
transmissions for cars: *4 speed*, *automatic*, etc.
texts for inscriptions: *a Webster's Third*, *a Guide Bleu*, etc.
painters for works: *a Picasso*, *a Derain*, etc.
containers for volumes of stuff: *She drank two glasses.*, etc.
writer for oeuvre: *fifty pages of Wordsworth*
place for inhabitants: *Indianapolis voted for the referendum.*
tree for wood: *The table is made of oak.*

That one is talking here about qualitatively identical phenomena is proved by the fact that they observe the same two constraints which govern the process of predicate transfer in the cases of type (1): there has to be a correspondence between the two properties in question and the transferred predicate has to be a noteworthy property for the bearer. Accordingly, the rule of "grinding", which converts a count noun into a mass noun denoting the stuff of which the countable entity consists, also has to meet both requirements. This explains why alongside of *Nous avons mangé du lapin.* ('We ate rabbit.'), we do not have, except in particular situations which are always possible, *Nous avons*

9 Called **occurrent metonymies** by Nunberg, because the relation between the two domains can only be used in a limited number of situations. As was similarly stated by Fauconnier (1985), this type of process needs a particular context: restaurant situation for *ham omelette*, hospital milieu for *the hepatitis in 3*, etc. In one note, Nunberg (1995: 116) very rightly emphasizes that this amounts to saying that the information one needs comes not from the representation attached to the lexeme *ham omelette* but from the representation associated with the situation or particular activity in question. It is in the *restaurant* scenario or frame that one finds knowledge about customers and not within *ham omelette.*

mangé du géant des Flandres. ('We ate giant of Flanders.'): the fact of having eaten a rabbit of a particular breed is not, by default, gastronomically relevant.

That there are lexical specificities, cases of idiomatic transfer,[10] cannot be denied –Nunberg talks about **lexical licenses** (Nunberg & Zaenen 1992) –, but does not justify refusing to see in them occurrences of a general transfer process. As Nunberg correctly states (1995: 119), it is a mistake, well-spread in the circles of lexical polysemanticians, to think that transfer is itself something intrinsically lexical: "Even when a rule like grinding has been explicitly lexicalized, what is conventionalized is not the mechanism involved, but only the particular semantic domains the mechanism is allowed to operate on."

3.2.2. Transfer and Semantic Analysis

If it allows one to integrate all cases of metonymy, whether lexical or not, the extension effectuated by Nunberg from NPs to NPs or arguments has the consequence of posing a completely new problem, that of the choice of the transferred expression. An utterance like (27):

(27) *Fred noue ses souliers.*
'Fred is tying his shoes.'

theoretically gives place to two possible predicate transfers: it is either the predicate *nouer* ('to tie') that is its object and thus denotes a new relation between Fred and his shoes, or it is *souliers* ('shoes') that has a transferred sense to refer to the shoes' laces. The conjunction tests used by Nunberg speak in favour of the first solution. Only a copredicate that applies to *chaussures* ('shoes') is possible:

(28) *Les chaussures de Fred sont mal nouées et sales.*
'Fred's shoes are badly tied and dirty.'

(29) ??*Les chaussures de Fred sont mal nouées, car trop court(e?)s.*[11]
'Fred's shoes are badly tied because too short.'

The commentary to this example is very interesting: if it is *nouer* ('to tie') that has a transferred reading, that happens in virtue of a more general correspondence between the corresponding activities: to perform an action on something which fixes or supports an object is very often to perform an action on the object itself: cf. *verrouiller la porte* – 'to bolt the door', etc. If it is not *shoe* that has a transferred sense, namely to apply to

---

[10] In French, for example, there is no *une poire/une pomme* ('a pear'/'an apple') for cider, but there is for alcohol.

[11] Nunberg's examples are the following:
Billy's shoes were neatly tied but dirty.
??*Billy's shoes were neatly tied but frayed.*

shoelaces, it is because this kind of figure involves presuppositions which are not very appropriate. This would indeed mean that the speaker is interested in things which support, rather than in things which are supported, and the "supporters" are better classified in virtue of their correspondence with things than denoted by their function of "support".

In other contexts, it is rather the argument instead of the functor which has a transferred sense. It may even be that it is both of them and that one thus encounters bi-directional transfer, as in the example borrowed by Nunberg from Langacker (1984):[12]

(30) *We heard the piano.*

where, according to Nunberg, the possibility of having sequence (32) as well as sequence (31), and the impossibility of having the combination of the two prove that it is not only the predicate *heard* which can have a transferred sense and signify the relation that is established between listeners and objects when the former hear the sounds produced by the latter, but that *piano* can also be the object of predicate transfer and denote 'piano music':

(31) *We saw, touched, and heard the piano.*
We heard the piano, which was sitting on the terrace.

(32) *We heard the piano, which came drifting across the lake.*

(33) ??*We heard the piano, which was sitting on the terrace and came drifting across the lake.*

3.2.3. Dense Metonymy and General Sense

A supplementary stage thus leads Nunberg to postulate the notion of **dense metonymy** for cases like newspaper, magazine, review, etc., which are doubly particular: 1) they are polysemous in that they can refer to either a token of the publication, or an edition of the publication, or else the publishing organization itself, and 2) the properties which apply to one of these entities can also be applied to any other of these entities, because the different entities they refer to are in the relation of interdefinition: "equivalence

---

12 Another case of bi-directionality invoked by Nunberg is: *Yeats is still widely read* which gives place to the transfer of the predicate's meaning if the sequence is about the poet (cf. *Yeats is widely read, though he has been dead for more than 50 years*) and the transfer of the argument *Yeats* if it takes his works as subject of discourse (cf. *Yeats is still widely read, even though most of it is out of print*). A situation like this with pronoun change does not seem possible in French (cf. *George Sand est beaucoup lue, mais? il est pour la plus grande partie épuisé.* – 'George Sand is widely read but most of it is out print.'). One will notice that if one can have *George Sand est beaucoup lue, mais elle n'est plus éditée.* ('George Sand is widely read, but she is not published any more.'), one does not, on the other hand, have *George Sand est beaucoup lue, mais? elle est épuisée.* ('George Sand is widely read, but she is out of print.').

classes of copies and editions are individuated in large part by reference to the distinguishing properties of the organizations that produce them, and vice versa" (Nunberg 1995). That is to say, one can have, on the one hand, (34):

(34) *Which newspaper did Mary burn? – The one John works for.*

and, on the other hand, (35):

(35) *Which newspaper does John work for? – The one Mary burned.*

A densely metonymous word is defined as follows (Nunberg 1995: 126):

(36) Given several disjoint sorts of things *A*, *B*, ... and several classes of predicates *F*, *G*... such that members of *F* literally apply only to things of sort *A*, members of *G* literally apply only to things of sort *B*, and so on, a word *W* is densely metonymous iff:

(a) *W* has distinct uses to refer to things of sorts *A*, *B*... and
(b) When *W* is applied to something of sort *A*, it often happens that predicates belonging to *G* can be applied to *W* under transferred readings, and when *W* is applied to something of sort *B* it often happens that predicates belonging to *F* can be applied to *W* under transferred readings, and so on.

This category of words is, however, pertinent only if one differentiates it from **general sense** words. In fact, the identification of general sense words similarly rests on tests which place in the foreground phenomena of coordination and relative clause. To distinguish an ambiguous term from a general sense term, we address sentences of the type:

W is F and G
W which is F is G
W which is G is F

where *W* is a word that can refer to two sorts of things *A* and *B*, and where *F* is a predicate which only refers to *A*, and *G* is a predicate which only refers to *B*. If these sentences are well-formed, as is sequence (37) of Cruse (1986: 61):

(37) *My cousin, who is pregnant, was born on the same day as Arthur's, who is the father.*

then the word tested is not ambiguous, but has a general sense – such is the case of *cousin* used as an example by Cruse in (37).

One sees immediately that the notion of dense metonymy risks being confused with the notion of general sense, as it is based on identical sequences of predicate combination. Thus the word *bill* in (38):

(38) *He paid the bill and threw it away.*

that Robins (1987) analyses as a general sense word, having a single "semantic range" whose uses for referring to abstract and concrete things are different subdivisions, might well be described as a densely metonymous word which has as its referent either the physical inscription or the content of the inscription, and which, in all cases of predicate transfer, is accompanied by one of the verbs: either it is *paid* which has a transferred sense – then it denotes a relation between a person and a physical object – or, a more probable case, it is *throw away* which experiences predicate change and denotes a relation between a person and a financial obligation. The important point, as Nunberg notes, is that coordination tests do not allow one to decide the status of the word. This kind of situation is not rare, as it concerns a whole group of words such as *book*, for example, often cited as a typical case of polysemy:[13]

(39) *J'ai acheté le livre de Paul, mais je l'ai trouvé difficile.*
'I bought Paul's book, but I found it difficult.'

To separate the two types of semantic phenomena, and thus to identify the cases of densely metonymous words, Nunberg makes use of the noteworthiness condition put forward for predicate transfers. Because predicate transfers are not free, and because densely metonymous words accompany predicate transfer, it is sufficient to verify if there are any restrictions on the predicates, and one thus obtains a criterion for recognizing when a predicate has been "transferred" and so of knowing whether a word is general or polysemous:

(40) Let's suppose that we have an acceptable sentence of the form *W is F and G*, where *F* and *G* apply respectively to *A* and *B*. Thus, to show that *W* is in fact general with regard to *A* and *B*, we must show that neither *F* nor *G* has here a transferred sense. And we can do so by showing that the choice of predicates of the same type as *F* and *G* is relatively free and is not constrained by considerations of salience.

Applied to the term *book*, this criterion concludes in favour of its general sense – it denotes complex objects which at the same time have a physical extent and an intentional content –, whereas applied to terms like *pamphlet* or *memoir* it indicates that they represent cases of polysemous terms with sense transfer. This difference which scarcely appears in (41):

[13] It is important to note that Kayser (1987 & 1989) takes precisely the word *book* as his example to show that "one-way streets lead to dead-ends" („les sens uniques conduisent à des impasses" – the title of Coulon & Kayser's article, 1983). See our response in Kleiber (1990); Kleiber & Riegel (1989, 1991).

(41) *She published a 90-page book {pamphlet, memoir} which critics found hilarious.*

where the three nouns seem to have the same type of referents, follows from the comparison of (42), (43) and (44):

(42) *?She published a handsome {?offset, paperback} memoir, 90 pages long.*

(43) *?She published a slangy {?euphonious, ?poorly-spelled} 90-pages pamphlet.*

(44) *She published a paperback {offset, glossy} book, which was slangy and poorly-spelled.*

It is necessary to emphasize that Nunberg strives to make it precise that these tests have certain limits, that the dividing line between polysemy and generality is not as clear as it is drawn by the test and that generality is in fact only a limited case of dense metonymy: it is the case where a word denotes two (or more) sorts of things and where one can always apply to it all predicates that apply to each of them.

This final relaxation, however, should not make us lose sight of the importance of the general picture of lexical and non-lexical polysemy outlined by Nunberg. Putting forward the notion of predicate transfer not only regulates the referential problem posed by the analysis of utterances of type (1) and (2), but ultimately applies to all situations, including metaphor,[14] where the same linguistic expression refers to two distinct things. In the domain of metonymy, it constitutes, thanks to the new notions like dense metonymy and the criterion of polysemy recognition, a considerable change with regard to Nunberg (1978). It cannot thus be ignored and deserves to be examined with attention. This is what we will do in the next section.

4. Against Predicate Transfer

The most immediate advantage that Nunberg's solution offers is, indisputably, the fact that it surmounts all sorts of "anaphoric" difficulties which are engendered by the thesis of referent change. There is no need to resort to **divergent anaphora** to explain sequences like (13)(a) or (2)(h):

(13) (a) *Paul est garé sur la place. **Il** est venu jusqu'ici à pied.*
'Paul is parked in the square. **He** has come here on foot.'

(2) (h) *Marie **se** reboutonne.*
'Mary is buttoning (**herself**) up.'

---

14 The difference between metonymy and metaphor would consist in the following: predicate transfer in the case of metaphor is licensed by a direct correspondence between properties. In other words, predicate transfer which takes place in a metaphoric process does not correspond to the two types of instantiations (21)(a) and (b) postulated for metonymy.

As there is no change of referent, the pronouns *il* ('he') and *se* ('herself') remain here pronouns of coreference. Nunberg's analysis thus leads to the same anaphoric result as the one to which we were led by our re-examination of Fauconnier's connectors (Kleiber 1989).

The price that Nunberg paid for such a result seems to us too high. To maintain that the referent of *je* ('I') in an utterance like (1):

(1) *Je suis (garé) sur la place.*
'I am (parked) in the square.'

is the speaker and that it doesn't become the car, does one really need to postulate a change of predicate instead?

It seems to us that there are several reasons not to accept such a decision. First of all, there is the fact that Nunberg does not provide a clear and definitive argument in favour of predicate transfer. Unlike the thesis of referent change, that of predicate gliding rather runs against intuition. This obviously does not constitute a proof but the facts become more problematic when one observes that, with respect to the transferred property itself as well as the relation between the properties, the analysis remains much too vague.

We will thus note that we do not know very well what this new property obtained by derivation is like, whereas such imprecision does not exist at all for the thesis of referent change. Representing it with the same predicate but adorned on the right with an apostrophe – *to be parked in the square* becomes *to be parked in the square'* – does not throw much light on the real status of this new property. The glosses provided are no more instructive, as witness the paraphrases (45) and (46) intended to translate the sense of new predicates of an indefinite transfer like (1) and a definite transfer like *Je suis au Louvre* ('I am in the Louvre'):

(45) *Je suis dans la classe des gens dont la voiture ou les voitures est/sont garée(s) sur la place.*
'I am in the class of people whose car(s) is/are parked in the square.'

(46) *J'ai la propriété que l'on obtient lorsqu'un ou plusieurs de vos tableaux ont la propriété d'être au Louvre.*
'I have the property that one acquires when one or more of one's paintings have the property of being in the Louvre.'

The same fuzziness prevails with respect to the relation between the two properties, that is, with respect to the first condition on predicate transfer. Even though one clearly sees what sort of relation holds between the referents, assuming the thesis of referent change, one does not very well grasp what the transfer function would be which permits predicate transfer. Nunberg's formulation rests on the following very vague point: the properties must correspond "in a certain way" (cf. above). When is this the case? We have seen in example (1) that this happens when the two domains of properties correspond in an appropriate or useful manner: there is functional correspondence between the location of cars in a parking lot and the properties of their drivers. But if one looks at it more closely, one will see that in fact this appropriate or useful correspondence, the correspondence of functionality already meets the second condition, that of the salient character of the transfer function, which means that the transfer function is not defined in an independent way at all, prior to the restricting application of the **noteworthiness** condition.

Nor does it exist outside the relation which unites the two types of referent according to the thesis of referent change. It is, in fact, significant to observe that the rule of transfer (18), if it applies to phenomena of the metonymic order,[15] necessarily recognizes an instantiation, definite or indefinite, given in rule (21) which connects the two types of referent united by a metonymic relation: in other words, even if one postulates that *être garé sur place* ('to be parked in the square') said by a human being is a derived predicate or denotes a property different from the one it denotes normally, one has to introduce into one's account the metonymic relation between the owner or driver of a car and the car parked. More precisely, it is necessary that the car satisfy the non-derived predicate.

All these reasons lead us to believe that the solution of predicate transfer, however original and unexpected it may seem, does not have the substance necessary to serve as a solid theory for the explanation of referential phenomena like the ones exemplified in (1) and (2). It also seems to us that certain extensions and consequences it leads to ultimately speak against it, since they invite criticism.

Firstly, the assimilation of changes of type (1) and (2) to lexical polysemy, whether situational metonymy (cf. *L'omelette au jambon est parti sans payer* – 'The ham omelette left without paying') or cases of regular or systematic polysemy (cf. *un Picasso* – 'a Picasso') is involved, does not seem to us correct at all. Contrary to what Nunberg thinks, it is not exactly the same semantic mechanisms and the same pragmatic constraints that get employed there, even if the notion of salience or relevance appears to be appropriate in both cases, which should not come as a surprise. The fact that for the second type of cases it is the NP that is the place of change has important consequences that one does not find in the first type of cases. This is why one can indeed talk about referent change for the subject NP in (4)(a) and (47):

(4) (a) *L'omelette au jambon est parti sans payer.*
'The ham omelette left without paying.'

(47) *Un Picasso a été volé au Louvre.*
'A Picasso has been stolen from the Louvre.'

The fact that it takes place at a general level, that of referent types, and not at the level of particular referents in question – that which permits Nunberg to talk about **predicate**

---

15 As emphasized in the previous note, in the case of metaphor there is no instantiation of definite or indefinite transfer types.

transfer – is certain,[16] but it does not change anything in the end: in (4)(a) and (47) there surely is a referent different from the one normally designated by the expression *omelette au jambon* ('ham omelette') and the proper noun *Picasso*, namely the customer and a painting.[17] This result, as we have stressed above, is not obtained at the level of predicates in a situation like (1). Therefore, it seems inadequate to assimilate the two types of phenomena.

It also seems inadequate, on a larger scale, to move from predicates or functors to NPs or arguments, for this makes one conceive of utterances like (27) as theoretically ambiguous:

(27) *Fred noue ses souliers.*
'Fred is tying his shoes.'

whereas they seem to be open to two possible readings (the transfer of *nouer* – 'to tie' or the transfer of *souliers* – 'shoes') only because the system includes two types of possible transfers. We think that the best proof of this is that it is impossible to find utterances which really exemplify bidirectional transfer. We will not pass any judgement on the English utterances considered as truly ambiguous by Nunberg, such as (30) already cited above, and (48), presented in footnote 12:

(30) *We heard the piano.*

(48) *Yeats is widely read.*

but will simply observe that their French counterparts are not apparently open to two readings assigned by Nunberg (1995) to English utterances, as one can clearly show for (49):

(49) *Nous entendîmes le piano.*
'We heard the piano.'

the failure of the co-predication criterion:

(50) *Nous entendîmes le piano, qui se trouvait sur la terrasse.*
'We heard the piano that was on the terrace.'

---

16 There is a restriction, however, for the metonymy 'dishes ordered → customers': we do not have, at least not as naturally *C'est qui une omelette au jambon?/Je suis une omelette au jambon./Je suis une saucisse frites.* ('Who is a ham omelette?/I am a ham omelette./I am a sausage with French fries').

17 One will notice for *Un Picasso* ('A Picasso') that this change of referent is accompanied by the masculine gender. Whatever the gender of the name of the denoted work and the gender of the bearer of the proper name, it is always in the masculine (cf. *du Mozart, du George Sand*, etc. – du = de le (masculine) = 'of'). For more details on these metonymic proper names, see Kleiber (1994, ch. 5, 6 & 7).

(51) *?Nous entendïmes le piano, qui nous parvenait flottant par-dessus du lac.*
'We heard the piano that reached us floating over the lake.'

and for (52):

(52) *George Sand est lue par beaucoup de monde.*
'George Sand is read by many people.'

the failure of the pronominalisation of the works:

(53) *George Sand est lue par beaucoup de monde, bien qu'elle soit disparue depuis longtemps.*
'George Sand is read by many people, even though she has been dead for a long time.'

(54) *?George Sand est lue par beaucoup de monde, bien qu'ils ne soient plus édités.*[18]
'George Sand is read by many people, even though they are not published any more.'

Such facts question *ipso facto* the notion of **dense metonymy**. Terms like *journal*, *magazine*, *review*, etc. rather seem to us to depend on the notion of general sense as applied to *book*: they are nouns which denote heterogeneous objects, in multiple facets. One is tempted, to be sure, to invoke the identification test (40). But it hardly seems effective. This can be shown in two ways. On the one hand, by observing, as Nunberg does in one of his notes, that the English term *memoir*, which the test places among polysemous terms with sense transfer and not expressions with general sense (cf. (41) above), can be combined with predicates which impose a "concrete" reading (physical object), where one cannot see what the transferred sense could be:

(55) *She dropped the memoir she was reading on her toe.*[19]

On the other hand, if one takes a case like *Paul*, where (56):

(56) *Paul est grand, brun, bronzé et intelligent, calme, soucieux de plaire et d'apprendre la néo-linguistique alsacienne.*
'Paul is tall, brown-haired, tanned and intelligent, calm, anxious to please and to learn Alsatian neo-linguistics.'

---

[18] One will note that if one can have *George Sand est beaucoup lue, bien qu'elle ne soit plus éditée.* ('George Sand is widely read even though she is not published any more.'), one does not, on the other hand, have *George Sand est beaucoup lue, bien qu'elle soit épuisée.* ('George Sand is widely read even though she is out of print.').

[19] Nunberg's (1995) comment: "It is hard to see how this property could apply to a text in a transferred sense".

is catalogued as a general sense, and admits at the same time that one nevertheless comes across combinations like (57):

(57) *?Paul est bronzé et sec.*
'Paul is tanned and dry.' (for 'Paul's skin is tanned and dry')

one has to conclude that one is dealing here with a case of polysemy, which is the position that, as one knows, is generally adopted today.[20] These two kinds of data first of all weaken the thesis that the notion of predicate transfer cannot be identified by the criterion of there being restrictions on predicates, and then, together with other data against it, render invalid the very hypothesis of predicate transfer for referential phenomena of type (1) and (2).

5. Neither Referent Nor Predicate Change

It is clear that abandoning the thesis of predicate change puts us in an apparently uncomfortable situation, as we no longer have any metonymic recourse – neither referent change, nor predicate change – to explain the interpretation of utterances like (1):

(1) *Je suis (garé) sur la place.*
'I am (parked) in the square.'

Can one give an account of (1) without postulating that the referent of *je* ('I') is no longer the same or that the predicate expresses a new property? We have already given a positive answer to this question in our previous work in the same field (Kleiber 1987, 1989, 1990, 1991, 1992a, b, 1994) by introducing a pragmatic principle of a very general application, the **principle of integrated metonymy**, as the driving force of the desired interpretative inference. Although not false, our analysis of cases of type (1) was incomplete, and today we propose a second principle that intervenes in the computation of the sense of (1), a principle that we have soberly baptised, observing a lucid and playful distance from etiquette-setters, **principle of meronomisation** or **principle of meronomic integration**.

5.1. Application of the Principle of Integrated Metonymy

We will begin by going back to our definition of the principle of integrated metonymy:

(58) Certain characteristics of certain parts can characterize the whole.

---

20 See Kleiber (1994: ch. 8).

and by showing why, where and how it works. Let us take utterances like (59), (60) and (61):

(59) *Les Américains ont débarqué sur la lune en 1969.*
'The Americans landed on the Moon in 1969.'

(60) *Le pantalon est sale.*
'The trousers are dirty.'

(61) *Paul va à l'école à pied.* (in the usual reading)
'Paul goes to school on foot.'

One can observe that their truth does not imply that, respectively, all the Americans landed on the Moon, the whole surface of the trousers is dirty, and that Paul goes to school on foot each and every time he goes to school. In the first case, one single American is sufficient for us to be able to say about all the Americans that they landed on the Moon, just as in (60) a small stain on the trousers is enough to declare them dirty. (61) similarly does not demand that Paul go to school on foot every (pertinent) time. One can uniquely infer that Paul goes to school on foot in the majority of cases and that he only exceptionally uses other means of transport. If we want to translate it into quantificational terms – a mathematical translation which does not correspond in any way to the sense of such an utterance, let us recall that (Kleiber 1987), but which is nevertheless inferable from such common utterances –, it means that he goes there at least a number of times which is higher than half of the occasions of going to school.[21] A predicate can thus be true of an ensemble of things without the whole ensemble verifying it. There is no reason to claim that the expressions in question, in (59) and (60) for example, *Les Américains* ('The Americans') and *le pantalon* ('the trousers'), change referent or that it is the predicate bearing upon them which is the object of transfer. However, it has to be explained how such a thing is possible, in other words, how a predicate which does not turn out to be verified by all members of a class or the whole surface of an entity can nevertheless be said to be true of that ensemble and of that entity. It is here that our principle of integrated metonymy comes in. It aims to provide an account of a major cognitive phenomenon, that is of the fact that a referent, in the most general sense of the word, can be applied to properties, events, etc. which in fact only concern some of its "parts". The usefulness of this principle is obvious, on the one hand, because in many cases it would be impossible to say which part exactly is selected by the predicate, and, on the other hand, because isolating the part from the whole would have the effect of obscuring the consequence that the property or event in question can have for the whole.

Thus, one can already see under what conditions this transition occurs: the characteristics in question must, in one way or another, be equally salient for the whole. The American who first put his foot on the Moon did it representing all the Americans. As the normal state of trousers is to be clean, the fact of being stained, no matter how little,

[21] For a detailed study of this temporal domain see Kleiber (1987).

is a pertinent fact for the trousers as a whole. And if it is necessary that Paul go to school on foot on at least more than half the occasions for us to say in a pertinent way that *he goes to school on foot*, it is because, quantificational democratism obliging,[22] we reckon that in this case the most part constitutes the representative part: (61) would be judged misleading if Paul went to school on foot only two times out of six, for example. This part can obviously extend up to the whole, as shown by utterance (62):

(62) *Changez-moi les pneus.*
'Change the tires for me.'

which is used by a car driver to ask his mechanic to change, not only three tires out of four, but all four tires of the car.

The road to the solution of our referential problems is thus well-traced. It suffices to move from quantities or from homogeneous "parts" to "heterogeneous" parts that can constitute a complex referent, so we can go to the very heart of our problem. Let us first revisit examples of type (5)(a):

(5) (a) *Paul est bronzé.* (= la peau de Paul)
'Paul is tanned.' (= Paul's skin)

(b) *Marie est maquillée.* (= le visage de Marie)
'Mary is made-up.' (= Mary's face)

(c) *Paul est voûté.* (= le dos de Paul)
'Paul is bent.' (= Paul's back)

and add to them an example like (63):

(63) *Le stylo est rouge.*
'The pen is red.'

(a) the colour of the ink
(b) the exterior surface

Such examples, which have given rise to diverse analyses and denominations[23] of the sense and the reference of their subject NP, are to be dealt with, as we have shown several times elsewhere, with the help of the principle of integrated metonymy. To postulate here a change of referent for these subject NPs would mean to return to adopting an atomistic referential analysis which holds true the following principle:

---

22 The temptation to equate the notion of representative part with that of majority (cf. *Les français ont élu Mitterrand.* – 'The French elected Mitterrand.') is undoubtedly, as was remarked by the late Michel Galmiche, a cultural legacy of hellenic law.

23 In terms of **appropriated names (noms appropriées)**, elliptic NPs (**beheaded noun phrases**); indirect reference and **active zones** (see Kleiber 1991, 1994: ch. 8).

(64) If a part of an entity X is rendered salient (or activated) by a predicate Y, it is this part that becomes the true subject, that is to say, the referent of the predication XY. In other words, an assertion XY concerns X in its entirety only if it is the case that all parts of X verify Y.

Now, this principle is false: a predicate can be said to be true of an individual entity or an ensemble of individuals without all the parts necessarily satisfying that predicate. The principle of integrated metonymy allows us to explain here the referential phenomena in question without postulating a change of referent.

We have seen that this position is also Nunberg's position, and since he does not postulate predicate transfer for this type of expressions either (*book* is to be dealt with on the model of *pen*), one can think that his position is finally identical with ours. This is not quite so, however, to the extent that, as we have just seen above, when there is a complex object and thus general sense, the condition of "noteworthiness" need not apply, since there is no transfer and, consequently, no constraint on the predicates. Our own analysis in terms of integrated metonymy, on the contrary, predicts a condition of salience: if a property of the part is not judged salient enough for the whole, the principle of integrated metonymy does not apply, and we cannot extend to the whole those predicates which are valid for the part. This is why, even in those cases where one cannot talk about transfer, a pragmatic constraint of relevance nonetheless prevails, as we have already noted above for (57)

(57) ?*Paul est bronzé et sec.* (pour 'la peau de Paul est bronzée et sèche')
'Paul is tanned and dry.' (for 'Paul's skin is tanned and dry')

which shows that, except in special contextual conditions – Paul can get dressed again after the bath because he is no longer wet – it is difficult to say *Paul is dry*.

It is hardly necessary to emphasize why such a constraint is satisfied in the case of (5)(a), (b) and (c) and of (63). Let us simply recall here our analysis of (5)(c):

> The predicate *bent*, even if it refers exclusively to the back, in fact concerns the whole silhouette of the individual by giving him a crooked shape. It thus seems to be one of the fundamental features of the perception that one has of such an individual. The difference from the expression with the explicit active zone is quite striking here: *Paul's back is bent* rather tends to be used in the situation where the bend is not immediately perceptible. To this we can add the fact that to have a bent back is a physical defect, distinctive compared with the normal shape of the body. (Kleiber 1991, 1994: ch. 8, 156)

We will also understand why there are no utterances like (65) and (66), although (5)(b) is possible: make-up transforms not only the face of the person using it but also the appearance of the person as a whole.

(65) ??*Marie est rouge.*
'Mary is red.'

(66) ??*Marie est vernie.*
'Mary is varnished.' (to say that Mary has red varnish on her fingernails)

5.2. Application of the Principle of Integrated Metonymy

One may be tempted to apply this analysis directly to "the referential shift" of (1) and (2) and to neglect, as we were able to do in our works of 1991, 1994 (ch. 8), the major fact that distinguishes such uses from the ones of the type *Paul is tanned*, namely, that from the ontological point of view the relation between *car* and *driver* is not a part-whole relation as is the relation between *Paul's skin* and *Paul*, but a contiguity relation. This difference is primordial as it apparently prohibits here the use of the principle of integrated metonymy. It is, however, sufficient to postulate, as we suggested in our response to the question *But who is then on the left shelf?* (1992b), that the "alienated" entities in question can be transitorily conceived of as being in a part-whole relation so that integrated metonymy could operate there.

It seems that this is exactly what is required by such uses. We will start with clothes and example (2)(h):

(2) (h) *Marie se reboutonne.*
'Mary is buttoning (herself) up.'

It is significant to note that (2)(h) is possible only if Mary is wearing her blouse. Let us assume that it is placed on a chair and also that Mary in in fact buttoning it up again: such a situation cannot be described by (2)(h), because the blouse cannot be considered as being a "part" of Mary. If she is really wearing it, the blouse becomes in some sense **inalienable**, losing in a certain way the autonomy it has when not being worn.

The same goes for the car versus its owner or driver. It needs to be perceived as having become a "part" of the driver. This seems clear when the driver is behind the wheel of the car. And this is why when, with Jean behind the steering wheel, the car starts, goes at the speed of 100 km per hour, overtakes another car, slows down etc., one can express it by saying that it is Jean who goes at the speed of 100 km, overtakes another car, etc. (Kleiber 1992b). On the contrary, if Jean's car starts on its own, for a reason only linguists and the Martians can imagine, one evidently cannot say any longer *Jean starts, goes at the speed of 100 km per hour*, etc., even if it is Jean's car.

The use of (1) *I am (parked) in the square* poses a supplementary problem, as manifestly there is no person behind the wheel, and thus one cannot invoke the driving to make the car a "part" of the driver. The decisive point here, which is ignored by those who cite such examples (Borkin 1972; Deane 1988), is the parking place of the car with regard to the driver. A situation of parking must be such that the driver would retain his driver's status, even if he is on foot, and the car would thus remain a "part" of his state of being a driver. Similarly, if he leaves the car to go shopping or to go to the cinema or a restaurant, for example, the driver does not nonetheless lose his driver's status because he will get into the car again to .... go home (Kleiber 1992b). If the car is, on the contrary, in the garage and he is quietly watching TV, it will be difficult for him to say (67):

(67) ??*Je suis (garé) dans le garage.*
'I am (parked) in the garage.'

because having put his car in the garage, he ceases to be its driver and the car *ipso facto* ceases to be his part, as clothes once taken off do not any longer constitute part of the individual who has been wearing them.

It thus seems to us that Jackendoff scores a point against Nunberg concerning the restriction that has to be postulated to explain the use of (2)(d):

(2) (d) *Paul a été heurté à l'aile par un camion.*
'Paul was hit in the fender by a truck.'

Such a use is only possible if Paul is driving or has his car parked in a parking lot, as it is only in this situation that the car can be considered as a "part" of Paul.[24]

We could multiply the explanations to give an account of uses (2)(b) and (2)(c) or even (2)(a) and (2)(f) as well. We will leave it to the reader to figure out how and under what conditions the works of a creator (novelist, painter, etc.), or the name of an individual can be considered as relevant parts of the inventor and the individual.[25] The essential thing for us is to have shown that their uses just as that of (1) call for a new pragmatic principle, a principle of meronomic integration, which we will formulate as follows:

(68) Principle of meronomisation or principle of meronomic integration:
The relation of contiguity between two entities X and Y can in certain situations be transformed into the relation of part (X) -whole (Y).

It is obviously only in those situations where (68) applies that the principle of integrated metonymy also turns out to apply and that one can thus explain, without postulating referent or predicate change, the interpretations of (1) and (2). Our two-level analysis gives an account of the rhetoric effect that one very often associates with these referential phenomena and allows us both to bring them together with uses of type (5)(a) and to separate them from these uses at the same time. If the principle of integrated metonymy is valid to explain in both cases how that which is only right for a part can nevertheless be applied to the whole, the principle of meronomic integration is only necessary in (1) and (2) to explain the promotion to the status of part of one of the entities in contiguity relation. The condition of salience or "noteworthiness" remains in place in both cases equally, but for the cases of meronomic integration, it obviously

24 Jackendoff's analysis (1992: 7) is slightly different. For him, it is the part of the car that was brushed against that is considered as a part of Ringo, whereas for us, it is the car that is considered as a part of Ringo.

25 Elements of this explanation are given in Kleiber (1992b).

gets activated only inside the situation at the source of the meronomisation process, which often makes it difficult to distinguish between that which has to do with the principle of integrated metonymy and that which is due to meronomic integration.

6. Conclusion

We obviously will not conclude, conscious of it though we may be, that the principle of meronomic integration poses more problems than it resolves, and that consequently we should, as we have done for the principle of integrated metonymy, show its relevance in domains other than that of uses of type *I am (parked) in the square* and delimit in a more precise manner its conditions of application. Still, it seems to us that with these two driving forces of pragmatic inference we have attained the goal we fixed at the beginning of this paper, namely to show, on the one hand, that Nunberg's explanation is not totally satisfactory, and on the other hand, to pave the way for a new analysis of certain polysemy phenomena, which does not look to transfer as an explanatory mode. The phenomenon of **coercion** of Pustejovsky (1991) illustrated by:

(69) *J'ai commencé le livre.*
'I began the book.'

deserves, in our opinion, to be approached from this angle, and not from that of the change of the type of *book*, even if it is true that the two most natural readings of (69) are factual: 'I began reading the book' and 'I began writing the book'.[26] But this is already another program, which is not on our agenda today.

References

Borkin, A. (1972): Coreference and beheaded NP's. *Papers in Linguistics* 5, 28-45.
Coulon, D. & Kayser, D. (1982): Les sens uniques conduisent à des impasses. *Domaines et objectifs de la recherche cognitive*. Actes du 1er Colloque de l'A.R.C, 1-32.
Deane, P.D. (1988): Polysemy and cognition. *Lingua* 75, 325-361.
Fauconnier, G. (1984): *Espaces mentaux*. Paris: Seuil.
Fauconnier, G. (1985): *Mental spaces*. Cambridge: MIT Press.
Godard, D. & Jayez, J. (1993): Le traitement lexical de la coercion. *Cahiers de linguistique française* 14, 123-149.
Jackendoff, R.S. (1992): Mme. Tussaud meets the binding theory. *Natural Language and Linguistic Theory* 10, 1-31.
Kayser, D. (1987): Une sémantique qui n'a pas de sens. *Langages* 87, 33-45.
Kayser, D. (1989): Réponse à Kleiber et Riegel. *Linguisticae Investigationes* XIII/2, 419-422.
Kleiber, G. (1984): Polysémie et référence: la polysémie, un phénomène pragmatique? *Cahiers de lexicologie* 44, 85-103.
Kleiber, G. (1987): *Du côté de la référence verbale: les phrases habituelles*. Berne: Peter Lang.

26 For a critique of this analysis, see Godard & Jayez (1993).

Kleiber, G. (1989): Référence indirecte ou de la divergence sur les anaphores divergentes. *Cahiers de praxématique* 12, 51-74.

Kleiber, G. (1990): Sur la définition sémantique d'un mot: les sens uniques conduisent-ils à des impasses?. In: Chaurand, J. & Mazière, F. (éds.): *La definition*. Paris: Larousse, 125-148.

Kleiber, G. (1991): *Paul est bronzé* versus *La peau de Paul est bronzée*. Contre une approche référentielle analytique. In: Stammerjohann, H. (ed.): *Analyse et synthèse dans les langues romanes et slaves*. Tübingen: Gunter Narr Verlag, 109-134. Also in Kleiber (1994), ch.8.

Kleiber, G. (1992a): *Le drapeau est rouge et bleu* ou Comment "flotte" la quantité. In: Fontanille, J. (éd.): *La quantité et ses modulations qualitatives*. Actes du Colloque *Linguistique et Sémiotique II*. Limoges-Amsterdam-Philadelphie: NAS, Pulim/Benjamins, 143-162. Also in Kleiber (1994), ch. 9.

Kleiber, G. (1992b): Mais qui est donc sur l'étagère de gauche? ou Faut-il multiplier les référents? *Travaux de linguistique et de philologie* XXX, 107-124.

Kleiber, G. (1994): *Nominales*. Paris: A. Colin.

Kleiber, G. & Riegel, M. (1989): Une sémantique qui n'a pas de sens n'a vraiment pas de sens, *Linguisticae Investigationes* XIII/2, 405-417.

Kleiber, G. & Riegel, M. (1991): Sens lexical et interprétations référentielles: un écho à la réponse de D. Kayser. *Linguisticae Investigationes* XV/1, 181-201.

Langacker, R.W. (1984): Active zones. In: Brugman, C. & Macauley, M. (eds.): *Proceedings of the tenth Annual Meeting of the Berkekey Linguistic Society*. Berkeley: Berkeley Linguistic Society, 172-188.

Nunberg, G. (1978): *The pragmatics of reference*. Bloomington: Indiana University Linguistic Club.

Nunberg, G. (1995): Transfers of meaning. *Journal of Semantics* 12, 109-132.

Nunberg, G. & Zaenen, A. (1992): Systematic polysemy in lexicology and lexicography. In: Varantolu, K. et al. (eds.): *Euralex II*. Tampere.

Pustejovsky, J. (1991): The generative lexicon. *Computational Linguistics* 17, 409-441.

Quine, W. v. O. (1971): The inscrutability of reference. In: Steinberg, D. & Jakobovits, L.A. (eds.): *Semantics: an interdisciplinary reader in philosophy, linguistics and psychology*. Cambridge: Cambridge University Press, 142-156.

Robins, R.H. (1987): Polysemy and the lexicographer. In: Burchfield, R. (ed.): *Studies in lexicography*. Oxford: Oxford University Press.

PART III

FROM WORDS TO CONSTRUCTIONS

Systematic Polysemy of Verbs in Hungarian[*]

Mária Ladányi

Eötvös Loránd University of Sciences (ELTE), Department of Applied Linguistics,
H-1088 Budapest, Múzeum krt. 4/D
E-mail: ladanyi@ludens.elte.hu

1. A General Overview of Polysemy; Polysemy of Nouns and Verbs

Although the principle of "biuniqueness" – the one-to-one correspondence between form and meaning – is a preferred principle in universal grammars, it is a fact that polysemy, which contradicts this, is observable in human languages in general. The reason for the existence of polysemy is, on the one hand, linguistic parsimony/economy. But on the other hand, polysemy is a type of meaning relation that lends structure to the lexicon in a way similar to such semantic relations as subordination and superordination, synonymy and antonymy. Polysemy is capable of creating local structures or "bundles" whose components feature close and strong connections between them regardless of the position the individual meanings occupy in the lexical/conceptual hierarchy (cf. Sigman & Cecchi). Instead of discussing the more abstract issues of the interpretation and representation of polysemy directly, we will try to contribute to the discussion on these issues by providing a detailed analysis of specific polysemy phenomena connected to verbs in Hungarian.

Although the proportion of verbs in the lexicon is considerably lower than that of nouns, polysemy is present in the former class to a higher degree than in the latter (cf. the data in Fellbaum 2000).[1] At the same time, it is unanimously noted in the lit-

[*] Publication of the present paper was supported by the Research Group for Theoretical Linguistics of the Hungarian Academy of Sciences at the Universities of Debrecen, Pécs and Szeged. This study is connected to the research project 'OTKA T 042687' (Structural Grammar of Hungarian vol. IV, The Structure of the Lexicon; led by Ferenc Kiefer). I wish to thank Gergely Pethő for his useful comments and suggestions regarding an earlier version of this paper. This text was originally written in Hungarian. It was translated into English by Éva Kardos, and the translation was then revised by Gergely Pethő. I would like to thank both of them for their help in preparing this English version.

[1] This can be substantiated by examining the 500 most frequently occurring verbs in the Hungarian National Corpus (Magyar Nemzeti Szövegtár, a very large electronic corpus of Hungarian texts; I would like to thank Viktor Nagy for compiling this frequency list). *Van* 'be', the first verb on this list, has more than 60 distinctive meanings classified into 9 main groups, according to *A magyar nyelv értelmező szótára* (the most comprehensive, multi-volume dictionary of Hungarian, commonly abbreviated as ÉrtSz.). Similarly, the majority of the 20 most frequent items (e.g. *tart* 'hold', *ad* 'give', *kap* 'get', *kér* 'ask for') are characterised by multiple meanings. This is also true of many of the top 100

erature on this subject that the polysemy of verbs is more difficult to grasp than that of nouns, since it is not as regular or predictable as the latter, and lends itself less to generalisation. According to Fellbaum, one reason for the difference between the scopes of verbal and nominal polysemy is that in the case of nouns, change of meaning is typically based on the relation 'IS A' (the appearance of a new meaning of a noun is connected to the recognition of a superordinate category), whereas the extension of the meanings of verbs is determined by the notion of 'MANNER' (this is called troponomy by Fellbaum 1990 and 1998).

Hungarian linguist János Zsilka and his research group (Zsilka 1973, 1981, 1975, 1978; Ladányi 1993a, b and the publications of the research group "Dialectics of the Motion Forms in Language", volumes 1-11, 1982-1994) had reached partly similar and partly different conclusions. According to their view, extension in the meaning of verbs indeed proceeds (usually by metaphorical processes) in most cases along the lines of the notion of 'MANNER' by a process called 'meaning integration'). In addition, verbs or rather verb meanings are reclassified together with the appearance of a new meaning.

The reclassification of verbs can proceed in two ways. On the one hand, it may be based on a new superordinate semantic category that is added as a component to the meaning of a verb. Or, on the other hand, it can be based on the fact that a superordinate semantic category that is already present as a component becomes central in the derived meaning of a verb. For example, the meaning of the predicate *őröl* 'crush' in the expression *gabonát őröl* 'crush grain' is based on the meaning component 'transform' (in other words, *őröl* belongs to the group of verbs designating 'transformation'), whereas in the expression *lisztet őröl* 'crush flour', which is derived from the former, the central meaning component of the same verb is 'creation'. Thus, when *őröl* is used in this latter sense, it becomes a member of another semantic category of verbs. In other words, there is a correspondence between the meaning components of a verb and the superordinate categories of verb meaning. Frequently, the reclassification of a verb is connected to the syntactic environment of the verb as well, i.e. the change of meaning is concomitant with syntactic alternation, e.g. in the example above *gabonát őröl (lisztté/lisztnek)* 'crush grain (into flour)' – *lisztet őröl (*gabonából*)* 'crush flour (from grain)' in Hungarian.[2]

Later (see section 3.3.1) we will see that the reclassification of the verbs (according to a derived meaning that is the result of an alteration of the basic meaning of a verb) is an important distinctive feature, which differentiates between 1) systematic polysemy in verbs that is connected to syntactic alternation and 2) verbs that exhibit

---

verbs, and even several of the last 20 items (in this list of 500) are verbs that have 4 to 6 different meanings in the dictionary.

2 Translator's note: Throughout the paper we have tried to provide English paraphrases for the Hungarian expressions that are as close to literal translation as possible, in order to convey not only the meaning of the original phrases, but their structures as well, wherever the structure as such is relevant. We opted for a solution along this line even in cases where such "direct" paraphrases do not sound quite perfect in English, but are (at least more or less) comprehensible. For examples where we judged the literal paraphrase to be seriously incomprehensible or misleading, we also added a "true" idiomatic translation next to the literal paraphrase, which we marked accordingly (often abbreviated as 'lit.').

syntactic alternation without a change of meaning. Verbs belonging to this latter group do not undergo such reclassification.

The aim of this chapter is to search for systematic patterns in verbal polysemy – even though this phenomenon is only systematic to a relatively low degree – and make generalizations about this phenomenon.

2. Some General Issues of the Systematic Polysemy of Verbs

2.1. Systematic Polysemy and the Semantic Classification of Verbs

According to Apresjan's definition (1974: 16, cf. Pethő 2003: 75), we talk about systematic (or regular) polysemy if the relationship between two meanings of a word (e.g. a verb) can be observed in at least one other word as well. Talmy, Levin, Rappaport Hovav and others emphasise that regular polysemy – when examined independently of context – is a paradigmatic relation; it is a relation between the meanings of verb classes that is primarily connected to the semantic classification of lexical items (cf. Talmy 1985, Levin 1993, Levin & Rappaport Hovav 1995, 1996). The members of a semantic class behave in the same way regarding their (potential) polysemy[3] and, as a consequence, their syntactic behaviour. The analysis of (potential) polysemy may therefore contribute to a more refined classification of verbs. Semantic classification entails the layering of the verbal lexicon, cf. Stockinger (1989), and Zsilka's organic model (studies by Zsilka and his research group mentioned above), and Ladányi (1993a).

From the point of view of semantic classification, a verb manifests polysemy if (on the basis of its multiple meanings) it belongs to several different verb classes at the same time. In the case of systematic polysemy, under specific (structural and/or contextual) conditions, even every single member of one class may show behaviour identical to that of members of another class (cf. Levin 1993; Levin & Rappaport Hovav 1996).

2.2. Alternations, Context, Synonymy – and the Polysemy of Verbs

2.2.1. Alternations

Verb semantics has several aspects: it can be described in terms of lexical content, event structure, and argument structure. The question arises as to which aspects of verb meaning are affected by polysemy, or whether polysemy always affects all of its aspects. For example: is a difference in syntactic structures (syntactic alternation) always accompanied by a change of meaning, and is it possible for a verb appearing in the same syntactic structure to have a different meaning? We will touch on this ques-

---

[3] The term 'potential polysemy' was coined by Stein (1999). Pethő (2003 and this volume) refers to basically the same concept when noting (in connection with the polysemy of nouns) that some of the possible polysemic meanings become lexicalised, whereas others have an odd feel to them, and also where he introduces the semantic concept of lexical blocking (by analogy to morphological blocking) in order to constrain polysemy.

tion in section 3.3.1, in connection with cases of verb polysemy which are accompanied by syntactic alternation.

Variations in event and argument structure (e.g. causative and other alternations) belong to the most frequently studied types of the polysemy of verbs. In Hungarian, however, it is debatable whether alternations like these can be considered instances of verbal polysemy, since in this language such alternations involve replacement of the base verb by a verb form that is often the result of morphological processes (derivation or prefixation), as opposed to purely syntactic changes. We will return to this problem later.

2.2.2. Context

In connection with, or in addition to, semantic classification and possible syntactic alternation of a verb, systematic polysemy also depends on context. This entails (among other things) that "the description of verb meanings is dependent on the description of noun meanings and vice versa" (as Pethő 2003 puts it, writing about polysemy in nouns).[4]

The same is true of the systematic polysemy in verbs, which requires the availability of certain contextual relations, in addition to, or instead of, structural relations. We will see that even in those cases where the polysemy of a verb is accompanied by syntactic alternation, the verb's meaning depends not only on the type of the syntactic construction it appears in, but also on the semantic characteristics of the nouns that occur in the syntactic environment of the verb. For example, in the alternation *ki*-*pakolja az árut a ládából* 'unpack the goods out of the box' – *ki*-*pakolja a ládát* 'unpack the box' it is not only the syntactic alternation **prefix('out')-V(meaning.1) *x*(ACC) *y*(ELATIVE) – prefix ('out')-V(meaning.2) *y*(ACC)** that is important,[5] but also the semantic characterisation of the nouns: the goods (*x*) must be a collection of homogeneous entities in some sense (things to be sold, in this case), and their original location is a box (*y*), which is some kind of container.

It is essential in this respect to distinguish clearly between structures with compositional and non-compositional meanings, since verbs in non-compositional structures do not have an independent meaning of their own. Accordingly, the meaning of these structures is not connected to the meanings of the base verb, either. For example, lexically bound expressions (in other words, idioms) that contain a verb and have (i.e., the whole expression as a unit) a metaphorical meaning, cannot be related to the phenomenon of verbal polysemy, since the lexicalised meaning in this case is indivisible, non-compositional. For instance, the idiomatic meaning of the expression *ajtót nyit*

---

4 For example, in certain Hungarian transitive constructions (if the object is a singular bare noun that precedes the verb), the meanings of the verb and the object are inseparable and designate some 'institutionalised' activity. These constructions may reach beyond verbal polysemy, since they may have a special (institutionalised → lexicalised) meaning that may belong to a special, lexically bound structure.

5 The stems of the nouns in this example are *ládá-* 'box' and *áru-* 'goods'. Accusative (ACC) case is marked by the case suffix *-t*, and elative (ELAT) case by *-ból/-ből* (depending on vowel harmony), meaning 'out of'.

vminek, lit.: 'open door for something (e.g. for a certain idea)' does not belong to the possible meanings of *nyit* 'open' per se.

On the other hand, the semantics of verbs occurring in constructions designating a so-called institutionalised activity is different. Institutionalised activities are also referred to by lexically bound constructions, but the meaning of the latter always allows a compositional interpretation. For example, the activity expressed by *ajtót nyit vkinek,* lit.: 'open door for somebody', indeed belongs to the category of 'opening'. It is a special subtype within this category which is specified by the non-referential (bare noun) object.

2.2.3. Polysemy of Verbs and Selection Restrictions

Let us turn to the question whether different selection restrictions that apply within a uniform and very general schematic meaning serve as factors distinguishing between several separate meanings within the general scheme, or in other words, as evidence for polysemy. And vice versa: is it possible for the meaning schema within **one** meaning to be so general that it can disregard selection restrictions?

Let us consider the following examples for the verb *töm* 'stuff': a) *dohányt töm a pipába* 'stuff tobacco into the pipe', b) *iratokat töm a fiókba* 'stuff papers into the drawer', c) *ételt töm magába/a hasába* 'stuff food into oneself' ~ *tömi magát/a hasát étellel* 'stuff oneself/one's stomach with food', d) *tömik a fejét (vmivel)* 'they stuff his head (with something)', e) *szóvirágokkal tömi mondatait,* lit.: '(s)he stuff his/her sentences with flowers of speech (= uses florid language excessively)', f) *gazdag szülei folyton pénzzel tömik,* lit.: 'his/her rich parents stuff him/her with money all the time (= give him/her a lot of money)'. On the basis of these we can establish a uniform and generalised meaning schema: 'put a relatively large amount of *x* into *y*, which is some kind of container', which suggests that the verb *töm* has the same meaning in all these examples.

However, this meaning schema for the verb *töm* is too general and ignores certain structural and semantic differences, including different selection restrictions. If we assume that the general meaning schema only specifies that *y* has to be a container-like element and *x* something of which there is too much, one could imagine that these restrictions are not defined by the verb *töm* as such, but that it is the nature of the container instead that decides what kind of thing *x* can be. However, by examining the examples and their meanings, we find that selection restrictions (specified for the verb *töm* or rather the structure that is built on it) do indeed apply to both elements, *x* and *y*.

In examples b) to f) *töm* is used differently than in its proper meaning 'stuff' in a). These uses can be characterised by their paraphrases: b) 'put', c) 'eat', d) 'communicate', e) 'compose', and f) 'give something as a present in a special way' (similar to "stuffing" in some sense). In these examples the selection restrictions are different as well. Therefore it seems to be a reasonable assumption that *töm* has not one but several meanings and that selection restrictions applying to both *x* and *y* are specified by the different meanings of *töm* (based on the proper meanings of the verbs listed above).

While in a) (where *töm* is used in its proper meaning 'stuff') *x* can only be a material that is not rigid (e.g. paper, clothes, or feathers), in b) (where *töm*'s meaning is 'put something into something in a special way') *x* can only be a solid physical object, cf. *könyveket töm a fiókba/a táskájába* 'he stuffs books into the drawer/his bag'; but: **pépet/*lekvárt/*tudást töm a fiókba/a táskájába* 'stuff *pulp/*jam/*knowledge into the drawer/his bag'. In c) (where *töm*'s meaning is 'eat something in a special way') *x* must be some relatively solid food that can be eaten (not some kind of drink), e.g. *kenyeret/gyümölcsöt töm magába/a hasába* 'stuff bread/fruit into himself/into his stomach ~ *kenyérrel/gyümölccsel tömi magát/a hasát* 'stuff himself/his stomach with bread/fruit'; but: **bort/*vizet töm magába/a hasába* 'stuff *wine/*water into himself/ his stomach'~ **borral/*vízzel tömi magát/a hasát* 'stuff himself/his stomach with *wine/*water). In d) (where *töm*'s meaning is 'communicate something in a special way') *x* can only be a piece of information or knowledge that can be understood and verbally communicated, cf. *vad történetekkel/nehéz leckékkel/fárasztó szövegekkel/rímekkel tömik a fejét* 'they stuff his/her head with wild stories/difficult material/tiring texts/rhymes'. In e) (where *töm*'s meaning is 'compose something in a special way') *x* can only be a device for linguistic/stylistic embellishment: *barokkos jelzőkkel/hasonlatokkal/rímekkel tömi mondatait/szövegeit* 'stuff his sentences/texts with baroque expressions/similes/rhymes', but: **nehéz leckékkel/*történetekkel tömi mondatait* 'stuff his sentences with *difficult material/*stories'. Finally, in f) (where *töm*'s meaning is 'present somebody with something in a special way') *x* can only be something that can be given as a present, typically something that is not necessary or luxurious: *gazdag szülei folyton ékszerekkel/pazar ruhákkal/jobbnál jobb cuccokkal/pénzzel tömik* 'his/ her rich parents keep stuffing him/her with jewellery/lavish clothes/really good stuff/ money', but: **adósságokkal, *hitelekkel, *rongyos ruhákkal tömik* 'they stuff him/her with *debts, *loans, *ragged clothes'.

Similar restrictions could be derived from the different meanings of *töm* ('put/ eat/communicate/compose/present something in a special, "stuffing" way') for *y* (different types of containers) as well.

Therefore, the existence of selection restrictions in fact suggests that the different uses of *töm* outlined above represent different meanings, i.e. the verb is polysemous. The uniform meaning schema for *töm* ('put a relatively large amount of *x* into *y*, which is some kind of container') is a generalisation that combines several meanings which are both connected to and partly different from one another. This general schema ignores crucial meaning differences and so it can at best only highlight the fact that these meanings of *töm* are relatively closely grouped together within the lexical item, and that they represent one type of its meanings (the above examples do not represent all the possible uses of this verb). It is not, however, suitable for describing even the above uses of *töm* as a single uniform meaning.

Differences among selection restrictions show that although general meaning schemata are useful, overgeneralisation may be problematic in the lexical representation since we might not pay due attention to differences between the meanings, and therefore, we fail to represent instances of polysemy appropriately within a lexical item.

2.3. The Scope of Regular Polysemy and the Productivity of Regular Polysemy Types

As mentioned above, Apresjan states in his definition that we can talk about regular polysemy if the relationship between two meanings of a word is observable between two meanings of at least one other word as well. It is clear, however, that systematic polysemy types may differ in the extension of the range of verbs that are characterised by the semantic relation in question.

In works by Talmy, Levin, and Rappaport Hovav (see section 2.1), it is emphasised that systematic polysemy is a relation between the meanings of verb classes. If this relation is characteristic of the given classes in their entirety, it should be expected (if certain conditions are fulfilled that might be required) that any verb that is a member of one class must have a meaning on the basis of which it belongs to another verb class as well. In these cases, we can talk about the productivity of systematic polysemy types, which is an extension of the concept of productivity used in morphology (Dressler 1997; Dressler & Ladányi 2000; Kiefer 2003; Kiefer & Ladányi 2000a). Apresjan (1974: 18) also mentions the possible productivity of systematic polysemy:

> Regular polysemy is similar to word formation also in the sense that many of its types are productive; in other words, for any word which has a meaning of type 'A', it is true that it can be used in a meaning of type 'B' as well.

Regarding systematic polysemy, it is worth making a distinction between systematicity and productivity, since (as has been established in connection with productivity in morphology) productivity always presupposes systematicity, whereas the reverse is not true. Therefore, it makes sense to identify types of systematic polysemy that are productive as well. (In connection with the systematic polysemy of nouns, Pethő 2003: 78 also employs the notion of productivity in this sense.)

In the case of productive polysemy types among verbs (to use some of the components of the definition of productivity in morphology), a class that is characterised by polysemy must be definable by common properties (in other words, intensionally), and open. If a verb belongs to one class (or becomes a member of one class) because it has a meaning that is characteristic of that class, it must also possess – in a predictable way, and at least potentially – a second meaning that belongs to another class.

A type does not qualify as productive if, on the one hand, the regular meaning correspondence in question does not apply to all members of an intensionally definable class of verbs that are characterised by a certain pattern of systematic polysemy, or, on the other hand, if the intensionally definable class is not open.

2.4. Further Issues

As noted by Apresjan (1974: 25), the most problematic aspect of the regular polysemy of verbs is that "in a number of instances polysemy can be described as monosemy". In other words, it is questionable whether we can convincingly prove that there is indeed a difference between meanings that we consider to be separate.

Therefore, it is essential to decide on the basis of what criteria we can distinguish between meanings and delimit certain meaning types; that is, how we can establish a difference between meanings. As indicated earlier, examining the alternation pattern of the syntactic structure is probably not sufficient by itself, since we also need to identify, in the semantics of a verb, the new meaning component through which the verb becomes a member of a new class. If we accept this, the classification of verbs in terms of superordinate meaning categories becomes just as important as it is for nouns; accordingly, the categorising component similar to "IS A" is not exclusively characteristic of the polysemy of nouns (cf. section 1).

It also remains to be clarified what restrictions apply to potential polysemy (i.e. blocking phenomena, cf. Pethő 2003) and how lexicalisation processes can break up systematic polysemy. The former phenomenon is connected to productive types, whereas the latter is associated with non-productive systematic polysemy.

3. Regular Polysemy of Verbs in Hungarian

3.1. The Empirical Basis of Our Study

The theoretical background for identifying regular polysemy types of verbs in Hungarian has been provided by Apresjan and his polysemy types (1974: 25-29). However, this does not mean that all types have been adapted from Apresjan, since his typology that was worked out for Russian cannot be applied to Hungarian in its entirety due to typological and language-specific differences. In addition, there are some relations in Hungarian that are of types different from the ones in Russian.

When describing verb polysemy accompanied by syntactic alternation, it was even less possible to take polysemy types established for English into consideration, since – as we discuss in section 3.2 – the majority of types of meaning relations in English (cf. the above-mentioned works by Levin, Levin & Rappaport Hovav, and Goldberg 1995) are not connected to syntactic alternation and do not appear as polysemous verbs in Hungarian. Instead, in this language the derived meaning is associated with a new lexical item, which is either a derived or a prefixed version of the original verb. This can be explained by the fact that the two languages differ in their typological features and, compared to English, Hungarian has a much richer morphology. However, in section 3.3.1, we will examine a polysemy type that is present in English as well (the systematic polysemy of verbs of sound emission) and try to describe the special features of this type that are characteristic of Hungarian.

When analysing systematic relations in Hungarian, we have mainly relied on the structural and semantic relations described in Horváth (1983) – in connection with the systematic polysemy of verbs accompanied by syntactic alternation –, in addition to the criteria in Apresjan's classification. The relations that appear in Horváth (1983) represent a continuation of Zsilka's theory,[6] and the verbs she describes are taken from the most comprehensive dictionary of Hungarian, ÉrtSz. (see footnote 1).

[6] The theory of the late Hungarian linguist János Zsilka (1930-1999), the so-called organic-dialectic theory represents a uniform view of the linguistic system, including morphology, correlations of syntactic and semantic structures, the unity of synchronicity and diachronicity, and many other issues.

The material that we have used has mostly already been cited in Horváth's and/ or Apresjan's works mentioned above. We have also included further examples from ÉrtSz. and some of our own. We have analysed these examples according to our own criteria and classified them into polysemy types on the basis of the relations observed. We have also examined these types from the point of view of productivity.

Although certain syntactic-semantic groups of verbs in Hungarian have already been identified (e.g. Komlósy 1992, 2000, and Kiefer 2000), an exhaustive semantics-based classification of the verbs of this language is not *yet* available (which would be of considerable help when analysing their systematic polysemy). This study cannot undertake the task of classifying Hungarian verbs in their entirety, either. Not having an exhaustive or at least a relatively detailed classification of verbs at hand, it is not possible to provide an exhaustive description of the systematic polysemy of verbs. Instead, we had to content ourselves with working out some polysemy types that are characteristic of Hungarian, while being primarily interested in 1) whether the meaning relations associated with different types do in fact hold systematically for all verbs that belong to the same semantically defined class, 2) which types are not just systematic but also productive meaning relations, and 3) whether there is a parallel between the systematic differences among meanings and systematic syntactic differences.

3.2. Preliminary Notes

3.2.1. Alternations, Derived and Prefixed Verbs

As noted before, it is typical for Hungarian that multiple meanings that are expressed by a single verb in other languages are often connected to pairs of verbs, consisting of a verb without a prefix and its prefixed version, or of a base verb and its derived version (i.e. the same verb with a derivational suffix). These pairs, more specifically the meanings associated with these pairs, will not be considered as instances of polysemy in Hungarian (since polysemy presupposes that we are talking about a single form).

In the case of verb – derived verb pairs (since the latter are generally regarded as units having an independent lexical meaning) the notion of polysemy is definitely out of the question. The analysis of the semantic relationship between base verbs and their prefixed versions, on the other hand, is a more complex problem. If prefixes had aspectual meanings only, we could assume that prefixed verbs are not different from their base forms in lexical content per se – in this case we would have to take the prefixed versions into account as well when defining polysemy types for the base verbs. However, this is not the case. Verbs and their prefixed versions cannot be identified as a single lexical item since verb prefixation is a morphological process (different from both derivation and compounding; cf. Kiefer & Ladányi 2000b) in which prefixes pro-

---

We cannot describe these ideas here, and due to the nature of this chapter we can only take certain aspects of Zsilka's approach into account. The theory is presented in detail in the works written by Zsilka cited earlier, in publications by the research group "The Dialectics of Forms of Linguistic Motion", and in the above-mentioned works by Horváth, as well as Horváth (1993) and Ladányi (1993b) (unfortunately, most of these are only available in Hungarian).

vide verbs with an aspectual value as well as an Aktionsart and lexical content (with the exception of the prefix *meg-*).[7]

Accordingly, we will not consider cases in which a base verb alternates with its prefixed version as signs of the polysemy of the base verb, despite the fact that there is without doubt not only a structural alternation between the members of the verb pair, but their meanings are related as well. For example, we will not discuss the relationship between the meanings of verbs in pairs of constructions like *levegőt fúj a labdába* 'blow air into the ball' and *felfújja a labdát (levegővel)* 'prefix(lit. 'up')-blow the ball (with air)' in connection with the polysemy of the base verb (*fúj* 'blow' in this case), whereas pairs of constructions such as *szappanhabot fúj (buboréknak)* 'blow soap (for bubbles)' – *(szappanhabból) buborékot fúj* 'blow bubbles (from soap)' will be considered.

Similarly, we do not regard as polysemy those cases in which the alternating pair consists of the same verb with different prefixes (e.g.: *megfeji a tehenet* 'prefix-milk the cow' – *lefeji a tehenet* 'prefix-milk the cow')[8] to be instances of polysemy. What we are interested in with respect to the polysemy of verbs are only those syntactic structures that contain the same verb (either a base form only, or a verb occurring with one particular prefix), regardless of whether the type of syntactic structure is the same for different occurrences of the verb. Nevertheless, – as we will see this later – syntactic alternation is not always accompanied by systematic polysemy, and systematic polysemy can occur without syntactic alternation.

3.2.2. Primary and Derived Meanings

We have to ask ourselves which members of a set of related meanings should be considered to be primary or derived relative to the others, and whether this distinction makes any difference from the point of view of synchronic semantic relations at all.

It seems that in Apresjan's study it is always the simpler verbal meaning (which can be described as having fewer semantic components) that is selected as the primary one and the more complex meaning, the one that has more semantic components, is seen as derived (e.g. 'action' → 'causation of action': *a gyűrű csattog* 'the ring clinks' → *vki csattog a gyűrű(jé)vel* 'someone clinks with (his) ring'). However, Apresjan does not usually elaborate on the derivability of meanings (i.e. which meaning is primary relative to the other) in connection with the specific relations he describes. In the transformational groups worked out by Zsilka and Horváth, on the other hand, synchronic relations between structures and meanings (in transitive constructions) always reflect a diachronic relation (on the basis of their hypothesis about the historical development of transitive constructions). The construction that contains a more detailed and

7 Although the prefix *meg* is considered to express mainly an aspectual value (perfectivity), even it can introduce several meaning elements related to aktionsarten to the lexical content of the verb (iterative, resultative, semelfactive, ingressive – cf. Kiefer & Ladányi 2000b: 477-479).

8 Both prefixes in these examples render the event telic, i.e. when the event is finished, the cow is seen as not having any milk anymore. As has already been mentioned, the prefix *meg-* has no lexical meaning (it only carries an aspectual content), whereas *le-* in the second example literally means 'down'.

specific object, the so-called inherent object, is always considered to be primary in comparison with the object that is more general and has a wider scope, the so-called accusativus obiectivus. In other words, the point of departure is always the meaning that reflects a more concrete perspective. These two approaches do not always yield identical results.[9]

When examining the alternation of transitive constructions, we will rely mainly on Zsilka's view (although we will not discuss the historical aspects of meaning correlations) since we are convinced that this perspective allows us to analyse the semantic relations more precisely and in more detail. In the alternation of transitive constructions we will consider the more specific and detailed structure that is built around an 'inherent object' (in Zsilka's terminology) to be primary, e.g. *letörli a port (a bútorokról)* 'wipe off the dust (from the furniture)'. On the other hand, we regard as derived those structures that are built around a more general, wider-scope object ('accusativus obiectivus' in Zsilka's approach), e.g.: *letörli a bútorokat* 'wipe off the furniture'.

The question whether the primary or derived status of meanings is of any importance is also related to the issue of the productivity of types. In the case of productive types (where regular correlation between meanings implies that if a verb has a particular meaning as a member of one class, then – under the right conditions – it must also possess a predictable meaning belonging to another class), the aspect of derivability (and therefore the aspect of the relative ordering of meanings) may become significant. After all, only those verbs that possess a particular basic meaning in their original class will receive the predictable potential meaning (if the relevant conditions are fulfilled).

From a practical point of view, the question from which direction it is easier to describe the meaning relation can also play a role in choosing the direction of the derivation. For example, in the case of verbs of 'causation', it is easier to consider the verb meaning that contains the meaning component 'cause' as derived, irrespective of which one among the examined meanings may in fact underlie the other. For instance, in the case of the type *a bárka kiköt* 'the barge lands' – *vki kiköti a bárkát* 'someone lands the barge', it indeed makes sense to use Apresjan's solution for the sake of descriptive simplicity: We consider the meaning 'the barge lands' to be primary, and the meaning expressing 'causation of movement', i.e. 'someone lands the barge', to be derived, even though the structure meaning 'the barge lands' probably came into being secondarily, on the basis of an anthropomorphic view of the situation described.

---

9 For example, on the basis of Apresjan's pattern 'to treat in a particular way' – 'to remove by treating in this way': *learatja a táblát* 'harvest the field' – *learatja a gabonát* 'harvest the crops'. However, in Zsilka's approach, the derivation proceeds in the opposite direction, since the construction *learatja a gabonát (a tábláról)* 'harvest the crops from the fields' follows the pattern of the first line of the original transformational group (*törli a port a cipőről* 'wipe the dust off the shoes'), which contains a more concrete, narrower-scope, detailed 'inherent' object, whereas *learatja a táblát* 'harvest the field' follows the pattern of the second line – *letörli a cipőt (a portól)* 'wipe the shoes (of the dust)' – of the original transformational group, which contains a more general, wider-scope accusativus obiectivus. Note that alternations containing prefixed verbs are always considered to be secondary in comparison with the relations in Zsilka's original transformational group, where the prefix only appears in the second line: *aratja a gabonát a tábláról* 'harvest the crops from the field'→ *learatja a táblát (a gabonától),* lit. 'prefix(down)-harvest the field (from the crops)'.

In the case of relations that are systematic but not productive, what counts is only the fact that there is a correlation, and the simplicity of the description. It is unimportant which meaning is derived from another, related one.

3.3. Types of Systematic Polysemy in Hungarian

3.3.1. Systematic Polysemy Accompanied by Syntactic Alternation

As noted earlier, although syntactic alternation may be concomitant with systematic polysemy of verbs, the latter may also occur without syntactic alternation (cf. 3.3.2). Moreover, syntactic alternation does not necessarily lead to systematic polysemy.

Since systematic polysemy concerns the lexical meaning of verbs, this notion can only be relevant if the lexical meaning of the verb that occurs in alternating constructions changes (i.e. a difference in constructional meaning that follows from syntactic differences is not sufficient to warrant talking about polysemy). Therefore, we do not claim that the verbs *ken* 'spread' and *locsol* 'sprinkle' manifest regular polysemy in expressions such as *zsírt/lekvárt ken a kenyérre* 'spread lard/jam on the bread' – *zsírral/lekvárral keni a kenyeret,* lit.: 'spread the bread with lard/jam' or *vizet locsol a virágokra* 'sprinkle water on flowers' – *vízzel locsolja a virágokat* 'sprinkle flowers with water'. After all, we can define the meaning of *ken* 'spread' in both constructions as 'put some substance on a surface', and *locsol* 'sprinkle' as 'make some liquid go somewhere'.[10] In contrast, the verb *őröl* 'crush' is polysemous in syntactic alternations of the type *búzát őröl (lisztnek)* 'crush wheat (for flour)' – *lisztet őröl (búzából)* 'crush flour (from wheat)', since the meaning of the verb in the first case belongs to the semantic category 'transform something (for some purpose)', whereas in the second case it belongs to the category 'create something (from something)' (see section 1 on the reclassification of verbs).

On the basis of the material analysed we have identified the following types of systematic verbal polysemy accompanied by syntactic alternation:

(1) '**transform** something into something (for some purpose)' – '**create** something (= something else) (from something)'

This type combines two more specific alternations introduced by Apresjan: a) 'to deform in a definite way' – 'to cause by deforming in this way' and b) 'to treat, process in a definite way' – 'to cause by treating in this way'. Combining meaning relations a) and b) and subsuming these under a common type is justified because:

---

[10] In contrast to the common meanings identified in the above syntactic alternations, we can observe a change of meaning in the constructions *megkeni a kenyeret,* lit.: 'prefix-spread the bread' and *meglocsolja a virágokat,* lit.: 'prefix-sprinkle the flowers', which contain prefixed verbs. These structures mean 'put some kind of substance on its surface' + 'perfective', and 'make some liquid go somewhere' + 'perfective'. In these constructions, it is the prefix *meg-* that adds to the meanings of the verbs; the component of perfectivity that appears here does not belong to the range of meanings of *ken* 'spread' and *locsol* 'sprinkle' as such.

- verbs belonging to these two types display identical patterns of syntactic alternation (see below);
- the verbs' second (derived) meaning involves 'creation' in both cases;
- it is often difficult to distinguish between what Apresjan calls 'deformation' on the one hand, and 'treating' or 'processing' on the other hand.

This type of polysemy can be associated with transformational group IV in Horváth (1983). Horváth claims that in the course of the activities that are referred to by these verbs, the thing that is denoted by the 'inherent object' changes, both in terms of its shape and qualitatively. By the end of the work process, a result (a new object) comes into being, which had been previously (before the work began) planned (imagined) by the subject (Horváth 1983: 32).

A) *Typical syntactic alternations for this type:*

a) V(meaning.1) *x*(ACC) (<u>for</u> *y*) – V(meaning.2) *y*(ACC) (<u>into</u>/<u>on</u> *x*)[11]

falat tör (nyílás<u>nak</u>) – nyílást tör a fal<u>ba</u>/a fal<u>on</u>
'smash the wall (for a hole)' (i.e. 'in order to create a hole') – 'smash a hole into the wall/on the wall'

jeget vág (lék<u>nek</u>) – léket vág a jég<u>be</u>
'cut ice (for a hole)' – 'cut a hole into the ice'

földet ás (árok<u>nak</u>/gödör<u>nek</u>) – árkot/gödröt ás [a föld<u>be</u>][12]
'dig the ground (for a hole/pit)' – 'dig a hole/pit [into the ground]'

b) V(meaning.1) *x*(ACC) (<u>for</u> *y*)[13] – V(meaning.2) *y*(ACC) (<u>from</u> *x*)

vasat kovácsol (kard<u>nak</u>, patkó<u>nak</u>) – kardot, patkót kovácsol ((a) vas<u>ból</u>)
'hammer iron (for a sword/horseshoe)' – 'hammer a sword/horseshoe (from (the) iron)'

fát aprít (gyújtós<u>nak</u>) – gyújtóst aprít [(a) fá<u>ból</u>]
'cut wood (for firewood)' – 'cut firewood [from (the) wood]'

gabonát őröl (liszt<u>nek</u>) – lisztet őröl [(a) gaboná<u>ból</u>]
'crush grain (for flour)' – 'crush flour [from (the) grain]'

fát éget (szén<u>nek</u>) – szenet éget [(a) fá<u>ból</u>]
'burn wood (for coal)' – 'burn coal [from (the) wood]'

---

[11] Accusative case (ACC) is marked by the case suffix *-t*. The equivalent of the English preposition *for* that appears in these examples is the (dative) case suffix *-nak/-nek*. The equivalent of *into* is the (illative) case suffix *-ba/-be*, and that of *on* is the suffix *-on/-en/-ön*. In structures b) and c), to be introduced below, *from* corresponds to the (elative) case suffix *-ból/-ből*. All of these case suffixes are attached to the relative stem of the noun, which may contain further inflectional morphemes (like the plural marker) following the noun stem.

[12] The round brackets indicate the omissibility of the elements, whereas the square brackets show that these elements are unusual, their meaning usually only appears implicitly.

[13] In some cases a different suffix can also appear instead of *-nak/-nek* 'for', namely, the (translative) case suffix *-vá/-vé/-Cá/-Cé* (C stands for a consonant equal to the final consonant of the stem).

fát, követ farag (szobornak) – szobrot farag ((a) kőből/fából)
'carve stone/wood (for a statue)' – 'carve a statue (from (the) stone/wood)'

c) V(meaning.1) *x*(ACC) (into *y*) – V (meaning.2) *y*(ACC) (from *x*)

gyöngyöket fűz (láncba) – láncot fűz ((a) gyöngyökből)
'string beads (into a necklace)' – 'make (lit.: 'string') a necklace (from (the) beads)'

virágokat köt (csokorba) – csokrot köt ((a) virágokból)
'bind flowers (into a bouquet)' – 'make (lit.: 'bind') a bouquet from the flowers'

Note: In the alternations above, structures with V(meaning.1) contain an affected object. It either precedes the verb and is used without an article (representing indefiniteness or genericity), or follows the verb and occurs with a definite article (*töri a falat* 'smash the wall', *kovácsolja a vasat* 'hammer the iron' etc.). The first of these two constructions often designates an 'institutionalised' activity (e.g. *gabonát őröl* 'crush grain', *fát aprít* 'cut wood'). On the level of V(meaning.2) there is an indefinite effected object, which occurs without an article and precedes the verb. In this latter case, too, the transitive construction often designates an institutionalised activity (e.g. *kenyeret dagaszt* 'knead bread'). On this level, the element referred to as *x* – which appears as a direct object on the level of V(meaning.1) and as an adverbial on the level of V(meaning.2) – can often be omitted, because it is the creation of some new quality that is salient in this meaning of the verb.

In group b), the prefixed versions of some verbs also take part in an alternation. For instance, *felaprítja a fát* 'prefix('up')-cut the wood' – *felaprítja a gyújtóst* 'prefix('up')-cut the firewood', *megőrli a gabonát* 'prefix(perfective)-crush grain' – *megőrli a lisztet* 'prefix(perfective)-crush flour', *kikeveri a vajat* 'prefix('out')-stir the butter' – *kikeveri a krémet* 'prefix('out')-stir the cream'. However, these correlations are unique and cannot be extended to further cases.

B) Typical semantic characteristics of this type:

- V typically denotes a physical activity that is intended by the agent and driven by a specific goal;[14]
- V(meaning.1) is based on the meaning component 'transform';
- V(meaning.2) is based on the meaning component 'create';
- *x* = some substance or a multitude of homogeneous things (cf. Horváth 1983: 32);
- *y* = the new entity (substance or thing) that is created as a result of the transformation of some substance or a multitude of homogeneous things.

---

[14] In some irregular cases V can mean something other than a physical activity, e.g.: *gyerekeket nevel utánpótlásnak,* lit.: 'bring up children for successors', meaning approximately: 'bring up children with the purpose of providing fresh blood for the future' – *utánpótlást nevel* 'bring up successors'.

Note: Certain verbs whose lexicalised meanings include characteristics of the created substance/thing do not exhibit this type of syntactic alternation and accordingly, they do not manifest this type of polysemy. For example, the semantic component 'from thread/wool' has become an implicit part of the verb meanings *köt* 'knit', *horgol* 'crochet', *sző* 'weave' in the lexicon. Therefore, it is not possible anymore to say **fonalat köt/horgol (pulóvernek, sapkának),* lit.: 'knit/crochet wool (for a sweater/hat)', or **szálakat sző (szőnyegnek),* lit.: 'weave threads (for carpet)'. Instead, *you* say *pulóvert, sapkát köt/horgol* 'knit/crochet a sweater/hat' and *szőnyeget sző* 'weave a carpet'.

C) Productivity of this type:

Groups a) and c) include a relatively small number of verbs. Apart from the examples mentioned above, we can find only a few more cases in the reference material that we have used. The pattern found in group b) is characteristic of a large number of verbs (there are many relevant examples in addition to the ones cited above). However, the fact that the number of affected words is relatively large does not enable us to decide by itself whether this type of polysemy is productive.

On the one hand, we have to verify whether the class of physical actions that belong to the category 'transform something into something' is open (this is a major requirement from the point of view of productivity). On the other hand, we have to examine whether the relation 'transform' – 'create' is applicable (in accordance with the above-mentioned syntactic alternations) to new members that might be added to the class. Obviously, the class of physical actions that belong to the category 'transformation' is in fact open, since it can be extended with new lexical items that have been derived from names of tools, and also with ones that originate from other languages. However, we could not find any other verbs that show the alternations mentioned in a) and c), therefore they cannot be considered productive. In the case of b), not every new verb of the category 'transform' shows the alternation and meaning relation presented above. For example, *képeket montíroz (plakátnak)* 'arrange pictures (into a poster)' – *plakátot montíroz* 'arrange a poster', but *tupírozza a haját (frizurának)* '(s)he backcombs his/her hair (for a hairstyle)' – *??frizurát tupíroz* 'backcomb a hairstyle', *krumplit passzíroz (pürének)* 'mash potatoes (into mash)' – *??pürét passzíroz* 'mash some mash'. So we can conclude that the productivity of group b) is questionable as well.

(2) '**put** some substance/thing into a hole or opening' – '**close** and/or **eliminate** a hole or opening by filling it with the substance/thing[15]

A) Typical syntactic alternation for this type:

***be*('into')-V(meaning.1) *x*(ACC) <u>into</u> *y* – *be*('into')-V(meaning.2) *y*(<u>ACC</u>) with *x*[16]**

---

15 Apresjan introduced a similar type in a more comprehensive way: **'to transform in a certain way' – 'to eliminate by transforming in this way'**. This type, however, is not justified in Hungarian since it is not possible to collect a sufficient number of examples to support the rule.

16 The prefix *be-*, meaning 'into' is added to the verbs in question. Note that this local relation ('goal') is expressed twice in the first construction: both by this prefix and by the (illative) case suffix

betömi a rongyot a résbe – betömi a rést (a ronggyal)
'prefix('into')-stuff a rag into a gap' – 'prefix('into')-stuff a gap (with a rag)'

betapossa a földet a lyukba – betapossa a lyukat (a földdel)
'prefix('into')-tread sand into the hole' – 'fill the hole by treading sand into it', lit.: 'prefix('into')-tread the hole (with sand)'

bedugja a vattát/az ujját a fülébe – bedugja a fülét (a vattával/az ujjával)
'prefix('into')-plug cotton wool/his finger into his ears' – 'prefix('into')-plug his ears (with cotton wool/his finger)'

betömi a zsebkendőt a szájába – betömi a száját (a zsebkendővel)
'prefix('into')-stuff tissue paper into his mouth' – 'prefix('into')-stuff his mouth (with tissue paper)'

Note: In this and many other types to be introduced later on we find alternations that involve prefixed verbs. (It is worth noting that the prefix *meg-*, which primarily indicates perfectivity, appears in only a few cases among the alternating prefixed verbs.) On the level of V(meaning.1) the verb prefix expresses directionality and is used instead of or in addition to a directional adverbial (with a corresponding case suffix). On the level of V(meaning.2) this correspondence or parallel behaviour is no longer present; the constituent that appeared as a directional adverbial in the previous structure functions as the direct object of the predicate. This is connected to the fact that the prefixed verb on the level of V(meaning.2) does not designate directionality, but rather indicates that the action affects the object in its entirety.

B) *Typical semantic characteristics of this type:*

- V typically denotes a physical activity that is intended by the agent and driven by a specific goal;
- *be*-V(meaning.1) is based on the meaning component 'put into';
- *be*-V(meaning.2) is based on the meaning component 'close' and/or 'eliminate';
- *x* = some substance or thing;
- *y* = a hole or some space into which the substance or thing is put.

C) *Productivity of this type:*

This pattern does not even apply to all verbs expressing the meaning 'put something into something' (e.g.: *beszórja a földet a gödörbe* 'prefix('into')-throw sand into the pit' – **beszórja a gödröt,* lit.: ' prefix('into')-throw a pit'), nor could we find any new verbs that function according to this type. Therefore, this pattern cannot be considered productive.

The following polysemy types (3)-(6) show some similarity to two of Apresjan's types (**'to treat, process in a definite way'** paired with **'to eliminate by treating in this way'** and **'to remove by treating in this way'**, respectively). How-

---

-ba/-be (which we have already encountered, see footnote 11). This phenomenon can be regarded as similar to clitic doubling in other languages, and is essentially identical to the redundant expression of local relations (by a verb particle and a preposition at the same time) in languages like German.

ever, in Hungarian it is possible to identify significantly richer semantic relations on the basis of the transformational groups established by Zsilka and Horváth. The meaning relations below are related to the structural and meaning relations of group II in Horváth (1983) and describe in more detail the possible polysemic semantic connections among her data. As above, we ignore cases of verbs that can only alternate with their prefixed versions (although this is relatively uncommon in this type). Following the findings of Zsilka and Horváth, our main guiding principle is that we consider structures that are built around a more detailed, relatively narrow-scope inherent object to be the underlying structures. Therefore, in contrast to Apresjan's semantic relations above, the meaning component 'remove' will be considered primary in our three corresponding groups, (3) to (5). This component is represented and highlighted on level V(meaning.1) by the verb prefixes *ki-* 'out', *le-* 'off', and *fel-* 'up', which are attached to the verbs that take part in the alternations, and the suffixes *-ból/-ből* 'out of', and *-ról/-ről* 'off/from' at the end of the adverbials of prefixed verbs.

(3) '**remove** things or some substance in its entirety from (the inside or the surface of) something' – '**empty** (the inside or the surface of) something'

A) *Typical syntactic alternations for this type:*

a) ***ki*('out')-V(meaning.1) *x*(ACC) (out of *y*) – *ki*('out')-V(meaning.2) *y*(<u>ACC</u>)**

kiborítja a szemetet (a vödör<u>ből</u>) – kiborítja a vödr<u>öt</u>
'pour out the garbage (out of the bucket)' – 'empty (lit.: 'pour out') the bucket'

kiissza a vizet (a pohár<u>ból</u>) – kiissza a pohar<u>at</u>
'drink up the water (out of the glass)' – 'empty (lit.: 'drink out') the glass'

kipakolja az árut (a ládá<u>ból</u>) – kipakolja a ládá<u>t</u>
'unpack the goods (out of the crate)' – 'unpack the crate'

b) ***le*('down')-V(meaning.1) *x*(ACC) (<u>off/from</u> *y*) – *le*('down')-V(meaning.2) *y*(<u>ACC</u>)**

learatja a gabonát (a táblá<u>ról</u>) – learatja a táblá<u>t</u>
'harvest (lit.: 'harvest down') the crops (from the field)' – 'harvest the field'

lelegeli a füvet (a rét<u>ről</u>) – lelegeli a rét<u>et</u>
'graze (lit.: 'graze down') the grass off the pasture' – 'graze down the pasture'

lenyalja a mézet (a kenyér<u>ről</u>) – lenyalja a kenyer<u>et</u>
'lick the honey off the bread' – 'lick off the bread'

B) *Typical semantic characteristics of this type:*

- V denotes a physical activity that is intended by the agent and driven by a specific goal;
- *ki-/le-*V(meaning.1) is based on the meaning component 'remove';
- *ki-/le-*V(meaning.2) is based on the meaning component 'empty';

- x = substance or a multitude of homogeneous things;
- y = the original place of x, some surface or container-like object which becomes empty after the removal of x.

Note: On the level of V(meaning.1), the prefix is used in addition to a case suffix marking the adverbial of source (*-ról/-ről,* meaning '(down/away) from/off the surface of', or *-ból/-ből,* meaning 'out of'). The selection of the prefix and the suffix depends on whether y is a surface or a container. The prefix ***ki-*** **'out'** is used for containers along with the case suffix *-ból/-ből,* whereas ***le-*** **'off'** is used for surfaces along with *-ból/-ből.*

C) Productivity of this type:

Within this semantic relation, we consider (3) a) to be possibly productive, since appropriate verbs can be formed by productive processes of derivation. For example, from the noun *lapát* 'shovel' it is possible to derive the verb *lapátol* 'shovel', which can be combined with the prefix in question, i.e. *ki- + lapátol,* as in *kilapátolja a szenet a vagonból* 'shovel out the coal from the railway carriage' – *kilapátolja a vagont* 'shovel out the railway carriage'. Similarly: *kanál* 'spoon (noun)' > *kanalaz* 'spoon (verb)'; *kikanalazza a levest a tányérból* 'spoon the soup out of the bowl' – *kikanalazza a tányért* 'spoon out the bowl' etc.

(4) **'remove/extract**[17] **moisture** from something' – **'reduce the moisture content** of something **or remove it completely'**[18]

A) Typical syntactic alternation for this type:

***ki*('out')-V(meaning.1) *x*(ACC) (out of *y*) – *ki*('out')-V(meaning.2) *y*(ACC)**

kipréseli a levet (a szőlőből) – kipréseli a szőlőt
'squeeze out the juice (out of grapes)' – 'squeeze out the grapes'

kifacsarja a levet (a citromból) – kifacsarja a citromot
'squeeze out the juice (out of a lemon)' – 'squeeze out the lemon'

kicsavarja a vizet (a ruhából) – kicsavarja a ruhát
'wring out the water (out of clothes)' – ' wring out the clothes'

---

[17] On the level of V(meaning.1), if the goal of the activity described by the verb is to obtain some liquid, it makes sense to use Apresjan's formulation 'extract (something from something)'.

[18] In the case of structures that contain verbs without a prefix, and express some institutionalised activity, we could in theory make use of Apresjan's more comprehensive types **'to treat in a definite way' – 'to eliminate/remove by treating in this way'** to account for the alternation. For example: *szőlőt présel (mustnak)* 'squeeze grapes (for grape juice)' – *mustot présel (a szőlőből)* 'squeeze grape juice (from grapes)'. This more comprehensive type of Apresjan's cannot be adapted to Hungarian directly, since some alternation types that exhibit this kind of semantic variation cannot be regarded as polysemy, e.g.: *megfeji a tehenet* 'milk a cow' – *kifeji a tejet* 'milk out some milk' (in this case, the alternating verbs are different, since their prefix changes; see section 3.2.1 for discussion).

B) *Typical semantic characteristics of this type:*

- V denotes a physical activity that is intended by the agent and driven by a specific goal;
- *ki*-V(meaning.1) is based on the meaning component 'remove/extract moisture from something';
- *ki*-V(meaning.2) is based on the meaning component 'reduce the moisture content of something or remove it completely';
- *x* = moisture/liquid;
- *y* = the thing that contains *x*; its moisture content is reduced or eliminated completely by removing *x*.

Note: In this type there is a semantic connection between *x* and *y*, since *y* contains *x*, cf. *olajbogyó* 'olive' (literally: 'oil-berry') and *vizes ruha* 'wet (lit.: 'watery') clothes'. As a result of this relation of containment, on the level of V(meaning.1) only verbs with the prefix *ki-* 'out' and source adverbials with the (elative) case suffix *-ból/-ből* 'out of' may fall into this type.

C) *Productivity of this type:*

The productivity of this group is somewhat uncertain. We can, on the one hand, find new alternations whose syntactic structure and meaning correspond to the pattern described above, as in *kiszívja a levet a citromból* 'sip the juice out of the lemon' – *kiszívja a citromot* 'sip out the lemon', *kicentrifugálja a vizet a ruhából,* lit.: 'spin the water out of the clothes' – *kicentrifugálja a ruhát* 'spin out (i.e., spin-dry) the clothes'. On the other hand, in certain cases the availability of a derived structure and/or meaning is at least questionable, e.g.: *kitapossa a levet a paradicsomból* 'tread the juice out of the tomatoes' – *?kitapossa a paradicsomot* 'tread out the tomatoes'. However, this phenomenon is most probably motivated by cultural peculiarities as opposed to linguistic features in the sense that there are different preferred, usual ways (in different communities) to extract moisture or juice. The fact that expressions become conventional constitutes a counterargument against the assumption of productivity.

(5) '**remove** some substance or thing that is unnecessary, harmful or dirty (from or off something)' – '**clean** something (its surface or the inside of the thing)'

A) *Typical syntactic alternations for this type:*

a) ***ki*('out')-V(meaning.1) *x*(ACC) (<u>out of/off</u> *y*) – *ki*('out')-V(meaning.2) *y*(<u>ACC</u>)**

kiveri a port (a szőnyeg<u>ből</u>) – kiveri a szőnyege<u>t</u>
'beat out the dust (out of the carpet)' – 'beat out the carpet'

kiégeti a kormot (a kémény<u>ből</u>) – kiégeti a kémény<u>t</u>
'burn out the soot (out of the chimney)' – 'burn out the chimney'

kifőzi a szennyet (a ruhá<u>ból</u>) – kifőzi a ruhá<u>t</u>
'boil out the dirt (out of the clothes)' – 'boil out the clothes'

b) ***le*('off')-V(meaning.1) *x*(ACC) (off/from *y*) – *le*('off')-V(meaning.2) *y*(ACC)**

ledörzsöli a homokot (a kezéről) – ledörzsöli a kezét
'rub off the sand (off his hand)' – 'rub off his hand'

letörli a port (a cipőről) – letörli a cipőt
'wipe off the dust (off his shoes)' – 'wipe off his shoes'

lesöpri a havat/a leveleket (az útról) – lesöpri az utat
'sweep off the snow/the leaves (off the road)' – 'sweep off the road'

c) ***fel*('up')-V(meaning.1) *x*(ACC) (off/from *y*) – *fel*('up')-V(meaning.2) *y*(ACC)**[19]

felsöpri a morzsákat/piszkot (a padlóról) – felsöpri a padlót
'sweep up the crumbs/dirt (off the floor)' – sweep up the floor'

felsúrolja a foltot/a piszkot (a konyhakőről) – felsúrolja a konyhakövet
'scrub up the stain/the dirt (off the floor tiles in the kitchen)' – 'scrub up the floor tiles in the kitchen'

felporszívózza a morzsákat/koszt (a parkettáról) – felporszívózza a parkettát
'hoover up the crumbs/dirt (off the parquet floor)' – 'hoover up the parquet floor'

Note: Similarly to the previous patterns, on the level of V(meaning.1) the prefixes *le-* 'off' and *fel-* 'up' correlate with the case suffix referring to the surface of a thing, *-ról/-ről* '(down) from/off', whereas the prefix *ki-* 'out' correlates with the suffix referring to the inside of a container, *-ból/-ből* 'out of'.

B) Typical semantic characteristics of this type:

- V denotes a physical activity that is intended by the agent and driven by a specific goal;
- *ki-/le-/fel-*V(meaning.1) is based on the meaning component 'remove';
- *ki-/le-/fel-*V(meaning.2) is based on the meaning component 'clean';
- *x* = unnecessary, harmful or dirty substance or thing;
- *y* = the original place of *x*, the thing to be cleaned.

C) Productivity of this type:

The assumption of productivity cannot be justified for this group for semantic reasons. For example, the meanings of the alternating pairs *lekaparja a festéket az asztalról* 'sand the paint off the desk' – *lekaparja az asztalt* 'sand off the desk', *lefújja a homokot az asztalról* 'blow the sand off the table' – *lefújja az asztalt* 'blow off the table' do

[19] There is also a further pair of structures, namely, ***fel*('up')-V in *x* – *fel*('up')-V *x*(ACC)**, e.g.: *felsúrol a konyhában* 'scrub up in the kitchen' – *felsúrolja a konyhát* 'scrub up the kitchen'; *felporszívóz a szobában* 'hoover up in the room' – *felporszívózza a szobát* 'hoover up the room'. This cannot be considered an instance of polysemy because the verb expresses the same meaning ('clean') in both structures.

not correspond to the pattern we have proposed earlier (i.e. the meaning of the structure built on **pref.-V *y*(ACC)** is not necessarily 'clean *y*').

(6) '**open** something (on something)' – 'make something (= something else) **accessible**'[20]

A) *Typical syntactic alternation for this type:*
***ki*('out')-V(meaning.1) *x*(ACC) (on something) – *ki*('out')-V(meaning.2) *y*(ACC)**[21]

kioldja a madzagot (a zsákon) – kioldja a zsákot
'untie the string (on the bag)' – 'untie the bag'

kibontja a papírt (az ajándékon) – kibontja az ajándékot
'unwrap the paper (on the present)' – 'unwrap the present'

kinyitja a szoba ajtaját/a (szoba)ajtót – kinyitja a szobát
'open the door of the room/the (room's) door' – 'open the room'

B) *Typical semantic characteristics of this type:*
- V typically denotes a physical activity that is intended by the agent and driven by a specific goal;
- V(meaning.1) is based on the meaning component 'open';
- V(meaning.2) is based on the meaning component 'make something accessible';
- *x* = some substance or thing that closes or hides something;
- *y* = something that is closed, or completely covered and hidden by *x*.

C) *Productivity of this type:*
This type applies only to the verbs listed and *kiköt* 'untie', therefore it is not productive.

The following types (7)-(9) are characterised by the semantic relation 'action' – 'causation or control of action'. In Hungarian, the majority of examples that could be considered in connection with this type are not instances of polysemy, since the rela-

---

[20] This meaning relation is parallel to the following two types of Apresjan's: 'to attach' – 'to cause contact between two objects by attaching' and their antonyms, and 'to shut off' – 'to block access by shutting off' and their antonyms. In Hungarian, however, the meanings of the alternating verb pairs expressing **'to attach' – 'to cause contact between two objects by attaching' and their antonyms** cannot be considered instances of polysemy since they are connected to alternation either between base verbs and their prefixed versions, or between different prefixed verbs. For example: *kötelet köt a lóra* 'fasten/tie a bridle onto the horse' – *odaköti a lovat a kerítéshez* 'prefix('there')-tie the horse to the fence' – *megköti a lovat* 'prefix(perfective)-tie the horse'. Apresjan's second type **'to shut off' – 'to block access by shutting off' and their antonyms** do not apply in Hungarian either, since the relevant verb pairs mostly do not follow a consistent alternation pattern (except for a few examples: *kiköti/ beköti a szalagot* 'untie/tie the ribbon' – *kiköti/beköti a zacskót* 'untie/tie the bag'; *kinyitja az ajtót* 'open the door' – *kinyitja a szobát* 'open the room' etc.). This can be explained by the fact that the use of certain prefixes can be restricted by the semantic content of the verb. For instance, verbs inherently expressing 'opening' like *bont* 'unwrap/untie' can occur with the prefix *ki-* 'out', but not with prefix *be-* 'in'.

[21] The first structure in this alternation shows further variation as well, but we will ignore this here.

tion in question is mostly not expressed by different meanings of the same verb, but by pairs of verbs (one of which is a simple agentive verb, and the other is factitive). In connection with relations of the type 'action' – 'causation or control of action', we only find a single polysemous verb if the subject of the verb is the instrument of the event or the human being using the instrument (7),[22] or a body-part of the human being/animal, or the human being/animal itself (8; part-whole relationship), or a vehicle, or the human being controlling the vehicle (9).

(7) **'sound emission' – 'causation of sound emission'**

A) *Typical syntactic alternation for this type:*
'y's *x* V (meaning.1)' – 'y V (meaning.2) <u>with</u> his *x*'

(vkinek) a gyűrűje csattog – vki csattog a gyűrűjé<u>vel</u>
'(someone's) ring clinks' – 'someone clinks with his ring'

(vkinek) a sarkantyúja kopog – vki kopog a sarkantyújá<u>val</u>
'someone's spurs jingle' – 'someone jingles with his spurs'

(vkinek) a papucsa csattog – vki csattog a papucsá<u>val</u>
'someone's flip-flops are tapping' – 'someone is tapping with his flip-flops'

B) *Typical semantic characteristics of this type:*

- V belongs to the class of verbs expressing sound-emission;
- V(meaning.1) is based on the meaning component 'emit sound' (it is not connected to the agent and is not controlled);
- V(meaning.2) is based on the meaning components 'cause' and 'emit sound' (it is connected to and controlled by the agent);
- *x* = the object owned/used by *y*, the instrument of sound emission;
- *y* = a person, the owner or the user of *x*; sound emission by *x* (possibly) depends on *y*'s intention.

Note: In this type the verb's structure and meaning (as indicated above) represent sound emission as either 1) an uncontrolled event focusing on the instrument or 2) an event controlled by the agent. As the instruments in question are not independent sources of sound emission, and among the thematic roles it is typically the agent role (rather than the instrument role) that surfaces as the subject, in this type we might as well reverse the order of derivation (in contrast to Apresjan's categorisation): 'someone emits sound with something' – 'something emits sound'. In this case we would not regard this semantic relation as one of 'cause and effect', but rather as one reflecting

---

[22] We cannot include the type *a kés vág* 'the knife cuts' – *vki vág a késsel* 'someone cuts with the knife' in our list since the expression *a kés vág* 'the knife cuts' is to be interpreted as 'the knife cuts well ~ it is possible to cut with the knife efficiently, i.e. the knife is sharp' (similarly, *a kés nem vág* 'the knife does not cut' means 'the knife does not cut well ~ it is not possible to cut with the knife efficiently, the knife is blunt'). Accordingly, we do not consider *a kés vág* 'the knife cuts' and *vki vág a késsel* 'someone cuts with the knife' to be corresponding structures, since the latter expression cannot mean 'someone cuts well with the knife'.

an anthropomorphic view, according to which an unintentional participant in the event of sound emission is represented as an agent. However, this does not seem a viable option since sound emission may occur without the external control or intention of an agent, e.g.: *Ahogyan vitték, lelógó keze odaütődött a bútorokhoz, gyűrűje kellemetlenül csattogott.* 'As he was being carried, his hand was hanging in the air and hit the furniture, his ring was clinking annoyingly.' The observations in connection with group (2) further suggest that the originally proposed cause and effect relation is to be preferred.

C) *Productivity of this type:*

This type can be considered productive since it is possible to derive a syntactic structure with the meaning 'causation of sound-emission' for every verb of sound emission that possesses the syntactic and semantic characteristics described above.

(8) **'motion/sound emission' – 'the causation of motion/sound emission'**

'V(meaning.1) *y*'s *x*' – 'y V(meaning.2) <u>with</u> his *x*'[23]

hunyorog vkinek a szeme – vki hunyorog a szemé<u>vel</u>
'someone's eyes squint' – 'someone squints with his eyes'

csikorog vkinek a foga – vki csikorog a fogá<u>val</u>
'someone's teeth make a 'gnashing' sound' – 'someone is gnashing with his teeth'

B) *Typical semantic characteristics of this type:*

- V belongs to the class of verbs of motion or sound emission;
- V(meaning.1) is based on the meaning component 'move' or 'emit sound' (unintentional/uncontrolled motion or sound emission);
- V(meaning.2) is based on the meaning components 'cause' plus 'move' or 'emit sound' (intentional/controlled motion or sound emission);
- *x* = *y*'s body-part that is actually involved in motion or emits sound;
- *y* = human being or animal whose body-part is *x*; motion or sound-emission by *x* (possibly) depends on *y*'s intention.

Note: Similarly to type (7), it is intention/control or the lack of it that plays a role in 8). In this type it is not possible to reverse the relation since here it is even more obvious than in type (7) that the event of motion or sound emission may occur without the control (intention/volition) of the agent.

---

23 In the first structure, the possessive construction "*y*'s *x*" functions as the subject (i.e. its head *x* is a nominative form), i.e. the correct paraphrase should in fact be "*y*'s *x* V" (as in *his eyes blink*). The order given in the schema above reflects the word order in Hungarian: in this construction, the subject NP typically follows the verb (according to the order above), or only its head *x* is postverbal and the possessor appears preverbally, i.e. "*y*'s V *x*".

C) Productivity of this type:

This type is not productive: in Hungarian these semantic relations are typically expressed not by different uses of a single polysemous verb, but by verb pairs. If the primary verb is transitive, the difference between controlled/intentional and uncontrolled/ unintentional events is expressed by using a transitive and a (derived) unaccusative version of the same verb, respectively. For example, it is possible to say (using the transitive verb *összehúz* 'pull together') *összehúzza a szemöldökét* 'frown (literally: 'pull his eyebrows together')', but the corresponding structure with the same verb is ungrammatical: **összehúz a szemöldökével,* lit.: 'pull together with his eyebrows'. Instead an unergative version of this verb with a derivational suffix is used (*összehú-zódik,* approx.: 'being pulled together') if the speaker wants to express that the facial expression is unintentional: *összehúzódik a szemöldöke* 'frown' (literally: 'his eyebrows are being pulled together'). We can observe the same correlations in connection with a number of similar (essentially idiomatic) subject-verb combinations as well, e.g. *összecsapja a kezét/bokáját* 'clap his hands/ankles together', *félrefordítja a fejét* 'turn his head around', *behúzza a hasát* 'pull his stomach in'.

If the primary verb is unaccusative, the semantic difference is not expressed by polysemy, either. For instance, *remeg a feje/a hangja* 'his head/voice trembles', *reszket a keze* 'his hands tremble', *vibrál a szeme* 'his eyelids flicker', but **remeg a fejével* 'tremble with his head', **reszket a kezével* 'tremble with his hands', **vibrál a szemével* 'flicker with his eyelids'. In some contexts describing acting or pretence, the proper intentional event can be expressed by the causativisation of the verb, e.g.: *megremegteti a fejét/hangját* 'make his head/voice tremble' (the prefix *meg-* expresses the Aktionsart semelfactive in this case).

(9) **'motion' – 'control over motion'**

A) Typical syntactic alternation for this type:

x V(meaning.1) – *y* V(meaning.2) {with *x*/*x*(ACC)}

a bicikli megáll – vki megáll a biciklivel
'the bicycle stops' – 'someone stops with the bicycle'

a teherautó elindul – vki elindul a teherautóval
'the truck starts' – 'someone starts with the truck'

a busz lefékez – vki lefékez a busszal/vki lefékezi a buszt
'the bus brakes' – 'someone brakes with the bus/someone brakes the bus'

B) Typical semantic characteristics of this type:

- V(meaning.1) is based on the meaning component 'move';
- V(meaning.2) is based on the meaning components 'control' and 'move';
- *x* = vehicle;
- *y* = person controlling the movement of *x*.

Unlike types (7) and (8), this type does not include cases in which the motion event can occur independently of the agent's control (intention/volition). As far as the history of the structures and the corresponding meanings is concerned, the transitive verb phrase or the one containing an instrumental adverbial, or in other words, the level of V(meaning.2) almost certainly underlies the intransitive use, i.e. V(meaning.1). Synchronically, however, it is easier to describe the regular semantic relation if we treat 'motion' itself as the primary, simple meaning, and 'control over motion' as complex and derived.

C) *Productivity of this type:*
Whereas the alternating pair *x* **V(meaning.1) –** ***y*** **V(meaning.2) with** ***x*** applies to all verbs that indicate some kind of motion performed by a vehicle, the pattern ***x*** **V(meaning.1) –** ***y*** **V(meaning.2)** ***x*****(ACC)** cannot be considered productive as the given correspondence is not compatible with all types of verbs describing movement by a vehicle. In Hungarian, such relations (i.e. an intransitive verb alternating with its transitive version taking an accusative object) mostly involve either an unergative-causative or an unaccusative-causative verb pair, e.g.: *a kocsi megáll* 'the car stops' – *vki megállítja a kocsit* 'someone stops the car', *a busz elindul* 'the bus starts' – *vki elindítja a buszt* 'someone starts the bus'. However, this is not always possible, e.g. *a kocsi bekanyarodik* 'the car turns' – **vki bekanyarítja a kocsit* 'someone turns the car'.

(10) **'non-autonomous locomotion' – 'autonomous locomotion'**

A) *Typical syntactic alternation for this type:*
x **V(meaning.1) on *y*/by *y* –** ***y*** **V(meaning.2)**[24]

az ember megy a kocsin, vonaton/a kocsival, vonattal – a kocsi/a vonat megy
'someone travels on the car/train/by car/train' – 'the car/train travels'

az utasok elrepülnek a repülőgéppel – a repülőgép elrepül
'the passengers fly away with the plane' – 'the plane flies away'

az utasok elindulnak/megérkeznek a repülőn/repülővel – a repülő elindul/megérkezik
'the passengers depart/arrive on the plane/with the plane' – 'the plane departs/arrives'

B) *Typical semantic characteristics of this type:*
- V(meaning.1) is based on the meaning component 'move/travel';
- V(meaning.2) is based on the meaning component 'move/transport';
- *x* = typically a human being (as a passenger)
- *y* = a vehicle (as a carrier)

On both levels the meaning of the verb is based on the meaning component 'move' (directed motion), i.e. the verb belongs to the same core meaning category in both

24 In the first construction, two versions are indicated in the paraphrase. According to the first, the constituent *y* is marked by a locative (more precisely, superessive) case suffix *-n/-on/-en/-ön*, meaning 'on'. According to the second, it is marked by the (comitative-instrumental) case suffix *-val/-vel/-Cal/-Cel* meaning 'with' or 'by' (for a brief explanation of C, see footnote 13).

meanings. Although there is no difference between the types of motion in any of the example pairs listed above, the selection restrictions of the verbs that apply to the subject show systematic differences in the constructions: in the case of 'non-autonomous locomotion' the subject of the event is typically a human being as a passenger, whereas in the case of 'autonomous locomotion' it is a vehicle used as a means of transport.[25] The verbs in question are able to carry the meaning of 'non-autonomous locomotion' only if this characteristic pattern (e.g.: 'someone moves **on something/by something**') applies. The distinction between 'non-autonomous' and 'autonomous' locomotion is the only reason for claiming that these verbs are polysemous. Nevertheless, this type is somewhat out of place on this list: this is a case where Apresjan's statement according to which polysemy can often be described as monosemy is quite appropriate.

C) *Productivity of this type:*
This type is not productive. Moreover, we can find only a few examples that exhibit the systematic behaviour indicated in the examples above: for example, although the rule is applicable to the verbs *megy* 'go, travel', *repül* 'fly' (which are ways of travelling), and *elindul* 'depart', *megérkezik* 'arrive' (which are subevents of travelling), it is not compatible with the verb *utazik* 'travel'.

(11) **'manner of motion' – 'directed motion'**

A) *Typical syntactic alternation for this type:*
x V(meaning.1) – *x* <u>to *y*</u> V(meaning.2)[26]

a kislány táncol – a kislány <u>az ablakhoz</u> táncol
'the little girl dances' – 'the little girl dances to the window'

a labda pattog – a labda <u>a kapuhoz</u> pattog
'the ball bounces' – 'the ball bounces to the goal'

B) *Typical semantic characteristics of this type:*
- V refers to motion;
- V(meaning.1) expresses manner of motion;
- V(meaning.2) expresses directed motion;
- *x* = animate or thing;
- *y* = the animate being or thing towards which the motion is directed.

---

25 Motion performed by the vehicle is considered autonomous in comparison with the non-autonomous motion carried out by the passengers. Otherwise, the activity is assumed to be directly or indirectly controlled by a human being.

26 As in type 8), the structure for V(meaning.2) above, and also in type 12) below, is supposed to reflect the word order of the Hungarian construction instead of being a proper English paraphrase: it indicates that the goal adverbial 'to *y*' normally directly precedes the motion verb in Hungarian. The interpretation of the structure is, of course, '*x* V(meaning.2) to *y*'.

C) Productivity of this type

This type is productive since the pattern applies to all verbs describing manner of motion, provided that they occur in the syntactic construction in question.

Note: On the level of V(meaning.2), it is possible to use versions of the base verb that contain a directional prefix. This reinforces the semantic component 'directed motion', e.g. *az asztalhoz táncol* 'dance to the table' ~ *odatáncol az asztalhoz* 'prefix('to')-dance to the table', *a kapuba gurul* 'roll into the goal' ~ *begurul a kapuba* 'prefix('into')-roll into the goal'. However, such prefixed verbs expressing directionality do not take part in the syntactic alternation described above, their meaning only corresponds to the meaning of the base verb on the level of V(meaning.2). Regarding the polysemy of the base verb (in accordance with our principles described at the outset) we do not consider connections between a base verb and its prefixed versions as belonging to polysemy.

(12) **'sound emission' – 'directed motion accompanied by sound emission'**

A) Typical syntactic alternation for this type:
***x* V(meaning.1) – *x* to/into *y* V(meaning.2)**

a mozdony zakatol – a mozdony az állomásra zakatol
'the train engine rattles' – 'the train engine rattles to the station'

a szél süvít – a szél a kunyhóba süvít
'the wind howls' – 'the wind howls into the cabin'

a traktor berreg – a traktor az utcára berreg
'the tractor rumbles' – 'the tractor rumbles to the street'

B) Typical semantic characteristics of this type:

- V is a verb of sound emission;
- V(meaning.1) describes sound emission;
- V(meaning.2) describes directed motion;
- *x* = inanimate (thing/natural force), or animate entity (if the subject is an animate entity, there must be a tool or a vehicle that is connected with *x*'s motion, and it is this object that actually emits the sound);
- *y* = animate or inanimate entity towards which the motion is directed.

C) Productivity of this type:

This type is productive, although expressions formed according to the second pattern are still uncommon and strange lexically. It is more usual to use a prefixed version of the verb in these constructions. For example, *A villamos a sarokig csörömpölt/elcsörömpölt a sarokig.* 'The tram clanked (prefix: 'away') to the corner.'; *A traktor az utcára berregett/kiberregett az utcára.* 'The tractor rumbled (prefix 'out') to the street.'

Note: we have investigated this type in detail (primarily on the basis of Levin & Rappaport Hovav 1996) and presented our findings in a number of publications (Ladányi 2002, 2003, and to appear), so we will only briefly summarise the most important points concerning the polysemy of Hungarian verbs of sound emission.

Levin & Rappaport Hovav (1996) examine two semantic classes of verbs: the verbs of sound emission and those of manner of motion. They provide a detailed description of the variable syntactic behaviour of verbs of sound emission, claiming that this is due to their semantic shift resulting in two different semantic (sub)classes, one of which is based on their original meaning (emission of sound) while the other (derived from the first by a semantic shift) is built on their directed motion sense. The connection between the two (sub)classes can be characterised by the notion of regular polysemy. It is also shown by the authors that one can formulate a typological generalisation for English about a parallelism between verbs of sound emission and those of manner of motion concerning their regular polysemy.

According to our analysis, the framework introduced by Levin and Rappaport Hovav can be generally applied to Hungarian as well. In this language one can observe both the semantic shift and the regular polysemy of verbs of sound emission (and of manner of motion as well), cf. the types described above in (11) and (12). In other words, there are characteristic parallels regarding the polysemic behaviour of the verbs of these two classes in Hungarian as well.

Nevertheless, English and Hungarian show considerable differences concerning the conditions of meaning change and the structural justification of systematic polysemy. In English, in the case of verbs of sound emission, resultative constructions characteristically exhibit the above-mentioned semantic shift – proving that we are dealing with systematic polysemy (cf. Levin & Rappaport Hovav 1996: 493-494, 496) (e.g.: *bang* – sound emission, *The door banged shut* – directed motion). In Hungarian, there are no resultative constructions with a similar meaning; therefore we need another method to verify systematic polysemy by reference to structure. These complicated issues will not be discussed here, but are treated in Ladányi, to appear. The behaviour of verbs of manner of motion and that of verbs of sound emission show both similarities and differences in Hungarian. Since similarities are more numerous and of greater importance, the differences do not cast doubt on the typological generalisation that, in a way similar to English, a parallel can be drawn between the two classes in Hungarian as well.

3.3.2. Systematic Polysemy without Syntactic Alternation

(13) **'emit characteristic sounds (animal)' – 'produce speech that sounds like that (human being)'**

In Hungarian, there are quite a few verbs that are connected to the meaning pair 'sound emission by animals' – 'sound emission by human beings'. However, this type is not uniform and can be characterised in the following way:

1. In a metaphorical sense, verbs of animal sound emission do not always designate human speech; they can denote an act of human crying (*nyüszít* 'whimper', *vonyít* 'howl', *bőg* 'moo'), laughing (*nyerít* 'neigh', *nyihog* 'neigh'), singing (*zümmög* 'buzz') and other complex activities that include speech production by human beings (e.g.: *Folyton csak turbékolnak.* approx.: 'They are always kissing and talking softly.', approx. lit.: 'They are always billing and cooing.').

2. Verbs denoting sound emission by animals can rarely be described as onomatopoeic words when referring to human speech metaphorically, e.g.: *dörmög* 'speak with a deep voice' (lit.: 'growl like a bear'). Instead, most verbs belonging to this semantic field are generally associated with a special connotation when they are used to refer to human speech, which becomes conventionalised/lexicalised in the verb's semantic content. For example, *huhog* 'hoot' and *károg* 'cry like a crow' is used when the speaker being referred to predicts that something bad will happen; and similarly, *sziszeg* 'hiss' implies ill-will; *karattyol* 'croak' implies incomprehensibility, *béget* 'baa' and *gágog* 'honk' expresses that the speaker in question is considered stupid, *hápog* 'quack' implies that the speaker in question is surprised, *nyávog* 'miaow' is a synonym of 'complain', *sápítoz* 'wail' refers to fear, *makog* 'make monkey sounds' means 'talk gibberish'. Therefore, the meaning of these verbs cannot in fact be appropriately described as 'produce speech that sounds like that'.

3. When used in a metaphorical sense, verbs of animal sound emission referring to human speech are not necessarily onomatopoeic and they do not (or not only) generally describe distinctive characteristics of human speech objectively. They can express (positive or negative) evaluation by the speaker about the subject of the given verbal predicate (that may also be the interlocutor), e.g: *Ne pityeregj már.* 'Don't whimper.', and *Te ebbe ne ugass bele!* 'Don't interfere with this! (lit.: 'Don't bark into this!')', *Nem érdekel, mit brekeg.* 'I'm not interested in what he is saying (lit.: 'croaking')'.

On the basis of the observations above, it seems that in this group we are only dealing with systematic polysemy if animal sound emission refers to sound emission by a human being without having an idiosyncratic connotation specified in the lexicon. However, there are probably only a few such meaning pairs. We cannot consider this type productive, since when used in a metaphorical sense, meanings of this type are not predictable.

(14) **'make something the subject of depiction' – 'create by depiction'**

This relation applies only to the verbs *fest* 'paint' and *rajzol* 'draw' without prefixes: *rajzol/fest egy fát* 'draw/paint a tree' – *rajzol/fest egy portrét* 'draw/paint a portrait'. However, it is not just the fact that it contains very few members that makes this type problematic. The difference between the meanings of the verbs in the two constructions is also difficult to identify since both verbs take effected objects, i.e. the drawing of a tree as well as a portrait comes into existence as a result of the event. The only difference is that trees exist independently of the act of drawing, whereas portraits come into being as a direct consequence of the event. However, this results from the meaning difference between the nouns attached to the verb, rather than having to do with the verb itself. Therefore, we are dubious whether this relation should be considered systematic polysemy. At the same time, the above meaning difference is reflected by different prefixed versions of the verbs in question: the depiction of an independently given object is marked by the verb prefix *le-* 'down', whereas the creation of a depiction as such is marked by *meg-* (which has no lexical meaning, but usually perfectivises, as mentioned earlier). E.g. *lerajzolja/lefesti a fát* 'draw/paint the tree (i.e. the one that is standing over there)' vs. *megrajzolja/megfesti a portrét* 'draw/paint the portrait (i.e. create the portrait by painting)'. However, differences in meaning between verbs having different prefixes are independent of the issue of verbal polysemy.

4. Systematic Polysemy of Verbs in Hungarian – Conclusions

After having examined several examples of the systematic polysemy of verbs, we can conclude that it is true for Hungarian as well as for English and Russian that a systematic semantic variation involving a certain verb is usually accompanied by syntactic alternation. This is in accordance with the fact that the meaning of a verb is instantiated in syntactic structures even in cases when they are not parts of an idiomatic construction (i.e. in general, the meaning of a verb cannot be examined in isolation). The alternation of the syntactic structure is accompanied by verbal polysemy (i.e. a change of verb meaning) only if the verb undergoes semantic reclassification. Consequently, the meaning of verbs is extended along the lines of the rule 'ISA', just like that of nouns, although this process is more complex (especially in the case of non-systematic meaning variations) than in the case of nouns, since concerning meaning extension of verbs the feature of 'MANNER' plays an important role as well.

Most syntactic alternations connected to the polysemy of verbs which are found in other languages, such as English and Russian, are not present in Hungarian. Instead of polysemy with syntactic alternation, often a new verb is created by prefixation or derivation (by suffix); in other words, new lexical items are often derived instead of new verb meanings (i.e. polysemy). Regarding this phenomenon, we can reasonably assume that it may in part depend on typological features whether and in how many cases we encounter in a given language systematic verbal polysemy that is connected to certain syntactic structures; e.g. it may be a consequence of the morphological richness (more precisely, the richness of the word-formation system) of the language.

On the basis of the material analysed we can conclude that certain meanings/semantic relations can only come into being if the primary structure and its meaning meet a certain requirement (e.g. the material or other characteristics of the direct object or a locative element referred to in the syntactic structure, the starting point, direction, goal, intention of the event etc.).

We have found it useful to distinguish (within the systematic polysemy of verbs) between types that are merely regular and ones that are productive as well, by extending the concept of productivity used in morphology. In the case of productive types the direction of derivation is of some importance: it is worth making a distinction between the primary meaning and the predictable derived/secondary meaning.

References

Apresjan, J. D. (1974): Regular polysemy. *Linguistics* 142, 5-32.

Dressler, W.U. (1997): On productivity and potentiality in inflectional morphology. *CLASNET Working Papers 7* (Cross-Language Aphasia Study Network, Centre hospitalier Cote-des-Neiges, Montréal), 3-22.

Dressler, W.U. & Ladányi, M. (2000): Productivity in word formation (WF): a morphological approach. *Acta Linguistica Hungarica* 47 (1-4), 103-144.

Fellbaum, Ch. (1990): English verbs as a semantic net. *International Journal of Lexicography* 3 (4), 278-301.

Fellbaum, Ch. (1998): A semantic network of English verbs. In: Fellbaum, Ch. (ed.): *WordNet: An electronic lexical database*. Cambridge: MIT Press, 69-104.

Fellbaum, Ch. (2000): Autotroponymy. In: Ravin, *y*. & Leacock, C. (eds.): *Polysemy: theoretical and computational approaches*. New York: Oxford University Press, 52-67.

Goldberg, A.E. (1995): *Constructions: A construction grammar approach to argument structure*. Chicago: Chicago University Press.

Horváth, K. (1983): *Transzformációs csoportok a magyarban*. Nyelvtudományi Értekezések 115. Budapest: Akadémiai Kiadó.

Horváth, K. (1993): *A rész és az egész. A rész-egész viszony szerepe a nyelv működésében*. Budapest: Hungarian Academy of Sciences. Dissertation for attaining the degree of candidate. Manuscript.

Kiefer, F. (2003): Alaktan. In: É. Kiss, K., Kiefer, F. & Siptár, P.: *Új magyar nyelvtan*. Budapest: Osiris, 189-284.

Kiefer, F. (2000): *Jelentéselmélet*. Budapest: Corvina.

Kiefer, F. & Ladányi, M. (2000a): A szóképzés. In: Kiefer, F. (ed.): *Strukturális magyar nyelvtan 3. Morfológia*. Budapest: Akadémiai Kiadó, 137-164.

Kiefer, F. & Ladányi, M. (2000b): Az igekötőkről. In: Kiefer, F. (ed.): *Strukturális magyar nyelvtan 3. Morfológia*. Budapest: Akadémiai Kiadó, 453-518.

Komlósy, A. (1992): Régensek és vonzatok. In: Kiefer, F. (ed.): *Strukturális magyar nyelvtan 1. Mondattan*. Budapest: Akadémiai Kiadó, 299-527.

Komlósy, A. (2000): A műveltetés. In: Kiefer, F. (ed.): *Strukturális magyar nyelvtan 3. Morfológia*. Budapest: Akadémiai Kiadó, 215-292.

Ladányi, M. (1993a): Általános mozzanatok szerepe a metaforizációban és a szinonimitásban. (Az *eszik* ige és szinonimái). In: Hadas, E. (ed.): A metaforikus és hipotetikus jelentés további konkretizációja. A „Nyelvi mozgásformák dialektikája" kutatócsoport munkái 10. Budapest: ELTE BTK Általános és Alkalmazott Nyelvészeti Tanszék, 13-41.

Ladányi, M. (1993b): *Jelentés és szerkezet*. Hungarian Academy of Sciences. Dissertation for attaining the degree of candidate. Manuscript.

Ladányi, M. (2002): Igeosztályok – lexikai jelentés – szintaktikai szerkezet: a hangadást jelölő igék az angolban és a magyarban. *Modern Filológiai Közlemények* IV/1, 15-30.

Ladányi, M. (2003): A hangadást jelölő igék a magyarban: lexikai jelentés és szintaktikai struktúra. In: Kiefer Ferenc (szerk.): *Igék, főnevek, melléknevek. Előtanulmányok a mentális szótár szerkezetéről*. Budapest: Tinta Könyvkiadó, 44-56.

Ladányi, M. (to appear). Verb classes – lexical meaning – syntactic structure: Verbs of sound in Hungarian. In: Andor, J. & Pelyvás, P. (eds.): *Empirical, cognitive-based studies in the semantics-pragmatics interface*. CRiSPI, Elsevier.

Levin, B. (1993): *English verb classes and alternations: A preliminary investigation*. Chicago & London: The University Of Chicago Press.

Levin, B. & Rappaport Hovav, M. (1995): *Unaccusativity at the syntax – lexical semantics interface*. Cambridge: MIT Press.

Levin, B. & Rappaport Hovav, M. (1996): Lexical semantics and syntactic structure. In: Lappin, Sh. (ed.): *The handbook of contemporary semantic theory*. Oxford: Blackwell, 487-507.

Magyar Nemzeti Szövegtár [Hungarian National Corpus]. *http://corpus.nytud.hu/mnsz.*

A magyar nyelv értelmező szótára I-VII [A Comprehensive Dictionary of Hungarian I-VII]. (ÉrtSz.) (1959-1962). Budapest: Akadémiai Kiadó.

A „Nyelvi mozgásformák dialektikája" kutatócsoport munkái 1-11 (1982-1994). Budapest: ELTE BTK Általános és Alkalmazott Nyelvészeti Tanszék.

Pethő, G. (2003): A főnevek poliszémiája. In: Kiefer, F. (ed.): *Igék, főnevek, melléknevek. Előtanulmányok a mentális szótár szerkezetéről*. Budapest: Tinta Könyvkiadó, 57-124.

Sigman, M. & Cecchi, G.A.: Global organization of the lexicon. *http://asterion.rockefeller.edu/guille/Papers/lexicon.pdf*.

Stein, A. (1999): Describing verb semantics in a type hierarchy. Disambiguation of Italian verbs. *http://www.uni-stuttgart.de/lingrom/stein/pubs/pdf/stein99.pdf*.

Stockinger, P. (1989): From lexical meaning to conceptual meaning. *http://semioweb.msh-paris.fr/escom/resources_enligne/p_stockinger/1989/verbmodel.pdf*.

Talmy, L. (1985): Lexicalization patterns. In: Shopen, T. (ed.): *Language typology and syntactic description III. Grammatical categories and the lexicon*. Cambridge: Cambridge University Press, 57-149.

Zsilka, J. (1973): *Sentence patterns and reality*. The Hague: Mouton.

Zsilka, J. (1981): *Dialectics of the motion forms in language*. The Hague: Mouton.

Zsilka, J. (1975): *A jelentés szerkezete (A jelentés-mozgás egysége)*. Budapest: Akadémiai Kiadó.

Zsilka, J. (1978): *Jelentés-integráció*. Budapest: Akadémiai Kiadó.

Constructional Polysemy: the Applicative Construction in ChiShona[*]

Ronnie Cann/Patricia Mabugu

School of Philosophy, Psychology and Language Sciences, English Language and Linguistics, University of Edinburgh
Edinburgh EH8 9LL
E-mail: r.cann@ed.ac.uk

Department of Linguistics, University of Zimbabwe
MP167 Mount Pleasant, Harare
E-mail: pmabugum@uz.ac.zw

1. Introduction

The applicative construction in the Bantu languages has been the object of some considerable interest for many years, especially with respect to its syntactic properties.[1] The construction is traditionally characterised as involving the morphological extension of a verbal stem by an affix which syntactically increases its valency by one argument, the extra argument often being construed as a benefactive. In ChiShona, a Bantu language spoken in Zimbabwe, the applicative affix, *-ir-/-er*,[2] attaches to a verbal stem (itself also possibly derived), as exemplified in (1), where the non-applicative construction involving the transitive verb, *-bik-* 'cook', in (1)(a) is compared to its applicative (ditransitive) counterpart, with the extended verbal stem *-bik-ir-* in (1)(b).[3]

(1) (a) *Mayi* *va-ka-bik-a* *sadza*
1a mother 2aSM-PST-cook-FV 5 sadza
'Mother cooked sadza.'

(b) *Mayi* *va-ka-bik-ir-a* *mw-ana* *sadza*
1a mother 2aSM-PST-cook-APPL-FV 1-child 5 sadza
'Mother cooked sadza for the child.'

---

* Publication of the present paper was supported by the Research Group for Theoretical Linguistics of the Hungarian Academy of Sciences at the Universities of Debrecen, Pécs and Szeged. We are grateful to Jim Hurford, Lutz Marten, Marten Mous and Gergely Pethő for helpful and illuminating comments on earlier versions of the material reported in this paper.

1 See, especially, Trithart (1983), Baker (1988), Alsina & Mchombo (1992, 1993), Alsina (1994), Ngonyani (1996, 1998), Pylkannen (2000), Marten (2002), Mabugu (2001), amongst others.

2 The vowel change is phonologically conditioned.

3 Numbers in glosses refer to the noun classes. Other abbreviations used are: SM 'subject marker'; OM 'object marker'; PST 'past tense'; APPL 'applicative affix'; FV 'finite verb affix'.

Most discussions of this construction in Bantu have been concerned with the vagaries of its syntax. Since the applicative construction typically adds an extra argument to the verb, analyses have focused mainly on the relationship that exists between the applied object and the logical object.[4] In particular, we find emphasis laid on apparent asymmetries between the two objects, as in Bresnan & Moshi (1990) which defines applicatives in terms of two classes, **symmetric** and **asymmetric**.[5] Within the former type, both the applied object and the logical object behave as true objects with respect to passivization, word order and other tests, while with the latter type, only the applied object shows a full range of object properties. Applicative asymmetries have further been described in terms of the possibility of adding an applied object to a predicate with an implicit object. Adding an applied object is only possible with the symmetric type rather than the asymmetric type (see Pylkannen 2000; Bresnan & Moshi 1990; Machobane 1989 for more details).

Although the semantic (and/or pragmatic) aspects of the construction are less thoroughly studied, the fact that the applied object may be interpreted in a variety of ways is often noted. For example, while the applied object is prototypically interpreted as a benefactive in some way (as in (1)(b)), the relations that are introduced by the applicative affix may have a variety of interpretations: benefactive, locative, motive and others.

(2) (a)	*Baba*	*va-ka-uray-ir-a*	**v-ana**	*nyoka*	
	1a father	2SM-PAST-kill-APPL-FV	2-child	9 snake	
	'Father killed a snake for the children.'				
	BENEFICIARY				
(b)	*Baba*	*va-ka-uray-ir-a*	**pa-ruware**		*nyoka*
	1a father	2SM-PAST-kill-APPL-FV	16-11 flat granite		9 snake
	'Father killed a snake on the rock.'				LOCATIVE
(c)	*Baba*	*va-ka-uray-ir-a*	**mari**	*mu-rume*	
	1a father	2SM-PAST-kill-APPL-FV	9 money	1-man	
	'Father killed a man for his money.'				MOTIVE

Baker (1988), Ngonyani (1996) and others argue that the different thematic roles associated with the applied object induce different syntactic behaviour (again principally with respect to asymmetries between applied and logical objects). However, despite the fact that the applicative affix is generally regarded as the most productive derivational verbal affix in most Bantu languages, there have not been many detailed studies of the semantic heterogeneity of the suffix to date (see Port 1981), and those studies that do exist tend to concentrate on the differences rather than the similarities of the various interpretations. As a consequence of this (and the putative syntactic dif-

[4] Because the term 'direct object' is ambiguous in Bantu languages (as pointed out by Bentley 1994), we will refer to the introduced argument within an applicative construction as the **applied object** (AO). In contrast, the argument which corresponds to the direct object in transitive sentences like (1)(a) (e.g. *sadza* 'sadza') will be called the **logical object** (LO), borrowing the term from Marantz (1993).

[5] Pylkannen (2000) along the lines of Bresnan & Moshi (1990) defines applicatives in terms of **high** and **low** types.

ferences), the applicative construction is most often treated as ambiguous, and the applicative affix as homonymous. In this paper, we take issue with such an approach and, from an exploration of the various ways in which the construction can be interpreted within ChiShona, argue that the range of meanings conveyed by the construction indicates instead that it is polysemous and the interpretation of the applied object crucially depends on context, both linguistic and non-linguistic.

In many ways, the approach to be taken in this paper is in line with Marten (2000, 2002)'s dynamic analysis of the construction in Swahili. He argues that the applicative construction involves the Relevance-Theoretic notion of concept strengthening that indicates the ad hoc construction of a concept from the interpretation of a string of words uttered in some context (Carston 2002). However, Marten does not discuss how different meanings are arrived at, nor the constraints on the interpretation of the AO that appear to hold. Thus, although we accept his central idea that the applicative construction is semantically underspecified, we take issue with the apparent weakness of the idea of concept strengthening and argue that all the primary interpretations associated with the applicative suffix in ChiShona are derived from a single basic meaning, one that is underspecified but not empty of content.

In this paper, we develop a semantic-pragmatic account of the applicative construction that places the benefactive within a larger framework that embraces other applicative constructions such as MALEFICIARY, MOTIVE, PURPOSE and GOAL. We argue that an integrated description of the construction is possible and that all the primary meanings associated with the applicative suffix can be derived from an underspecified generalised GOAL relation. Specific semantic interpretations are shown to involve progressive strengthening of this GOAL relation induced by the semantic and pragmatic properties of the predicate and the applied (and logical) object. In addition, we provide some discussion of the extension of the applicative construction to LOCATIVE and SOURCE applied objects, arguing that this results from a grammaticalisation of the affix to induce focus readings for non-argument expressions.

The purpose of the paper is descriptive rather than theoretical and so we do not tackle head-on the different theoretical approaches to the applicative that have been proposed; nor do we provide a precise theory that encapsulates our argument. However, a number of problems for extant theoretical approaches are noted and a possible theoretical account is indicated.[6]

2. The Canonical Meanings

We begin by discussing what may be called the (three) canonical, or basic, meanings of the applicative construction with respect to the applied object which are generally held to be BENEFICIARY, MALEFICIARY and MOTIVE, as illustrated in (3)-(5).

(3) *Mw-ana* *a-ka-vak-ir-a* *va-bereki* *i-mba*
1-child 1SM-PST-build-APPL-FV 2-parent 9-house
'A child built a house for the parents.' BENEFICIARY

6 For a theoretical account couched within HPSG, see Mabugu (2001a).

(4)	*Ma-tombo*	*a-ka-donh-er-a*	*mu-soro*	*w-ake*
	6-5 stone	6SM-PST-fall-APPL-FV	3-head	POSS-3SG
	'Stones fell on his head.'			MALEFICIARY

(5)	*Va-nhu*	*va-no-vereng-er-a*	*ruzivo*
	2-person	2SM-PRES-read-APPL-FV	11 knowledge
	'People read for knowledge.'		
	'People read in order to eventually gain knowledge.'		MOTIVE

The question naturally arises as to how distinct these readings are in fact. In particular, are these meanings sufficiently far apart that they require the postulation of different homonyms of the applicative affix or can the different meanings be derived from the examples themselves?

2.1. BENEFICIARY Readings

Consider first the apparently most straightforward cases of the benefactive interpretations of the AO. The nature of the beneficiary relation in each case is dependent on the semantic properties of the LO and the main verb. In general, the examples provided above can be interpreted in one of two ways: as involving the creation or construction of some object which itself will be to the benefit of the AO, a reading based on the interpretation of the direct object found in the construction; or, more generally, as involving the execution of some event which is to the benefit of the AO, a reading inferred from the event being depicted by the verb.

Thus, in sentence (1)(b) the object is food and the normal (decontextualised) inference would be that the food that is cooked directly benefits the child and that such direct benefit involves the child obtaining (and eating) it. Hence, we have a recipient reading whereby the sadza ends up with the child. However, there is a second possible reading for this sentence which is that it is the event of making sadza that is to the child's benefit. In other words, the applicative affix signals that it is the cooking of the sadza (and not the foodstuff itself) that benefits the child, without the sadza necessarily being obtained by the child. Such an interpretation will be primed, for example, in a context in which the child has to prepare sadza as a school project. This relation can be further shown by instances of 'object deletion' as in (6) which just states that the named event was done on behalf of the child. In this reading, the child stands in a benefactive relation to the event of sadza-cooking but bears no relation to the object of cooking.

(6)	*Mayi*	*va-ka-bik-ir-a*	*m-wana*
	1a mother	2aSM-PST-cook-APPL-FV	1-child
	'Mother cooked for the child.'		

The ambiguity is more marked in (7). For example, in one context Muchaneta is the recipient of the essay, written by Pio. In another context in which Muchaneta is a pupil, and is ill, we can have the interpretation in which 'Pio wrote an essay on behalf of Muchaneta'. (7) can thus be disambiguated by extending the linguistic context as shown in (8) where it is clear that the latter interpretation is intended.

(7) *Pio* *a-ka-nyor-er-a* *Muchaneta* *rondedzero*
1a name 1SM-PST-write-APPL-FV 1a name 9 essay
'Pio wrote an essay for Muchaneta.'

(8) *Pio* *a-ka-nyor-er-a* *Muchaneta* *rondedzero*
1a name 1aSM-PST-write-APPL-FV 1a name 9 essay
a-ka-i-p-a *mu-dzidzisi*
1SM-PST-9OM-give-FV 1-teacher
'Pio wrote an essay for Muchaneta and she gave it to the teacher.'

Of course, not all examples are ambiguous. For example, (9) can be interpreted only as indicating that the *sadza* is for the street children and that the entire event benefits the queen, a relation between the applied object and the event denoted by the verb. Here the queen stands in a benefactive relation to the event of giving but bears no relation to the objects of giving sadza or *street children.*

(9) *Mayi* *va-ka-p-ir-a* *mambokadzi* *sadza* *ma*-street kids
1a mother 2aSM-PST-give-APPL-FV 1a queen 5 sadza 6-street kids
'Mother gave sadza to street children for the queen.'

The interpretation we give to a particular construction thus varies from context to context. Even with respect to the basic benefactive reading of the applicative construction, it is clear that actual interpretation of the thematic role of the applied object with respect to the predicate is determined by the semantic properties of the applied object, the logical object and the predicate and pragmatics of the whole clause. In effect, the recipient reading is an enriched interpretation of the benefactive reading whereby the referent of the LO is located at (or with) the AO. Thus, while in all cases the AO is a benefactive with respect to the eventuality denoted by the verb, its interpretation as a recipient is pragmatically determined according to whether the LO is something that can be received, whether the AO is in a position to receive the LO and arbitrary aspects of the context.

Having established that even with a beneficiary AO the precise interpretation of the applicative construction depends on the semantic and pragmatic properties of the verb and the LO, we consider whether the other basic relations, MALEFICIARY and MOTIVE, may be derived in a similar way.

2.2. MALEFICIARY

A maleficiary interpretation of the AO occurs when the relation marked is to the disbenefit/detriment of the recipient involved in the event being described. For example, the verb 'give' typically portrays a beneficiary situation, in which a recipient benefits from the situation of giving, but we can have an unfavourable situation expressed by the same verb as in *Tanga gave me a slap*. The examples in (4), repeated below, and (10) provide illustrations of this type of interpretation.

(4) *Ma-tombo a-ka-donh-er-a mu-soro w-ake*
6-5 stone 6SM-PST-fall-APPL-FV 3-head POSS-3SG
'Stones fell on his head.' MALEFICIARY

(10) (a) *Mu-dhebhe w-angu wa-ka-ndi-donh-er-a*
3-trousers POSS-1SG 3SM-PST-1SG-fall-APPL-FV
'My trousers slipped (off) on me.'

(b) *Mu-kadzi w-angu a-ka-ndi-nyep-er-a*
1-wife POSS-1SG 1SM-PST-1SG-lie-APPL-FV
'My wife lied on me.'

(c) *Va-ka-mu-sek-er-a mu-kadzi w-ake*
3PL-PST-1OM-laugh at-APPL-FV 1-wife POSS-3SG
'They laughed at his wife on him.'

The AO introduced in these examples conveys a sense of adversity or inconvenience befalling the referents in the construction (Humphreys 1999). In example (4)(b) above it is obvious that stones falling on someone's head affects them adversely. Similarly, in a null or minimal context the example in (10)(a) is interpreted negatively and the event of trousers falling down is taken to affect the speaker adversely. In (10)(b) similarly, the event of the wife's lying is taken to affect the husband negatively, just as it is the event of 'them laughing at wife' that is to the detriment of the husband in example (10)(c). In all these cases, we have a predicate that denotes an event that is typically interpreted negatively and the AO is thus construed as being the entity that is negatively affected, i.e. as a maleficiary.[7]

If, however, it is possible to construe the event positively, then the AO itself may also be construed as being positively affected by it, depending on the discourse, or wider, context. For instance, (10)(b) could be interpreted as 'My wife lied on my behalf.', in which case it may be to the benefit of the husband. It is not hard to think of contexts that could turn the other maleficiaries above into 'beneficiaries' (or more accurately positively affected participants). For example, falling trousers could be construed positively in a situation in which an overweight person is trying to lose weight and laughter need not always connote mockery. It thus appears again that it is the nature of the event denoted by the predicate, and contextual, possibly extra-linguistic information (such as cultural norms concerning e.g. the embarrassment or otherwise in-

[7] These maleficiaries can be likened to what are termed in Indo-European languages (like German and Greek) as 'ethical' datives, where the referent of the dative term is marked as somehow being ethically implicated in the event. It is also a widespread trait observed in Slavic languages (see Wierzbicka 1988) as well as in modern Hebrew (Berman 1982).

volved in a loss of trousers), that determines whether the AO is interpreted as being positively or negatively affected.

Considerations such as these show that the meaning of the verb stem and the context of utterance has a central role to play as to whether the predicate should be interpreted as beneficiary or maleficiary, just as it does in determining whether a beneficiary is interpreted also as a recipient or not. Thus, we may hypothesize that that the applicative affix itself signals only a single relation for the AO whose interpretation is pragmatically enhanced in various ways. Thus, we may define a participant role that includes MALEFICIARY and BENEFICIARY, which we will refer to as an ADFICIARY, based on the Latin verb meaning 'to affect'. This "macrorole" has two primary instantiations, differentiated by whether the predicate denotes an eventuality that may connote positive or negative effects on the denotatum of the AO. Additionally, both roles may be further pragmatically enhanced to being a recipient (positively or negatively) according to whether the LO may be construed as ending up with the AO or not, as illustrated in Figure 1:

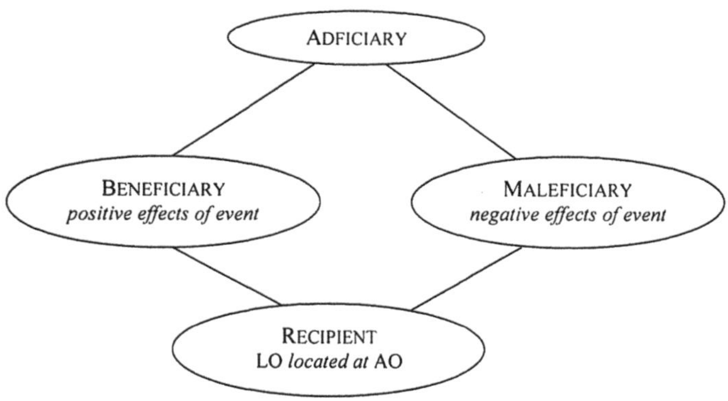

Figure 1: ADFICIARY applicative readings

2.3. MOTIVE

The third canonical interpretation of the applied object in ChiShona is that of MOTIVE. In the literature, MOTIVE is generally associated with two instantiations: PURPOSE (11) and REASON (12).

(11.) (a) *Ma-poachers* *a-no-vhim-ir-a* *mari* *chi-pembere*
6-poacher 6SM-PST-hunt-APPL-FV 9 money 7-rhinoceros
'Poachers hunt the rhinoceros for money.'

(b) *Ma-kororo* *a-ka-uray-ir-a* *u-pfumi* *mu-svetaupfumi*
6-robber 6SM-PST-kill-APPL-FV 14-wealth 1-one who sucks wealth
'Robbers killed the capitalist for his wealth.'

(12) (a)	*A-ka-pfek-er-a*	*mu-sangano*	*sutu*	
	3SG-PST-wear-APPL-FV	3-meeting	9 suit	
	'He wore a suit because of the meeting.'			
(b)	*A-ka-uy-ir-a*	*u-rwere*		
	3SG-PST-come-APPL-FV	11-ill		
	'S/he came because of the illness.'			
(c)	*Va-rwi*	*ve-rusunungulo*	*va-ka-rw-ir-a*	*i-vhu*
	2-fighter	2GEN-11-freedom	2SM-PST-fight-APP-FV	5-soil
	'The freedom fighters fought for/because of/in order to obtain land.'			

There are a number of factors that lead to the interpretation of an applied object as MOTIVE. The most obvious of these is where the AO is not animate as in the examples in (11) and (12). Inanimate and abstract objects cannot in general be interpreted as adficiaries[8] so they cannot directly be beneficially affected by a verb. Compare (11)(a) with (13)(a) and (12)(b) with (13)(b).

(13) (a)	*Ma-poachers*	*a-no-vhim-ir-a*	*mu-svetaupfumi*	*chi-pembere*
	6-poacher	6SM-PST-hunt-APPL-FV	1-capitalist	7-rhinoceros
	'Poachers hunt the rhinoceros for the capitalist.'			
(b)	*Ma-comrades*	*a-ka-rw-ir-a*	*va-nhu*	*ve-Zimbabwe*
	6-comrades	6SM-PST-fight-APP-FV	2-person	of-9 country
	'Comrades fought for the people of Zimbabwe.'			

Where the AO is animate, however, it may be interpreted as ADFICIARY or as MOTIVE, depending on contextual factors, as illustrated in the two different English translations of the example in (14).

(14)	*Mu-komana*	*a-ka-rwis-ir-a*	*John*	*mu-sikana*	
	1-boy	1SM-PST-fight-APP-FV	john	1-girl	
	'The boy fought John for the girl.'				BENEFICIARY
	'The boy fought John because of the girl.'				MOTIVE

The second interpretation of (14) indicates a second, and more important, factor that distinguishes MOTIVE from ADFICIARY. In the latter interpretations, the denotatum of the AO is interpreted as a direct participant of the event denoted by the verbal root: the fighting event is directly beneficial to the girl or the event of cooking sadza is directly beneficial to the children, etc. In the case of MOTIVE readings, however, the association of the AO with the main event is less direct and apparently mediated by another, implied, event. Thus, the translations of the examples in (11) and (12) could be given more verbosely as in (11'):

---

8 Except, for example, where a non-animate noun can be interpreted meronymically as standing for an animate object such as the name of a country standing for its people, etc.

(11')(a) 'Poachers hunt the rhinoceros to gain money.'
(b) 'Robbers killed the capitalist to obtain his wealth.'

The use of the purpose clauses to bring out the intended interpretations indicates that PURPOSE AOs are enriched in some fashion to provide a secondary event which serves as the GOAL of the primary event expressed by the verbal root. Such interpretations have been referred to in the literature as motivational goals, the contextual endpoints of predication (Frawley 1992), encoding the result or consequence of an event. Such an interpretation provides a useful link with the ADFICIARY interpretations, as beneficiaries (and maleficiaries) may be viewed as instances of GOALs of an event and this indicates that we may interpret the function of the applicative ending as introducing a GOAL argument. That GOAL may, however, be interpreted as a direct participant in the event denoted by the verb root (in ADFICIARY readings) or, indirectly, as providing an event that involves the AO which is itself the GOAL of the primary event. Thus, in (13)(a), the capitalist is the direct GOAL of the event of the poachers' hunting the rhinoceros while in (11)(a) the GOAL of the event is an event of obtaining money.

In the reason examples in (12), however, it might be argued that the AO does not obviously express a GOAL, the endpoint of the primary event, but its initial point. REASON interpretations focus on the **prior conditions** of a predication. Hence, the suit-wearing is motivated by the meeting in (12)(a), the coming to a particular place is motivated by illness in (12)(b), and in (12)(c) it is the lack of land that motivates the fighters to fight. Given this, Frawley (1992) has concluded that reasons can be referred to as motivational sources, the opposite of motivational goals: there is a prior condition that eventually leads to whatever action has to be done in the construction. If this is the correct way to view the semantic difference between reason and purpose, then we seem to be hard put to provide a unitary characterisation of these two sorts of motive. However, it is not obvious that reasons should be interpreted as **source** rather than as **goal.** We have suggested that the GOALS expressed by PURPOSE readings of AOs involve the enrichment of the nominal to express an event which itself acts as the goal argument of the verb. So we might paraphrase the translations of the examples in (12) as in (12'):

(12')(a) 'He wore a suit to attend the meeting.'
(b) 'She came to ease/cure/alleviate the illness.'[9]
(c) 'The freedom fighters fought to gain land.'

From these particular instances, it seems that reason AOs may also be interpreted as goals in the same way as purpose clauses. But there are other examples which are more difficult to reconcile with this such as (15), where it is precisely to be away from ill-fortune that the church elder goes to the diviner:

9 The precise interpretation of this sentence depends a lot on the context and could, in an appropriate situation, mean: 'She came to hasten the illness.'

(15)	*Madzi-baba*	*va-ka-end-er-a*	*mi-nyama*	*kun'anga*
	6-1a father	2aSM-PST-go-APPL-FV	4-ill-fortune	17 9 diviner

'A church elder visited a diviner because of ill-fortune.'

In this case, however, the goal is again an event enrichment of the AO whose interpretation, depending on context, is something like:[10]

(15') 'A church elder visited a diviner to get rid of/to understand/to find out the source of his ill-fortune.'

The important point here is that there is, in all cases, some GOAL of the event involving the AO. The precise goal that involves the AO may, thus, on occasion only be identified through further inference to do with real world knowledge. What is interesting here is that such further inference is often (but not always) induced by negative connotations of the AO, such as illness, ill-fortune or lack of land. So we have a parallel here with the two different ADFICIARY interpretations. The interpretation of REASON AOs as SOURCE is therefore a function of the pragmatic enhancement of the GOAL argument introduced by the applicative morpheme to alter in some way a (negative) situation that currently obtains. The difference between PURPOSE and REASON may thus be seen as a difference in the intended end result: for PURPOSE the GOAL is to achieve a situation in which the subject or the LO possesses or is somehow located with the AO while for REASON the GOAL is to achieve a situation in which the subject or LO does not possess the AO. In other words, the same property that distinguishes RECIPIENTs from Beneficiaries in general operates to distinguish PURPOSE from REASON.

As noted in the introduction, it is not our purpose here to provide a full theory of the applicative construction in ChiShona, but we pause at this point to sketch how the observations made above might be interpreted. It is clear in the cases so far considered that the applicative affix *-ir-/-er-* provides an additional argument to those introduced by the verbal stem that is interpreted as some sort of goal. Syntactically, that argument is both obligatory and expressed by a noun phrase that has the properties of a (direct) object (at least in ChiShona).[11] Semantically, we may view the applicative affix as introducing an argument that is specified as having a GOAL thematic relation to the event. This is illustrated in (16) which assumes a neo-Davidsonian event semantics where the verb introduces an event variable to which its arguments are bound by (possibly schematic) theta roles.[12] The applicative affix then appends (⊕) a GOAL argument linked to the relevant event:

---

10 Notice that similar interpretations apply to some of English translations of the ChiShona examples which use the preposition *for*:
(i) *He wore a suit for the meeting.*
(ii) ??*She came for the illness*. (cf. *She came for the food./She came because of the food.*)
(iii) *The freedom fighters fought for land.*
(iv) ???*A church elder visited a diviner for ill-fortune.* (cf. *A church elder visited a doctor for his ill-health.*)

11 See a.o. Mabugu (2002); Machobane (1989); Ngonyani (1998); Matambirofa (2003).

12 See Parsons (1990); Schein (1996), inter al.

(16) $V(e) \wedge \theta_1(e, a_1) \wedge \ldots \wedge \theta_n(e, a_n) \oplus \text{GOAL}\,(e, a_i)$ where $\text{AO} \leq a_i$

This argument is not, however, semantically necessarily identified with the referent of the AO directly, but as we have seen may be interpreted as an event to which the AO is directly linked.[13] Additionally, there may be an enrichment of the AO whereby it is interpreted as 'being at' (or possessed by) the subject or the logical object of the main predicate. So we can give schematic semantic representations to the two interpretations of (1) above (BENEFICIARY and RECIPIENT) as in (17) and to (11)(a) and (12)(a) as in (18) and (19), respectively.[14]

(17) (a) BENEFACTIVE:
Cook' (*e*) ∧ ACT (*e*, *Mother'*)

(b) RECIPIENT:
Cook' (*e*) ∧ ACT (*e*, *Mother'*) ∧ UND (*e*, *Sadza'*) ∧ BE-AT (*Sadza'*, *Child'*)

(18) *Hunt'* (*e*) ∧ ACT (*e*, *Poachers'*) ∧ UND (*e*, *Rhinoceros'*) ∧ GOAL (*e*, *e'*) ∧ *Obtain* (*e'*) ∧ ACT (*e'*, *Poachers'*) ∧ UND (*e'*, *Money'*) ∧ BE-AT (*Money'*, *Poachers'*)

(19) *Wear'* (*e*) ∧ ACT (*e*, *He'*) ∧ UND (*e*, *Suit'*) ∧ GOAL (*e*, *e'*) ∧ *Attend* (*e'*) ∧ ACT (*e'*, *He'*) ∧ UND (*e'*, *Meeting'*)

So far, we have identified two basic meanings for the applicative, ADFICIARY and MOTIVE, but shown that the interpretation of these is dependent on the semantics of the AO and the verb with regard to the ability of the AO to be interpreted as a direct participant in the event denoted by the latter. Within these two classes we differentiate subclasses of BENEFICIARY and MALEFICIARY on the one hand, and PURPOSE and REASON, on the other. We have argued that both adficiary and motive readings may be interpreted as pragmatically enriched instantiations of a potential goal Thus, it appears that the applicative morpheme can be treated as expressing, in its most common manifestations, an underspecified relation GOAL with polysemous interpretations induced by context, as summarised as in Figure 2.

[13] This is the intended effect of the condition $\text{AO} \leq a_i$. In a properly formulated theory this would be captured by some linking rule between syntax and semantics, the details of which we leave on one side in this paper.

[14] These representations use the "macroroles" of ACTOR (ACT) and UNDERGOER (UND) of Role and Reference Grammar (Foley & van Valin 1984).

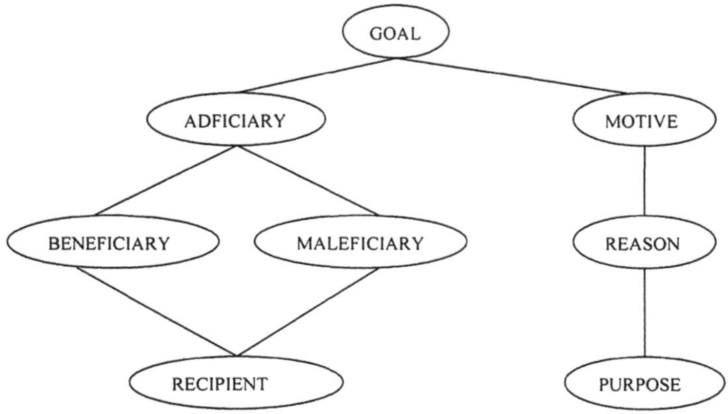

Figure 2: The canonical applicative meanings

2.4. True GOAL applicatives

We suggested at the end of the last section that the applicative construction should be construed as involving the specification of a "goal" of the event denoted by the verb, where this interpretation is more or less abstract depending on the semantic properties of the verb, the applied object and any associated logical object. If this is the case, then we might expect to find applicatives where the AO is interpreted as a real locative goal. Such is the case in ChiShona.

As expected, the interpretation of an AO as a true goal is dependent on the lexical meaning of the verb. In non-applicative verbs, GOALs are generally encoded as adjuncts with the use of a locative phrase headed by *kuna*.[15] Their applied counterparts, however, may internalise the adjunct phrase and this argument acquires all the properties of a direct object,[16] since it has to be obligatorily subcategorised for (see Khamisi 1985). Thus, (20)(a) shows the ditransitive base form *tuma* 'send', with one object and an optional locative adjunct *kuna mbuya*. (20)(b), on the other hand, shows the applied form *tumira* 'send to' with two objects *mwana* and *mbuya* the latter not being marked by *kuna* but still interpreted as the goal.

15 *Kuna* is an allomorph of *ku-*, a combination of the class 17 prefix and an associative marker, and appears with proper names and titles in class 1a. It has been argued to be a form of a preposition in ChiShona (Harford 1993). However, within most Bantu languages the category of preposition has been assumed not to exist. We do not go into detail here but just assume that *kuna* marks an oblique form within a goal oriented phrase and view it as a locative adjunct.

16 See Mabugu (2001b) and Hawkinson & Hyman (1974) for more details of the syntactic properties of the applied objects within ChiShona.

(20) (a)

Mai	*va-ka-tum-a*	*mw-ana*	*(kuna mbuya)*
1a mother	2aSM-PST-send-FV	1-child	to 1a grandmother

'Mother sent the child towards grandmother.'

(b)

Mai	*va-ka-tum-ir-a*	*mw-ana*	*mbuya*
1a mother	2aSM-PST-send-APPL-FV	1-child	1a grandmother

'Mother sent the child to grandmother.'

(21) (a)

Mw-ana	*a-ka-mhany-a*	*kuna mai*
1-child	1SM-PST-run-FV	to 1a mother

'The child ran towards mother.'

(b)

Mw-ana	*a-ka-mhany-ir-a*	*mai*
1-child	1SM-PST-run-APPL-FV	1a mother

'The child ran to mother.'

(22) (a)

Godhi	*a-ka-nyor-a*	*tsamba*	*(kuna Anatoria)*
1a name	1SM-PST-write-FV	9 letter	to 1a name

'Godfrey wrote a letter to Anatoria.'

(b)

Godhi	*a-ka-nyor-er-a*	*Anatoria*	*tsamba*
1a name	1SM-PST-write-APPL-FV	1a name	9 letter

'Godfrey wrote a letter to Anatoria.'

One of the differences between the applicative and non-applicative versions in the examples above relates to the endpoint of the event described. The sentences with adjunct goals marked by *kuna* do not carry the implication that the non-applicative object necessarily arrives at the goal, an 'unachieved goal' (as indicated by the use of 'towards' in English in Mabugu 2001). Thus in the (a) examples above, the action defined in the event does not necessarily culminate to the endpoint provided by the *kuna*-marked object, as indicated by the acceptability of sentence (23) which explicitly states this.

(23)

Mai	*va-ka-tum-a*	*mw-ana*	*kuna*	*mbuya*	*asi*
1a mother	2aSM-PST-send-FV	1-child	to	1a grandmother	but
haana	*ku-svik-a*				
NEG	15-arrive-FV				

'Mother sent the child to grandmother but she did not arrive.'

However, the applicative counterparts in the (b) examples above, carry a strong implication that the final destination is reached and this may be referred to as an 'achieved' GOAL which can be paraphrased as 'to the point of being at the GOAL'. The applicative suffix in this context focuses narrowly on the goal relation that exists between the two objects, the AO and the logical (or direct) object. What is highlighted in this context is the movement of the subject/object with its location at a specific endpoint, the applied object. The applicative thus serves to strengthen the concept of the goal of the event, yielding the implicature of actual relocation of the direct object. Querying whether the child reached its final destination in terms of acceptability is peculiar as shown by example (24).

(24) *#Mai* *va-ka-tum-ir-a* *mw-ana* *mbuya* *asi*
1a mother 2aSM-PST-send-APPL-FV 1-child 1a grandmother but
haana *ku-svik-a*
NEG 15-arrive-FV
'Mother sent the child to grandmother but she did not arrive.'

Thus, the LOCATIVE GOAL induces a pragmatic effect of emphasising the GOAL relation through the use of the applicative, as well as through the semantics of the verb, a double goal, if you like, an instance of what Marten (2002) refers to as concept strengthening. The effect is thus one of emphasis or focus on the GOAL itself, a hypothesis that is supported by the fact that the applicative verb can be used together with an explicit marking of the GOAL by *kuna* as in (25).[17]

(25) *Mai* *va-ka-tum-ir-a* *mw-ana* *kuna* *mbuya*
1a mother 2SM-PST-send-APPL-FV 1-child to 1a grandmother
'Mother sent the child to grandmother.'

This triple marking of the GOAL relation, through the semantics of the verb, the applicative affix and the goal marker *kuna* even further emphasises the endpoint of the GOAL and as such example (26) is even less acceptable than (24).[18]

(26) *??Mai* *va-ka-tum-ir-a* *mw-ana* *ku-na* *mbuya*
1a mother 2aSM-PST-send-APPL-FV 1-child 17-ASS 1a
grandmother
asi *haana* *ku-svik-a*
but NEG 15-arrive-FV
'Mother sent the child to grandmother but she did not arrive.'

Clearly, this use of the applicative morpheme can be connected with the adficiary and motive uses noted above: all involve the concept of GOAL. The difference between them is derived from the semantics of the verb. Where the verb is associated with a GOAL role through its lexical meaning, the internalisation of this role as an AO serves to

17 This according to Maarten Mous (pc) is also similar to the causative construction with a double agent.

18 Note in passing that the existence of examples like that in (20)(c) undermines syntactic analyses of the applicative that involves preposition incorporation (Baker 1988). The co-existence of the 'preposition' and the applicative morpheme indicates that they are not reflexes of the same syntactic position. The rather weak formulation of the semantic effect of the applicative affix given in (16) in the previous subsection, however, predicts that this should be possible. The append function encodes no requirement that the introduced argument is distinct from any other argument (or adjunct) of the verb. Hence, if an adjunct introduced by *kuna* adds a GOAL to the semantics of the verb this may unify with one introduced by the applicative affix.

specify that the endpoint is achieved. Hence, we have what we might call a LOCATIVE GOAL, differentiated from the GOAL underlying adficiary and motive readings by the semantics of the verb. Our hypothesis that the applicative morpheme denotes a GOAL relation is thus supported by these facts, underlining the idea that the precise interpretation of the role of an applied object is determined by semantic and pragmatic factors, not syntactic ones.

2.5. SOURCE and GOAL

A further piece of evidence in support of our hypothesis that the applicative affix introduces a GOAL argument can be found with certain verbs which, in their non-applied form, may have an expressed SOURCE, but which, in the applied form, are interpreted as taking a GOAL AO.

(27) (a)	*Beatrice*	*a-ka-dzok-a*	*(kubva)*	*ku-chi-koro*	
	1a name	1SM-PST-return-FV	from	17-7-school	
	'Beatrice returned from school.'				
(b)	*Beatrice*	*a-ka-dzok-er-a*	*ku-chi-koro*		
	1a name	1SM-PST-return-APPL-FV	17-7-school		
	'Beatrice went back to school.'				

(28) (a)	*Ma-war*	*veterans*	*a-ka-tiz-a*	*(kubva)*	*pa-purazi*
	6-war	veterans	6SM-PST-flee-FV	from	16-5 farm
	'War veterans fled from the farm.'				
(b)	*Ma-war*	*veterans*	*a-ka-tiz-ir-a*	*pa-purazi*	
	6-war	veterans	6SM-PST-flee-FV	16-5 farm	
	'War veterans ran onto the farm.'				

(29) (a)	*Grace*	*a-ka-tsvair-a*	*ma-rara*	*(kubva)*	*mu-mba*
	1a name	1SM-PST-sweep-FV	6-dirt	from	18-room
	'Grace swept dirt from the room.'				
(b)	*Grace*	*a-ka-tsvair-ir-a*	*ma-rara*	*mu-mba*	
	1a name	1SM-PST-sweep-APPL-FV	6-dirt	18-room	
	'Grace swept dirt into the room.'				

The SOURCE interpretation of the non-applicative verbs derive from the semantics of the verb (for instance, fleeing implies something one flees from, sweeping implies removing something from somewhere).[19] However, with applicatives, the AO is interpreted as a GOAL not a SOURCE, giving the effect of a reversal of the assumed role of one participant. The literature on Bantu applicatives is mainly silent about these examples, which Harford (1993) calls lexicalised or idiomatic, noting that they fall out-

---

19 In actual fact, the source argument is in most cases left out since it is implied.

side the purview of Lexical Mapping Theory (Bresnan & Moshi 1990, Alsina & Mchombo 1992), because the theta roles are not held constant, but change from SOURCE to GOAL. The verb still implies a SOURCE reading, of course, as part of the verbal semantics but where these participants explicitly appear, as in (30), they are no longer so closely associated with the verb:

(30) *Patricia* *a-ka-dzok-er-a* *ku-Harare* *a-chi-bv-a*
1a name 1SM-PST-depart-APPL-FV 17-Harare 1SM-FLPRE-come-FV
ku-Edinburgh
17-Edinburgh
'Patricia returned to Harare coming from Edinburgh.'

The importance of this example is to show that Edinburgh is interpreted as the SOURCE while Harare is the GOAL, despite both being identically marked with the locative affix *ku-*. It is thus the applicative object that provides the endpoint of the event (Harare) while the initial point is an adjunct.[20]

3. Non-Canonical Meanings

In the previous section, we argued that a single interpretation of the applicative construction is sufficient to account for the various basic interpretations of BENEFICIARY, MALEFICIARY, MOTIVE and GOAL readings of the applied object. In this section, we focus on two non-canonical interpretations denoting Location and SOURCE. In these roles, the generalised GOAL relation hypothesized to underlie the other interpretations is not obviously observable. We argue that these result instead from the grammaticalisation of the object position for purposes of information structure, possibly from the focus effects we have already observed in the GOAL interpretations.

3.1. LOCATIVE

As shown by Harford (1993) and Salkie (1994), locatives in ChiShona may appear in the clause with or without an applicative main verb. This gives rise to a situation in which we have minimal pairs such as those in (31)-(32):

20 The issue of the dual nature of locatives has occupied Bantu linguists for a while as to whether locatives should be treated as adverbs or as noun phrases. Perez-Harford (1983) argues that ChiShona locatives should be treated as adverbs since they are pseudo-subjects. Arguments have been postulated to treat locatives as prepositional phrases as argued for by Kashina (2000) when he analyses Silozi and claims that the locative classes of 15, 16, 17 and 18 within this language should be analysed as prepositions. Similarly, Dembetembe (1987) argues that the locative complements are distinct from real objects because we cannot question them using the same question word form as other nouns. However, in this paper, following Bresnan & Kanerva (1989) and Bresnan (1991), we adopt the position that distributional and morphological considerations indicate that locatives should be treated as noun phrases (see also Hyman & Duranti 1982).

(31) (a) *Yeso* *a-ka-chem-a* *pa-mu-chinjikwa.*
1a Jesus 1SM-PST-weep-FV 16-3-cross
'Jesus wept on the cross.'

(b) *Yeso* *a-ka-chem-er-a* *pa-mu-chinjikwa.*
1a Jesus 1SM-PST-weep-APPL-FV 16-3-cross
'Jesus wept [while he was] on the cross.'

(32) (a) *Baba* *va-ke* *va-ka-f-a* *mu-ma-oko* *a-ke*
1a father 2SM-POSS 2SM-PST-die-FV 18-6-hand 1SM-POSS
'His/Her father died in his/her hands.'

(b) *Baba* *va-ke* *va-ka-f-ir-a* *mu-ma-oko* *a-ke*
1a father 2SM-POSS 2aSM-PST-die-APPL-FV 18-6-hand 1SM-POSS
'His/Her father died in his/her hands.'

Although most native speakers agree that it is very difficult to differentiate the meanings of the applicative and non-applicative versions, there are subtle interpretational effects.

The non-applicative sentences in (31)(a)-(32)(a), which contain intransitive verb stems with an optional locative argument, have more than one interpretation. In sentence (32)(a), the preferred reading is that the dying of the father occurred literally in his child's hands. But there is another available reading in which the dying happened while father was generally in the child's hands (i.e. in the child's care). However, in the applicative construction, only one reading is available: (32)(b) can only mean 'the event of father dying' is located specifically in his child's arms. This strong implication that the applicative signals that the subject is located at the place where the AO is holds for the other example above: in (31)(a) Jesus wept whilst he was on the cross or when he just passed in the vicinity of the cross, while in (31)(b) in that the weeping of Jesus was located specifically on the cross, when he was being crucified. What then seems to be happening within applicative sentences is putting Jesus, and father respectively in a specific location where the event occurred and seem to be emphasising the location where the event happened.

Examples based on transitive verb stems are given in (33), (34). Again the function of the applicative suffix is to emphasise the event and where it specifically took place. The subject in these examples is restricted to being located in the same place as the applied object.

(33) (a) *Patrick* *a-ka-on-a* *va-sikana* *mu-gomo.*
1a name 1SM-PST-see-FV 2-girl 18-5 mountain
'Patrick saw the girls [while they were] on the mountain.'

(b) *Patrick* *a-ka-on-er-a* *va-sikana* *mu-gomo*
1a name 1SM-PST-see-APPL-FV 2-girl 18-5 mountain
'Patrick saw the girls [while he was] on the mountain.'

(34) (a) *Ramos* *a-ka-nzw-a* *mu-mhazi* *mu-chovha.*
1a name 1SM-PST-hear-FV 3-music 18-taxi
'Ramos heard music [while it was] in the emergency taxi.'

(b) *Ramos* *a-ka-nzw-ir-a* *mu-mhazi* *mu-chovha*
1a name 1SM-PST-hear-APPL-FV 3-music 18-taxi
'Ramos heard music [while he was] in the emergency taxi.'

The sentences (33)(a) and (34)(a) which have a non-applicative verb and an optional locative adjunct leave the location of the subject vague. Thus, (33)(a) is interpreted as locating the logical object, the girls, on the mountain when Patrick saw them but does not indicate anything specific about Patrick's location. Similarly, sentence (34)(a) has the preferred reading in which Ramos heard the music coming from the emergency taxi without indicating his location. These sentences could thus be interpreted with the subject in the same place as the locative adjunct, or not.

However, this is not the case with the applicative counterparts in (33)(b) and (34)(b). The former entails that Patrick's seeing the girls is true if and only if Patrick is also on the mountain. The latter example places both Ramos and the music within the emergency taxi. So an applicative locative in this context has the semantic function of restricting/constraining the location of an event as a whole to be in the same place as the locative AO, thus ensuring that subjects and any logical objects are also so located. As can be seen from the above, although both sentences in examples (33) and (34) encode the same proposition, the applied verb licenses an extra object and at the same time additional contextual effects which are not found with the non-applicative verb.[21] Notice that while this locative reinforcement does not appear to be derivable from any sort of GOAL relation, the inferential effect of 'x being located at AO' is one that we suggested as an enrichment of the applicative constructions involving RECIPIENT and PURPOSE, an emphasis on the endpoint of the event. In this case of LOCATIVE AOs, this provides the location of the event.

This specification of location of the event denoted by the main verb apparently introduced by the applicative affix may give rise to further inferential effects, such as inducing habitual readings or inducing contrastive focus interpretations. Consider the examples in (35)-(36):

---

[21] Note here that the locative marker in the locative object examples is retained when it becomes the applied object. If the locative marker is 'incorporated' (as Baker 1988) the sentence with an applicative verb is infelicitous as illustrated in (i) and (ii), which are marked as unacceptable rather than ungrammatical (#), as in the English translations, since it seems to be pragmatic infelicity rather than ungrammaticality per se that is at issue here. The introduction of an unmarked locative renders an inappropriate interpretation, at most giving a BENEFICIARY reading which is unacceptable. This shows that locative arguments within ChiShona should be treated as noun phrases which a verb can be obligatorily subcategorised for given appropriate modifications.

(i) *#Mu-biki* *a-no-bik-ir-a* *sadza* *moto*
1 cook 1SM-PRE-cook-APPL-FV 5 sadza 9 fire
'The cook is cooking sadza for an open fire.'

(ii) *#Margret* *a-ka-nyor-er-a* *tsamba* *tafura*
1a name 1SM-PST-write-APPL-FV 9 letter 9 table
'Margret wrote a letter for the table.'

(35) (a)	*Mu-biki*	*a-no-bik-a*	*sadza*	*pa-moto.*
	1-cook	1SM-PRE-cook-FV	5 sadza	16-9 fire
	'The cook is cooking sadza on an open fire.'			
(b)	*Mu-biki*	*a-no-bik-ir-a*	*sadza*	*pa-moto.*
	1-cook	1SM-PRE-cook-APPL-FV	5 sadza	16-9 fire
	'The cook is cooking *sadza* on an open fire.'			

(36) (a)	*Margret*	*a-ka-nyor-a*	*tsamba*	*pa-tafura.*
	1a name	1SM-PST-write-FV	9 letter	16-9 table
	'Margret wrote a letter on the table.'			
(b)	*Margret*	*a-ka-nyor-er-a*	*tsamba*	*pa-tafura.*
	1a name	1SM-PST-write-APPL-FV	9 letter	16-9 table
	'It was on the table that Margret wrote a letter.'			

The difference between (35)(a) and (35)(b) is that in the applicative form there is an emphasis on location indicates to the hearer that there is something significant about the event of cooking is taking place 'on an open fire'. One possible reading is that it is the subject's habit to cook sadza on an open fire.[22] A second reading is that the cook was cooking on an open fire instead of a stove because the sadza required a certain amount of fire heat. Similarly, in example (36)(a) we have the transitive use of *nyora* 'write', here with an optional adjunct, *pa-tafura* 'on the table'. In the applicative form in (36)(a), the adjunct has become an object (the AO) with extra contextual effects, that of contrastive focus: that Margret wrote the letter this time on the table, rather than on the floor, as indicated by the use of the English cleft construction in the translation. The point here is that the precise interpretation of the sentence depends on context interacting with the interpretation of the AO is indicating a strong locative relation with the event denoted by the main verb.

3.2. SOURCE

The section above has shown that the applicative suffix can have a locative interpretation emphasising the location at which an activity has taken place. Some applicatives, however, have an AO that is interpreted as a source, the initial point of some movement. The source interpretation is mainly determined by the lexical meaning of the verb.

(37) (a)	*Patricia*	*a-ka-simuk-a*	*(ku-Edinburgh)*
	1a name	1SM-PST-depart-FV	17-place
	'Patricia departed from Edinburgh.'		

---

[22] The habitual reading seems to be brought out not only by the applicative but the combination of the applicative and tense. More research needs to be done on the relation between tense and applicatives in Bantu.

(b)	*Patricia*	*a-ka-simuk-ir-a*	*ku-Edinburgh*
	1a name	1SM-PST-depart-APPL-FV	17-place
	'Patricia departed from Edinburgh.'		

(38) (a)	*Chi-tima*	*cha-ka-bv-a*	*ku-Harare*
	7-train	7SM-PST-come from-FV	17-place
	'The train came from Harare.'		
(b)	*Chi-tima*	*cha-ka-bv-ir-a*	*ku-Harare*
	7-train	7SM-PST-come from-APPL-FV	17-place
	'The train came from Harare.'		

The (a) and (b) sentences above are, like the locative examples in the previous section, truth conditionally equivalent, but most native speakers agree that they are subtly distinct. In the non-applicative form there is no implication that the source of the activity is exactly the initial point. So, in (37)(a) Patricia left from Edinburgh but Edinburgh might just have been a stopover in some longer journey and in (38) the train's point of departure is given as anywhere in Harare, but the train might have started its journey elsewhere. In the applicative forms, however, the point of departure is focused and there are implicatures that some definite place is intended (such as Edinburgh airport or the central train station in Harare) to constitute the **initial** source of the activity (Patricia's journey began at Edinburgh airport and the train starts out from Harare). The reading also gives rise to contrastive focus: due to some complication, Patricia's departure point ended up being Edinburgh instead of somewhere else; the train's point of origin ended up being Harare instead of Bulawayo for instance.

In section (2) it was hypothesised that GOAL, MOTIVE, MALEFICIARY and BENEFICIARY applied objects are essentially GOALs specifying a relation between the event denoted by the verb with the applied object. The specific interpretations were argued to depend on a number of contextual factors involving the semantics of the verb stem, the applied object and the logical object (if it is present) and pragmatic enrichment of location of some argument at the applied object and hence focussing on the completion (endpoint) of the event expressed by the clause. With SOURCE applicatives, the reading can thus be seen as a pragmatic effect of emphasising the **initial** point in a path not its endpoint, as with GOALs, giving rise to a focus reading in just the same way as some of the locative examples discussed in the previous subsection. The problem remains how to incorporate the locative and source roles into this hypothesis since the two seem to identify a **locative** relation.

There are two ways in which this position may be rectified. The first way would be to say that the applicative morpheme encodes a general LOCATIVE relation, one that may be interpreted as GOAL, SOURCE or LOCATIVE. While this seems to be a valid generalisation within ChiShona, it fails to account for the fact that the **default** interpretation is as a goal, of a more or less abstract sort, with the SOURCE and LOCATIVE AOs being less frequent.

The second is to explore the possibility that the SOURCE and LOCATIVE applied objects are the result of some process of grammaticalisation of the applicative construction. We have already seen that the locative examples seem to involve at least some of the effects of the GOAL interpretation by specifying the locative point of some entity as the AO. Unlike RECIPIENT but like PURPOSE, what is specified as at the AO is an event not an entity (denoted by the subject or logical object). Unlike PURPOSE, however, the event that is specified is that denoted by the verb stem. This as we have seen leads to the drawing of pragmatic inferences over the properties involved in the situation described (including tense) to give readings of habituality or contrast. The latter is a typical type of linguistic focus which, we suggest, provides the pragmatic bridge needed to explain the extension of the original GOAL features of the applicative construction to SOURCE interpretations.

Native speakers perceive applicative constructions involving these roles as emphasising or focusing the AO in some way. It is this that gives rise to the interpretations of locative examples as involving the actual location of an event **at** the AO, since the event is said to be located/being emphasised with respect to the applied object. This idea that the applicative morpheme involves focus can be seen in the appropriateness or otherwise of using an applicative form in reply to questions:

(39) (a) *Mw-ana* *a-ka-famb-(ir-)-a* *kupi?*
1-child 1SM-PST-walk-(APPL)-FV where
'Where did the child walk?'

(b) *??Mw-ana* *a-ka-famb-a* *mu-bindu*
1-child 1SM-PST-walk-FV 3-garden
'The child walked in the garden.'

(c) *Mw-ana* *a-ka-famb-ir-a* *mu-bindu*
1-child 1SM-PST-walk-APPL-FV 3-garden
'The child walked [while it was] in the garden.'

(40) (a) *Ndi-yani* *a-ka-famb-a* *mu-bindu?*
who 1SM-PST-walk-FV 18-garden
'Who walked in the garden?'

(b) *Mw-ana* *a-ka-famb-a* *mu-bindu*
1-child 1SM-PST-walk-FV 3-garden
'The child walked in the garden.'

(c) **Mw-ana* *a-ka-famb-ir-a* *mu-bindu*
1-child 1SM-PST-walk-APPL-FV 3-garden
'The child walked in the garden.'

(41) (a) *Patricia* *a-ka-simuk-(ir)-a* *ku-pi?*
1a name 1SM-PST-depart-APPL-FV 17-where
'Where did Patricia depart from?'

(b) *??Patricia* *a-ka-simuk-a* *ku-Edinburgh*
1a name 1SM-PST-depart-FV 17-place
'Patricia departed from Edinburgh.'

(c) *Patricia* *a-ka-simuk-ir-a* *ku-Edinburgh*
1a name 1SM-PST-depart-APPL-FV 17-place
'Patricia departed from Edinburgh.'

(42) (a) *Ndi-yani* *a-ka-simuk-a* *ku-Edinburgh?*
who 1SM-PST-depart-FV 17-place
'Who departed from Edinburgh?'

(b) *Patricia* *a-ka-simuk-a* *ku-Edinburgh*
1a name 1SM-PST-depart-FV 17-place
'Patricia departed from Edinburgh.'

(c) **Patricia* *a-ka-simuk-ir-a* *ku-Edinburgh*
1a name 1SM-PST-depart-APPL-FV 17-place
'Patricia departed from Edinburgh.'

This pragmatic explanation of the spread of the applicative from GOALs to SOURCEs is also supported by syntactic factors. The literature on the syntax (and semantics) of focus is vast and there is no intention of reviewing it here, but one of the things generally agreed about the phenomenon is that the focus of a sentence provides new information, or at least information that is currently of most relevance. Creissels (2004) in a discussion of the focus effects of the applicative construction in Tswana attributes these to the object properties of the AO, this being a position in many languages including the Bantu languages that provides new information. The association of object syntactic functions with the discourse interpretational effect of new information and focus provides a strong source in such languages for the using of objectivising constructions to put expressions in focus that would not otherwise receive straightforward stress. Ordinary SOURCE phrases are adjunct-like in ChiShona and do not interact with verbal complements in any obvious way (unlike LOCATIVEs and some GOALs, see Mabugu 2001). Therefore, extending the applicative construction which creates a new object to adjunctlike constructions is a natural move within the language, the locative nature of GOALs making them more likely to take part in initial grammaticalisation than non-locative roles such as Instrumental. That what is happening with the SOURCE examples is the internalisation of an adjunct (or promotion of adjunct to object) can be seen in examples such a those in (43) where the co-occurrence of *kubva* 'from' is required with non-applicative verbs but prohibited with applicative ones.

(43) (a) *Ma*-war veterans *a-ka-tor-a* *purazi* **(kubva)* *ku-mu-rimi*
6-war veteran 6SM-PST-take-FV 5 farm from 17-1-farmer
'The war veterans took the farm from the farmer.'

(b) *Ma*-war veterans *a-ka-tor-er-a* *(*kubva)*
6-war veteran 6SM-PST-take-APPL FV from
*(*ku-)mu-rimi* *purazi*
(17-)1-farmer 5 farm
'The war veterans took the farm away from the farmer.'

So what we have with SOURCE readings of an applicative object is a function of the grammaticalisation of the object function in ChiShona to mark sentential focus and the pragmatic enrichment of GOAL and LOCATIVE AOs to provide an explicit location for the event, subject or logical object.

4. Conclusion

We have in this paper argued that the basic applicative construction in ChiShona involves the introduction of an internal argument that is interpreted as involving a generalised GOAL relation with an event. If the identified event is that expressed by the main verb stem then, for events that do not lexically express a locative goal, the interpretation of the applied object is as an ADFICIARY. Negative connotations of the situation described by the clause normally lead to an interpretation as MALEFICIARY and positive ones as BENEFICIARY, but general linguistic context may alter this. Both roles may involve a pragmatic enhancement such that the AO is interpreted as being with (or at) either the subject or the logical object, yielding a RECIPIENT interpretation. Where the main verb stem lexically implies a locative GOAL and where the AO may be interpreted as a Location, then we derive instances of true (locative) GOALs. Where the AO is inanimate and not a possible location, the event with which the applied object is related is interpreted as an event GOAL of the main event, i.e. an inferred event that the main event is intended to bring out. In such cases, the AO is not itself the GOAL but merely a participant in some GOAL event determined pragmatically from context and thus interpreted as MOTIVE, either directly as REASON, or through enrichment of the BE-AT property, as PURPOSE. Animate AOs may also be so interpreted, depending on context. LOCATIVE and SOURCE AOs do not receive any sort of GOAL reading but are licensed in the applicative construction if they are focussed in the discourse. This development away from the basic GOAL applicative we suggest derives from the effect with true GOALs of emphasizing the actual location of the main event, subject or logical object at the place specified by the AO. This focuslike affect becomes associated with the general focus effects of objects and this leads to the development of other locative phrases coming into the domain of the applicative construction. Notice that in ChiShona, such non-canonical applicatives are restricted to locative relations, while in other Bantu languages (such as Swahili) instrumental, and perhaps other roles, may be marked by the applicative. This strongly implies that the applicative construction is continuing to undergo extensions from its canonical benefactive interpretation.[23] This development gives us a picture like that shown in Figure 3.

---

[23] See Trithart (1983) for a discussion of the historical development of the applicative construction that bolsters this view.

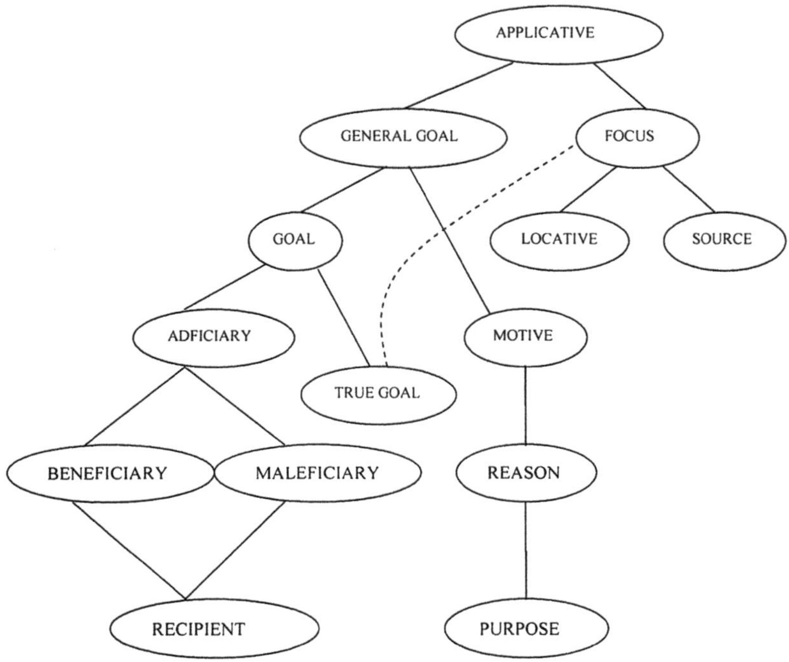

Figure 3: The applicative construction in ChiShona

References

Alsina, A. (1994): Bantu multiple objects: analyses and fallacies. *Linguistic Analysis* 24, 154-174.

Alsina, A. & Mchombo, S. (1992): The syntax of applicatives in Chichewa: problems for a theta theoretic asymmetry. *Natural Language and Linguistic Theory* 8, 493-506.

Alsina, A. & Mchombo, S. (1993): Object asymmetries and the Chichewa applicative construction. In: Mchombo (ed.), 17-45.

Baker, M. (1988): Theta theory and the syntax of applicatives in Chichewa. *Natural Language and Linguistic Theory* 6, 353-380.

Bentley, M.E. (1994): *The syntactic effects of animacy in Bantu languages*. Unpublished doctoral dissertation, Indiana University.

Bentley, M.E. (1998): The marking of grammatical relations in Swahili. *Studies in African Linguistics* 27, 177-197.

Berman, R. (1982): Dative marking of the effectee role: data from modern Hebrew. *Hebrew Annual Review* 6, 35-59.

Bresnan, J. (1991): *LOCATIVE case vs. locative gender*. Proceedings of 17th Annual Meeting of the Berkeley Linguistics Society.

Bresnan, J. & Kanerva, J. (1989): LOCATIVE inversion in Chichewa. *Linguistic Inquiry* 20, 1-50.

Bresnan, J. & Moshi, L. (1990): Object asymmetries in comparative Bantu syntax. *Linguistic Inquiry* 21, 147-185.

Carston, R. (2002): *Thoughts and utterances*. Oxford: Basil Blackwell.

Creissels, D. (2004): *Non-canonical applicatives and focalisation in Tswana*. Paper presented at Syntax of the World's Languages, Leipzig.

Dembetembe, N. (1979): A syntactic classification of non-auxiliary verbs in Shona. *Zambezia* 7, 471-484.

Fortune, G. (1984): *Shona grammatical constructions*. Volume 1. Mercury Press.

Foley, W.A. & Van Valin, R.D. (1984): *Functional syntax and Universal Grammar*. Cambridge: Cambridge University Press.

Frawley, W. (1992): *Linguistic semantics*. London: Lawrence Erlbaum.

Harford, C. (1993): The applicative in ChiShona and lexical mapping theory. In: Mchombo (ed.), 93-111.

Hawkinson, A. & Hyman, L. (1974): Hierarchies of natural topic in Shona. *Studies in African Linguistics* 5, 147-170.

Humphreys, R.L. (1999): Valency changing alternations. In: Brown, K. & Miller, J. (eds.): *Concise encyclopedia of grammatical categories*. Cambridge: Cambridge University Press.

Hyman, L. & Duranti, A. (1982): On the object relation in Bantu. In: Hopper, P. & Thompson, S. (eds.): *Syntax and Semantics 15: Studies in Transitivity*. New York: Academic Press.

Kashina, K. (2000): *Silozi constituent ordering and the theory of endweight*. Unpublished PhD dissertation. University of Edinburgh.

Khamisi, A. (1985): *Swahili verb derivation*. Unpublished doctoral dissertation. University of Hawaii.

Mabugu, P. (2001a): *Polysemy and the applicative verb construction in ChiShona*. Unpublished PhD dissertation. University of Edinburgh.

Mabugu, P. (2001b): A unitary description of the interpretations of ChiShona applicatives. In: Githiora, C., Littlefield, H. & Manfredi, V. (eds.): *Trends in African Linguistics* 5. Africa World Press.

Machobane, M. (1989): *Some restrictions of transitivising morphemes in Sesotho*. Unpublished doctoral dissertation, McGill University.

Marantz, A. (1984): *On the nature of grammatical relations*. Cambridge, MA: MIT Press.

Marantz, A. (1993): Implications of asymmetries in double object constructions. In: Mhombo (ed.), 113-150.

Marten, L. (2002): *At the syntax-pragmatics interface*. Oxford: Oxford University Press.

Matambirofa, F.A. (2003): *A lexical mapping theory account of the applicative and the causative extensions in Shona*. Unpublished PhD dissertation. University of Zimbabwe.

Mchombo, S. (ed.) (1993): *Theoretical aspects of Bantu grammar*. Stanford: CSLI Publications.

Ngonyani, D. (1996): *The morphosyntax of applicatives*. Unpublished doctoral dissertation. University of California.

Ngonyani, D. (1998): Properties of applied objects in KiSwahili and KiNdendeule. *Studies in African Linguistics* 27, 68-95.

Parson, T. (1990): *Events in the semantics of English*. Cambridge, MA: MIT Press.

Perez-Harford, C. (1983): LOCATIVE pseudo subjects in Shona. *Journal of African Languages and Linguistics* 5, 131-155.

Port, R. (1981): The applied suffix in Swahili. *Studies in African Linguistics* 12, 71-82.

Pylkkanen, L. (2000): What applicative heads apply to. *Penn Working Papers in Linguistics* vol. 6.4. University of Pennsylvania.

Salkie, R. (1994): *The applied extension in Shona and case theory*. 7th Niger-Congo Syntax and Semantics Workshop.

Schein, B. (1993): *Plurals and events*. Cambridge, MA: MIT Press.

Trithart, L.M. (1983): *The applied affix and transitivity: A historical study in Bantu*. Unpublished doctoral dissertation. UCLA.

Wierzbicka, A. (1988): *The semantics of grammar*. Amsterdam: John Benjamins.

Remarks on the Aspectual Polysemy of the Hungarian Verbal Particle *el* 'away/off'*

Balázs Szilárd

University of Szeged, Theoretical Linguistics PhD Program
H-6722 Szeged, Egyetem u. 2.
E-mail: szilardb@hung.u-szeged.hu

1. Introduction

It is a widespread assumption that the most important type of perfective motion event predicates describes the reaching of a goal. It is also well-known that verbal particles that surface preverbally usually – though not always – mark perfectivity in Hungarian. Thus, sentence (1) implies that a perfective event took place, at the end of which Péter was in the kitchen.

(1) *Péter* *be*$_{\text{PRT(=PARTICLE)}}$*ment* *a konyhá.ba.*
Péter PRT.went the kitchen.into
'Péter went in the kitchen.'

In this paper, my goal is to discuss aspectual phenomena related to the spatial uses of the Hungarian verbal particle *el* 'away/off'. (This particle has several non-spatial uses as well, but in this paper I disregard them.)

The particle *el* is to be found in contexts describing motion events implying the reaching of a goal, cf. (2), but also in contexts that do not imply arrival at a specific goal, cf. (3).

(2) (a) *Jani* *el*$_{\text{PRT}}$*.jutott* *a kapu.ig.*
Jani PRT.arrived the gate.to
'Jani arrived at the gate.'

---

* Publication of the present paper was supported by the Research Group for Theoretical Linguistics of the Hungarian Academy of Sciences at the Universities of Debrecen, Pécs and Szeged. It is an extended and revised version of a poster presentation presented at the *1st Central European Student Conference in Linguistics* (CESCL), Budapest, 29-31 May 2006. Many thanks to Károly Bibok, István Kenesei, Gergely Pethő, and Csilla Rákosi for their precious comments on issues discussed in this paper.

(b) *Jani* *el*$_{\text{PRT}}$*.jött* *hozzánk.*
Jani PRT.came to-us
'Jani came to us.'

(3) (a) *Péter* *el*$_{\text{PRT}}$*.hagyta* *a ház.at.*
Péter PRT.left the house.ACC
'Péter left the house.'

(b) *Péter* *el*$_{\text{PRT}}$*.lépett* *az ajtó.tól.*
Péter PRT.stepped the door.from
'Péter stepped away from the door.'

The predicates *eljutni* 'to arrive' and *eljönni* 'to come' demand an explicit goal adverbial, but they also allow insertion of an explicit source adverbial in the sentence. Semantically, these predicates imply the attainment of a specific goal associated with the syntactic goal argument of the sentence. On the other hand, the predicates *elhagyni* 'to leave' and *ellépni* 'to step away' demand an explicit source argument, and, furthermore, it is impossible to insert an explicit goal adverbial in sentences (3)(a) and (3)(b). (Note that it is possible for the predicates *eljönni* and *ellépni* to appear in sentences without an explicit goal argument or source argument, respectively – cf. *Jani eljött.* and *Péter ellépett.* –, but only in case a contextually salient place can be identified as the implicit goal or source argument, respectively.) On the basis of the presented data, I conclude that the Hungarian particle *el* is aspectually polysemous: it has two distinct perfective uses, one of which expresses an arrival event at a specific goal, while the other one expresses a departure event from a specific source.[1]

In addition to these two classes of *el*-verbs – i.e. the one demanding an explicit goal adverbial, and at the same time allowing an explicit source adverbial, as well; and the other one demanding an explicit source adverbial but at the same time excluding appearance of an explicit goal adverbial – there also exist other classes of motion verbs with *el.* First, the predicate *elindulni* 'to set forth to' allows an explicit source adverbial, and at the same time an explicit goal adverbial, as well. (Cf. *Péter el*$_{\text{PRT}}$*. indult otthon.ról a város.ba.* Péter PRT.left-for home.from the city.into 'Péter left home for the city'). Nevertheless, this predicate never implies arrival at the goal described by the explicit goal adverb. In other words, this predicate patterns syntactically with verbs belonging to the group in (2), but conveys different implications. Second, another class can be illustrated by the Hungarian predicate *elmenni* 'to go away', cf. (4).

(4) (a) *Ferenc* *el*$_{\text{PRT}}$*.ment* *az* *erdő.ig.*
Ferenc PRT.went the forest.to
'Ferenc went all the way to the forest.'

---

1 The term 'aspectual polysemy' is perhaps a little bit misleading, as at first sight the reader could expect that it covers cases where a linguistic description is ambiguous between a perfective and an imperfective reading.

(b) *Ferenc* *el*$_{PRT}$*.ment* *otthon.ról.*
Ferenc PRT.went home.from
'Ferenc left home.'

As the examples (4)(a) and (4)(b) show, the predicate *elmenni* can turn up in both contexts related to the two above-mentioned groups of *el*-verbs (cf. (2) and (3)). Thus, the question naturally arises whether the predicate *elmenni* is polysemous or it represents another natural class of *el*-verbs in Hungarian? In my opinion, the particle-verb *elmenni* is polysemous between a goal-reaching and a source-leaving reading, and, thus, its different uses fit into the two above-mentioned classes of *el*-predicates, cf. (2) and (3). Furthermore, having already established that the particle *el* is aspectually polysemous, I suggest that the polysemy of the motion verb *elmenni* – cf. 'to go away from a specific place' vs. 'to arrive at a specific place' – results from the polysemy of the spatial particle *el.* Note also that the predicate *elmenni* does not require obligatorily the presence of an explicit source argument, nor the presence of an explicit goal argument. Nevertheless, out of context, a missing source argument is always identifiable with a contextually salient place, while a missing goal argument usually is not, cf. *Ferenc el.ment* 'Ferenc went away' (from a specific place)(*to a specific place).

The structure of the paper is as follows. In section 2, I introduce the notions of goal-particle and source-particle. I will argue for the claim that most of the spatial uses of the Hungarian particles *be* 'into' and *el* 'away/off' can be taken as representatives of these two groups of particles, respectively, and that several syntactic and semantic asymmetries are observable between these two types of particle. Section 3 deals with the "goal-reaching" uses of particles. In this part, I will make use of related works of Tenny (1994), É. Kiss (2005), and Tschander (2003) who proposed detailed terminative analyses of motion events. The so-called terminative analysis claims that the perfectivity of motion events results from the attainment of a goal. Sections 4 and 5 deal with the "source-leaving" uses of the particle *el.* In section 4, I will introduce a system which is supposed to be an alternative to the terminative approach. This alternative system rests mainly on the mereo-topological analysis and the so-called Dominance Theory of Galton (2000). In section 5, I will apply this latter system to my Hungarian data: I will demonstrate that, on the one hand, this system can treat "source-leaving" uses of spatial particles more adequately than the more usual terminative approach, and, on the other hand, this system is also capable to furnish adequate analyses for "goal-reaching" uses of particles as well.

2. Verbal Particles

2.1. Hungarian Verbal Particles and Perfectivization Phenomena

Sentence aspect is more or less compositional in Hungarian, i.e. there are several tools to turn a lexically imperfective verb to a perfective predicate (cf. Kiefer 2000). Two of these tools are relevant to the subject matter of this paper: (i) particles positioned in the immediate preverbal position (cf. (5)(b)), and (ii) goal adverbials positioned in the immediate preverbal position (cf. (6)(b)):

(5) (a)	*Délután*	*Péter*	*ír.t*	*egy level.et.*
	In the afternoon	Péter	write.PAST	a letter.ACC
	'In the afternoon, Péter was writing a letter.'			
(b)	*Délután*	*Péter*	***meg***$_{\text{PRT}}$*.ír.t*	*egy level.et.*
	In the afternoon	Péter	**PRT**.write.PAST	a letter.ACC
	'In the afternoon, Péter wrote a letter.'			

(6) (a)	*Józsi fut.ott.*	
	Józsi run.PAST	
	'Józsi was running.'	
(b)	*Józsi* [***a szobá.ba***$_{\text{GOAL ADV}}$]	*fut.ott.*
	Józsi [**the room.into**]	run.PAST
	'Józsi ran into the room.'	

2.2. Source and Goal Particle Uses

I give the label 'goal particle' to those spatial uses of verbal particles that demand an explicit goal adverbial and imply the attainment of a specific goal associated with it – like presumably all the spatial uses of the Hungarian particle *be*, cf. (1), and at least some uses of the Hungarian particle *el*, cf. (2)(a) and (2)(b).

On the other hand, I label 'source particle' in advance those uses of the Hungarian verbal particle *el* that do not allow insertion of an explicit goal adverbial in the sentence, cf. (3)(a) and (3)(b). According to my intuitions, these uses of the verbal particle *el* do not require the goal of the motion to be identifiable with a specific place. (In section 5.2, I will introduce new definitions of goal particle use and source particle use, as well. However, these new definitions will not be in contradiction to the ones given in the current section.)

If we choose the spatial uses of the Hungarian particle *be* 'into', on the one hand, and some spatial uses of the particle *el* 'away/off' together with some spatial uses of the Hungarian particle *ki* 'out', on the other hand, as representatives of goal and source particles, respectively, then we can observe several syntactic and semantic differences in their behavior.

2.3. All the Spatial Uses of the Particle *be* 'into' Are Goal Particle Uses

As far as I know, all the spatial uses of the Hungarian verbal particle *be* show the typical syntactic and semantic characteristics of goal particles. Here, I will mention only a few of these characteristic features.

First, in the case of movement predicates containing the particle *be,* it is possible (or, more precisely, obligatory) to unequivocally reconstruct a goal with specific reference when the goal argument is not realized syntactically, cf. (7). Thus, in this case the implicit goal argument is referential.

(7) *Ferenc* *be.ment.* RECONSTRUCTABLE GOAL
Ferenc PRT.went
'Ferenc went in (*from a specific place)(to a specific place).'

Second, sentence (7) does not require the likewise implicit source argument to be unequivocally reconstructable. Note that the star in the English translation attached to the source adverbial in sentence (7) is not meant to exclude existence of contexts in which the source argument is unequivocally reconstructable. It states no more than the fact that out of context this sentence does not require the reconstructability of the source argument – as opposed to the goal argument. This means that in this example the source argument (as opposed to the goal argument) is not referential: it is only an existentially bound variable. Thus, sentence (7) conveys that Ferenc went from some unknown starting location into a specific place located in a conceptually closed region.

Third, the construction in which we put the goal argument in the preverbal position and omit the particle does not show any change in meaning when compared to the structure that contains both a preverbal particle and an explicit goal argument, cf. (8)(b) vs. (8)(a), borrowed from É. Kiss (2005).

(8) (a) *Péter* *be*$_{\text{PRT}}$*.gurította* [*a labdá.t*$_{\text{THEME}}$] [*a kapu.ba*$_{\text{GOAL ADV}}$].
Péter PRT.rolled [the ball.ACC] [the goal.into]
'Péter rolled the ball in the goal.'

(b) *Péter* [*a kapu.ba*$_{\text{TERMINUS}}$] *gurította* [*a labdá.t*$_{\text{THEME}}$].
Péter [the goal.into] rolled [the ball.ACC]
'Péter rolled the ball in the goal.'

2.4. Source Particle Uses of the Spatial Particles *el* 'away/off' and *ki* 'out'

As far as I know several spatial uses of the Hungarian verbal particles *el* 'away/off' and *ki* 'out' do not show the typical syntactic and semantic features of goal particles. However, the use types of these particles do not show as clear a homogeneity as the uses of the particle *be* (cf. section 2.3). In other words, while the uses of the verbal particle *be* were all to be classified as goal particle uses, in the case of the verbal particles *el* and *ki* it is possible to find source particle uses as well as goal particle uses. For example, (2)(a) and (2)(b) above are to be classified as goal particle uses of the particle *el*. On the other hand, in this section I deal with characteristic features of source particle uses of the verbal particles *el* and *ki*.

First, while sentence (7) is acceptable just in case the goal argument is reconstructable with a specific reference, the interpretation of its *el*-counterpart does not require this, cf. (9):

(9) *Ferenc* *el*$_{\text{PRT}}$*.ment.* RECONSTRUCTABLE SOURCE
Ferenc PRT.went
'Ferenc went away (from a specific place)(*to a specific place).'

Second, in the case of source particle uses it is possible to reconstruct a source argument with specific reference when this thematic role is not filled in by any of the overt syntactic arguments, cf. (9).

2.5. Goal Adverbials and the Verbal Particles *el* and *ki*

As I mentioned before, these verbal particles have goal particle uses, as well. Thus, there are examples in which these verbal particles co-occur with an explicit goal adverbial. Often, these goal particle uses match perfectly with the general picture of goal particle use presented in section 2.3. Nevertheless, there are some intriguing data in connection with some goal particle uses of *el* and *ki*.

First, if we try to analyze the sentence pair given in (10) on the basis of a presumed parallel with the sentence pair given in (8), then we should not expect any change in meaning if we put the goal argument in the immediate preverbal position and omit the particle. However, in fact, we do observe semantic changes.

(10)(a) *János* *ki*$_{\text{PRT}}$*.rakta* *[a könyvek.et]* *[a polc.ra]*.
János PRT.put [the books.ACC] [the shelf.onto]
'János put the books out of some closed space onto the shelf.'

(b) *János* *[a polc.ra]* *rakta* *[a könyvek.et]*.
János [the shelf.onto] put [the books.ACC]
'János put the books on(to) the shelf.'

Sentence (10)(a) implies that János first took the books out of a closed space (presumably out of a box), and then he put them on the shelf. On the other hand, sentence (10)(b) does not express any more than the fact that János put the books on the shelf. This means that the sentence variant containing the particle *ki* 'out' conveys extra information about the source of the motion, as opposed to the variant with a preverbal goal adverbial and a bare verb form.

Second, there is a syntactic structure, in which the particles *ki* and *el* naturally group together in a same class, as opposed to e.g. the particle *be*. While predicates like *elmenni* 'to go away' and *kimenni* 'to go out' tolerate a goal adverbial formed with the postposition *felé* 'towards', predicates like *bemenni* 'to go into' do not, cf. (11).

(11) A: *Mit csinált Péter tegnap?*
'What did Péter do yesterday?'

B: (a) *El*$_{\text{PRT}}$*.ment* *autó.val* *Makó felé.*
PRT.went car.with Makó towards
'He went (on a trip) towards Makó by car.'

(b) *Ki*$_{\text{PRT}}$*.ment* *autó.val* *Makó felé.*
PRT.went car.with Makó towards
'He went (out of the city) (on a trip) towards Makó by car.'

(c) **Be$_{PRT}$.ment autó.val Makó felé.*
PRT.went car.with Makó towards
*'He went into on a trip towards Makó by car.'

In my opinion, the examples (11)(a)-(c) confirm the claim that there exist two distinct use types of spatial verbal particles in Hungarian, one of which enforces a "goal-reaching" reading on the sentence, whereas the other one does not.

3. The Terminative Approach

As I already mentioned above, for example the uses of the particle *be* – and some of the uses of the particle *el* – are to be classified as goal particle uses. In this section, I survey the usual analysis of goal particle uses of particles: the so-called terminative approach.

According to Carol Tenny (1994: 4f.), perfectivization – 'measuring out' in her terms – of an event depends on the so-called aspectual role grid associated with predicates. The aspectual role grid is a special kind of theta grid: i.e. the sum of semantic roles associated with predicates.[2] Aspectual roles can be used in the same way as thematic roles have been used: a verb has a set of aspectual roles to assign to its arguments, and linking principles govern the mapping of aspectual roles onto syntax.

Arguments fulfilling aspectual roles can provide a gradable scale and/or an endpoint on that scale: if we go through the scale and reach the endpoint, the event will be perfective. It follows that not all the syntactic arguments of verbal predicates are supposed to be associated with aspectual roles.

The three kind of aspectual roles used by Tenny (1994: 94-106) are the following:

MEASURE: provides both a gradable parameter (scale) and the endpoint, cf. (12).
PATH: provides only the scale along which the event is measured out, cf. (13).
TERMINUS(= endpoint): marks the endpoint on an independently given scale, cf. (13).

(12) *John*$_{\text{SUBJECT}}$ *ate* [*an apple*$_{\text{MEASURE – DIRECT INTERNAL ARGUMENT}}$].

(13) *Bill*$_{\text{SUBJECT}}$ *climbed* [*the ladder*$_{\text{PATH – DIRECT INTERNAL ARGUMENT}}$] *to* [*the top*$_{\text{TERMINUS – INDIRECT INTERNAL ARGUMENT}}$].

[2] Levin and Rappaport Hovav (2005) claim that alternative argument realization patterns of a same verb result from alternative conceptualizations of a same event that are attached to different semantic argument role grids (cf. *Brett swept the floor* vs. *Brett swept the floor clean*). One major type of theory dealing with event conceptualization is the so-called aspectual approach, as represented by Tenny (1994).

According to Tenny, MEASURE and PATH take the form of direct internal arguments, while TERMINUS appears as an indirect internal argument (i.e. PP). The event described by the sentence is perfective if in the sentence (i) there is an argument with a MEASURE aspectual role or (ii) there are two arguments with a PATH and a TERMINUS role, respectively, (cf. (12) and (13)).[3] Furthermore, Tenny (1994: 69) claims that there is only one kind of indirect internal argument (i.e. PP), in terms of thematic roles, that does affect aspectual structure, and that is a goal expressing the TERMINUS of the event.

According to Katalin É. Kiss (2005: 64), a major type of delimited events denotes a change of location of the theme argument, and in these cases the endpoint of the motion is "expressed by an argument bearing a terminus role in the terminology of Tenny (1994)". Moreover, a predicate expressing a terminated motion event has a verbal particle of a terminative role, cf. the particle *be* in (8)(a) repeated just below. (The term 'terminative particle' refers to one of the two types of particles stipulated by É. Kiss 2005. While so-called terminative particles are supposed to mark the temporal endpoint of a perfective event, the so-called 'resultative particles' mark the result state following the event described by a perfective sentence. Resultative particles are supposed to have the same semantic effect as resultative secondary predicates: cf. *Mari kimosta a ruhákat* Mari PRT.washed the clothes.ACC 'Mari washed the clothes clean' as compared to *Mari tisztára mosta a ruhákat* Mari clean.to washed the clothes.ACC 'Mari washed the clothes clean'.)

(8) (a) *Péter* *be*$_{\text{PRT}}$.*gurította* [*a labdá.t*$_{\text{THEME}}$] [*a kapu.ba*$_{\text{TERMINUS=GOAL ADV}}$].
Péter into.rolled the ball.ACC [the goal.into]
'Péter rolled the ball in the goal.'

(b) *Péter* [*a kapu.ba*$_{\text{TERMINUS}}$] *gurította* [*a labdá.t*$_{\text{THEME}}$].
Péter [the goal.into] rolled [the ball.ACC]
'Péter rolled the ball in the goal.'

É. Kiss (2005: 64) claims that "[t]he particle bears the same type of relation to the terminus argument as an object clitic bears to the lexical object in a clitic doubling construction". (Clitic doubling constructions are well-known in Romance languages.) That is why the sentence meaning does not change in Hungarian when the terminus argument occupies the immediate preverbal position and the particle is omitted, cf. (8)(b) vs. (8)(a) above.

É. Kiss (2005: 65) noticed that there is a problem with this analysis: "[a] terminative verbal particle [sic!] sometimes co-occurs with a source argument: however, despite appearances, it is independent of the source argument; it is associated with the explicit or implicit terminus in such cases as well", cf. (14):

(14) *Péter* *ki*$_{\text{PRT}}$.*ment* *a szobá.ból.*
Péter PRT.went the room.from
'Peter went out of the room.'

---

[3] Sentences having PATH arguments but no TERMINUS argument are of imperfective aspect. On the other hand, if there is a TERMINUS argument but no PATH argument, the sentence is perfective, and the presence of an implicit PATH-argument is stipulated.

The problem noticed by É. Kiss (2005) in connection with sentence (14) is related to the fact that different particle-verbs composed of the same verb but different particles can convey different presuppositions. For example, the predicate *bemenni* 'to go into' expresses that the motion ended in a closed space, but conveys no precise information about the starting location. On the other hand, the predicate *kimenni* 'to go out' locates the starting point in a closed space, and puts no constraint on the endpoint. These presuppositional discrepancies among particles are challenges to theories treating all the spatial uses of particles as homogeneously referring to a specific end location of the moving entity. In my opinion, it is not necessary to maintain the claim that examples like (14) do also contain terminative verbal particles as É. Kiss suggests in the quotation.

Ladina Tschander (2003) presented an analysis of spatial verbal particles which is very similar to that of É. Kiss (2005). According to Tschander (2003: 422f.), in sentences containing complex verb constructions (i.e. particle-verbs) "the additional prepositional phrase identifies the goal given implicitly by the meaning of the particle". For example, in sentence (15) the PP *in das Wasser* 'in the water' clarifies the implicit goal expressed by the particle *ein* 'into'.

(15)	*Max ist*	*in das Wasser*	*ein*$_{\text{PRT}}$*.getaucht.*
	Max has	into the water	PRT.dived
	'Max has dived into the water.'		

However, Tschander (2003: 411) – as compared to É. Kiss (2005) – went a step further. Tschander, who assumes – like many other linguists – that particles are intransitive variants of existing prepositions, excluded the German particle *ab* 'away' from her analysis, because it is not absolutely clear what the corresponding preposition should be. Similarly, if we assume that Hungarian verbal particles are associated with full PPs (cf. É. Kiss 2005), it seems difficult to find a unique type of PP associated with the particle *el*, as it has two quite different use types.

In my opinion, the behavior of the particles Hung. *el* 'away/off', *ki* 'out' and Germ. *ab* 'away' can be accounted for, if we admit that there exist non-terminative directional spatial particles, as well. The first step towards this analysis would be to admit that source denoting expressions are also able to perfectivize motion events. In fact, this is what Joost Zwarts (2005) proposes: "there is no aspectual asymmetry between source prepositions and goal expressions". That is why sentence (16) is "telic even though *away from the accident* does not specify a particular endpoint" – note that sentence (16) contains a verbal particle:

(16) *Alex ran away*$_{\text{PRT}}$ *from the accident.*

4. The Alternative Approach

In what follows, I will propose an alternative analysis of directional spatial verbal particles. In this work, I will rely mostly on the mereo-topological system of Galton (2000). Galton's (2000) system makes use of the Regional Connection Calculus of

Randell et al. (1992) and supplements it with a so-called Dominance Theory. In section 4, I survey these systems, and in section 5, I will apply them to the investigated data.

4.1. The Reference Region Approach

Before presenting Galton's system, I make a short detour, and introduce a few general ideas of the so-called reference region approach.

According to Talmy (1975: 181), in a motion situation one object (the so-called Figure) is moving with respect to another object (the so-called Ground). Furthermore, Galton (2000: 157) claims that the reference object (= Ground) "may be regarded as generating a continuous field of locations in the space around and/or within it, which may be partitioned into zones of qualitatively similar locations". These "zones of qualitatively similar locations" are the so-called reference regions. The meaning of locative and directional prepositions, adverbs, particles etc. can be defined by locating the starting point and the endpoint, or some intermediate point(s) of the path in a particular region relative to the reference object (cf. also Zwarts 2005).

While this approach can be adequate when used to characterize locative expressions, we run into problems when trying to apply it to directional PPs, and to motion in general. A crucial problem that turns up in connection with source and goal particles is that the reference region approach cannot answer the following question on its own: Which subevent can perfectivize the whole motion event?

To answer this question we have to enrich our actual system with further tools. This will be done in sections 4.2-4.4.

4.2. Mereo-Topology: Mereology and Topology

According to Krifka (1998, 2001), we have to assume more general topological structures if we want to deal with movement predicates. Topological structures are richer than mereological structures. We need them because "temporal adjacency of movement events is reflected in spatial adjacency of the paths and vice versa", and adjacency cannot be captured in a pure mereological system. The basic relation in topological structures is connectedness. The mereological part relation as well as the adjacency relation can be defined on the basis of the connectedness relation.

The next notion we have to become familiar with is the notion of the topological space. A topological space is any system consisting of a set of points together with a specification of which sets of points are to count as neighborhoods of each given point. In a topological space, we can define the interior, closure, exterior and boundary of a set (Galton 2000: 48).

4.3. The RCC8 Theory

The Regional Connection Calculus was developed by Randell, Cui and Cohn (1992) in a topological background. The unique primitive relation of the system is connection (C), which is both reflexive and symmetric. Using connection as a primitive, RCC8 defines a set of eight mutually exclusive relations, such that any two regions of the same dimension and co-dimension must stand in exactly one of the eight relations (cf. number 8 in the name of the theory). The notion of co-dimensionality means that regions of the same co-dimensionality must be embedded in a space which is of the same dimensionality number (e.g. three-dimensional) as the regions themselves. Thus, RCC8 investigates situations in which, for example, two three-dimensional regions interact in a three-dimensional space.

The eight mutually exclusive relations of RCC8 are given in the lines written in boldface italic in Figure 1 (cf. Galton 2000: 75-79).

P(x,y): part-of	$\forall z[\mathrm{C}(z,x) \rightarrow \mathrm{C}(z,y)]$
PP(x,y): proper part-of	$\mathrm{P}(x,y) \wedge \neg\mathrm{P}(y,x)$
O(x,y): overlap	$\exists z\ [\mathrm{P}(z,x) \wedge \mathrm{P}(z,y)]$
DC(x,y): disconnection	$\neg\ \mathrm{C}(x,y)$
EC(x,y): external contact	$\mathrm{C}(x,y) \wedge \neg\mathrm{O}(x,y)$
PO(x,y): partial overlap	$\mathrm{O}(x,y) \wedge \neg\mathrm{P}(x,y) \wedge \neg\mathrm{P}(y,x)$
EQ(x,y): equality	$\forall z[\mathrm{C}(z,x) \leftrightarrow \mathrm{C}(z,y)]$
TPP(x,y): tangential proper part	$\mathrm{PP}(x,y) \wedge \exists z[\mathrm{EC}(z,x) \wedge \mathrm{EC}(z,y)]$
NTPP(x,y): non-tangential proper part	$\mathrm{PP}(x,y) \wedge \neg\mathrm{TPP}(x,y)$
TPPI(x,y): TPP-inverse	$\mathrm{TPP}(y,x)$
NTPPI(x,y): NTPP-inverse	$\mathrm{NTPP}(y,x)$

Figure 1

The first three relations in Figure 1 can be expressed as disjunctions of the eight RCC-relations, and thus they are only notational simplifications:

(i) $\mathrm{P}(x,y) = \mathrm{EQ}(x,y) \vee \mathrm{TPP}(x,y) \vee \mathrm{NTPP}(x,y)$

(ii) $\mathrm{PP}(x,y) = \mathrm{TPP}(x,y) \vee \mathrm{NTPP}(x,y)$

(iii) $\mathrm{O}(x,y) = \mathrm{PO}(x,y) \vee \mathrm{EQ}(x,y) \vee \mathrm{TPP}(x,y) \vee \mathrm{NTPP}(x,y) \vee \mathrm{TPPI}(x,y) \vee \mathrm{NTPPI}(x,y)$

There are several direct and indirect transition types between these eight relations: that is to say that starting from a given state characterized by a given RCC-relation we cannot reach all the states characterized by other RCC-relations in one step. To demonstrate this fact we can use a so-called conceptual neighborhood diagram, which shows how RCC-relations change between any two regions when the regions themselves undergo continuous spatial change (change in position, orientation, shape, size etc.). In what follows, I will restrict myself to continuous change of position, i.e. motion.

In the case of continuous motion, there are no instantaneous jumps from one state to a different state (Galton 2000: 305). According to Galton (2000: 19f.), the possibilities for variety of any property (e.g. location, size, color, temperature, speed) define a so-called space of variation (the so-called phase space) that can be characterized in terms of some set of numerical parameters. The phase space is mathematically (numerically ~ quantitatively) continuous, and is to be divided up into broad categories. As Galton writes "the range of each parameter is divided up into intervals at salient 'landmark' values", and any other values – apart from the landmark values – are abstracted away. (For example, the range of the parameter on a temperature scale is divided up into intervals at degrees Celsius, and any temperature level is classified as one of the distinct degrees Celsius.) After having made the partition of the phase space we obtain a so-called mode space, which is a qualitative (i.e. not quantitative) state space. A qualitative space – as opposed to a quantitative one – is not continuous, but discrete, i.e. categories in a qualitative space are supposed to have sharp boundaries.[4]

Galton (2000: 127) claims that "natural objects [...] tend to undergo continuous, rather than abrupt changes", and this goes for motion, as well. This means that a parallel can be drawn between the analysis of Galton (2000) and that of Jackendoff (1996). Jackendoff (1996: 316f.) encodes motion as a continuous change over time, instead of treating it as a finite sequence of states. In his words, "we conceptualize both the path over which motion takes place and the time period during which motion takes place as dense intervals – they map onto the real numbers". In other words, the phase space of motion is continuous, but it can be (conceptually) divided up into discrete regions (spatial categories).

Figure 2 shows the conceptual neighborhood diagram of RCC-relations and describes the possible transition types between them (note that the arrows are bidirectional):

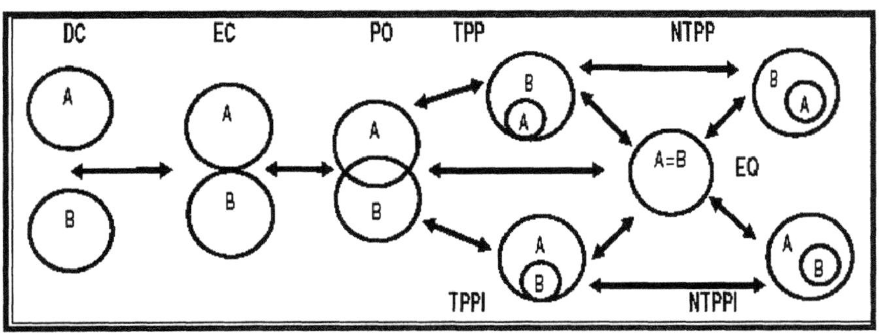

Figure 2

[4] The terms 'phase' and 'mode' are near-synonyms: they both refer to different subevents of a greater event (events like e.g. the warming up of a soup or the acceleration of a car). The difference is that the terms 'phase' and 'mode' are theoretically associated with the quantitative representational tier and with the qualitative representational tier, respectively.

The following example illustrates the use of the conceptual neighborhood diagram of RCC-relations. Assuming continuous motion, when someone enters a room we can observe the following relations between the region occupied by her body and that of the room, and in the given order: DC → EC → PO → TPP. (And, as Galton 2000: 168 writes, if afterwards she gets into bed and lifts her legs up the floor then her relation to the room becomes NTPP.)

An important property of Figure 2 is that there are three distinct situation classes summarized in it according to the following two parameters: (i) the regions can/cannot change their shape and/or size; (ii) the regions are/are not of equal size, cf. Figure 3. In this paper, I discuss situations including rigid regions only.

non-equal rigid regions	DC ↔ EC ↔ PO ↔ TPP ↔ NTPP, and DC ↔ EC ↔ PO ↔ TPPI ↔ NTPPI
rigid regions of equal size	DC ↔ EC ↔ PO ↔ EQ
non-rigid regions	EQ ↔ TPP(I), and EQ ↔ NTPP(I), and PO ↔ EQ, etc.

Figure 3

4.4. Galton's Dominance Theory

With the help of the RCC8 relations, Galton (2000: 282-86) discusses several motion types, such as the following ones (the numbers given in the lower indices refer to one and the same (1-1) or to two different regions (1-2)):

(17)(a) entering a region ($EC_1 \rightarrow TPP_1$),
(b) coming into contact ($DC_1 \rightarrow EC_1$),
(c) moving from one region to another-1 ($TPP_1 \rightarrow TPP_2$),
(d) moving from one region to another-2 ($EC_1 \rightarrow EC_2$).

The Dominance Theory of Galton (2000) enables us to distinguish punctual and non-punctual subevents from each other in a motion event. In the qualitative representational tier, subevents are called modes (cf. footnote 4). In the case of continuous spatial change sequences, Galton distinguishes more dominant modes and less dominant modes. According to Galton (2000: 378), more dominant modes (= landmark modes) are more unstable, existing as they do in the interstices between their less dominant neighbors. Furthermore, assuming continuous motion, less dominant modes (= non-landmark modes) correspond to open intervals, while more dominant modes[5] hold at isolated instants, i.e. at closed intervals (Galton 2000: 346).

[5] Of course, those modes named as landmark modes in certain examples by Galton can hold over open intervals, too, but just in case (i) the objects (regions) between which we observe the relations under discussion are not changing any of their spatial properties (e.g. their location), or in case (ii) the mode under discussion is a less dominant mode in the given situation. (We must note that a same mode can be a dominant mode or a dominated mode in different situations.)

What does it mean for a mode to dominate another mode? Galton (2000: 375) claims that a relation *r* dominates a relation *r'* if and only if it is possible for the relation which appears as *r* at a certain level of granularity to appear as *r'* at a finer level. Galton mentions that his approach to dominance coincides with the notion of downward granularity conversion used by Euzenat (1995). Euzenat (1995) uses downward granularity conversion in defining the above-mentioned conceptual neighborhood relation between relations. When applied to a given relation, the downward conversion operator provides a set of relationships at a finer granularity which represents what can be perceived potentially under this latter granularity. Euzenat gives us the following example: when you are standing far from a house you see a truck next to it, and they seem to meet (EC-relation). But approaching closer you notice a little space between them (DC-relation). So, for EC it is possible to turn into DC at a finer resolution level, and thus EC dominates DC.

5. Perfectivizer Subevents in Motion Events: A Case Study of the Spatial Particle *'el'*

5.1. The Punctual Subevent Approach

The approach to spatial verbal particles represented by É. Kiss (2005) and Tschander (2003) can be labeled 'goal-particle-analysis', as it treats spatial uses of particles as elements indicating the endpoints of motion events. On the other hand, I give the label 'punctual-subevent-analysis' to the alternative approach, that I argue for in this article. We can summarize the tools necessary for the punctual-subevent-analysis as follows.

First, RCC8 and the conceptual neighborhood diagram can determine the subevents (modes) of a continuous motion event. Second, Galton's Dominance Theory can differentiate landmark and non-landmark modes. Third, in case of continuous motion, landmark modes hold at isolated instants. And fourth, I accept Ferenc Kiefer's (2000: 303) claim, according to which a sentence is of perfective aspect just in case its event structure contains a punctual subevent. Kiefer (2000) assumes that non-punctual perfective events[6] always contain at least one punctual subevent. (As he writes: the moments of having written the letter or of having reached the top count as punctual subevents, cf. *Peter wrote a letter* and *Peter climbed the mountain*).

5.2. Case Study

Now we can apply the above-mentioned tools to the investigated data. I will demonstrate how this system works with the help of some source particle uses of the Hungarian particle *el* 'away/off'. But if we go through the four steps mentioned in section

---

[6] Kiefer (2000: 276) uses the notion of perfective aspect in much the same way as Krifka (1998) uses the notion of quantized predicate: an event is perfective if and only if there is no such proper part of its temporal domain that the event could also be predicated of that subdomain. Zwarts (2005), as opposed to Krifka, argues that the relevant property distinguishing perfective and imperfective events is not quantization, but cumulativity. In this paper, I ignore this issue.

5.1, we can obtain adequate analyses of other source particles (e.g. Hung. *ki* 'out') and of goal particles like Hung. *be* 'into' as well.

I will analyze the following three examples:

(18)	*Ferenc*	*el*$_{PRT}$*.ment*	[*otthon.ról*].
	Ferenc	PRT.went	[home.from]
	'Ferenc left home.'		

(19)	*A labda*	*el*$_{PRT}$*.pattant*	[*az asztal.ról*].
	The ball	PRT.bounced	[the table.from]
	'The ball bounced away from the table.'		

(20)	*A repülő*	*el*$_{PRT}$*.hagyta*	[*a magyar légteret*].
	The airplane	PRT.left	[the Hungarian airspace]
	'The plane left the Hungarian airspace.'		

As I mentioned earlier, we have to go through the four steps of the analysis.

In step one, we have to carry out the RCC8-translations of the examples (18)-(20). The translations are as follows:

Example (18):	EC → DC (or: TPP → PO → EC → DC)
Example (19):	DC → EC → DC
Example (20):	NTPP → TPP → PO → EC → DC

In the case of example (18), we can imagine two different situations with respect to the location occupied by Ferenc at the beginning of the situation described: (i) Ferenc was at the front door next to his apartment (standing in EC relation with his apartment), (ii) Ferenc was inside his apartment (TPP-relation).

In step two, we have to differentiate landmark modes from non-landmark ones. If we apply the test of granularity conversion, then we see that the relation EC can potentially turn into PO or DC (cf. Euzenat's truck-and-the-house example), and TPP can potentially turn into PO or NTPP when changing to a finer resolution level. On the other hand, the inverse conversions (PO > EC, or DC > EC, or PO > TPP, or NTPP > TPP) are impossible when we change from a coarser resolution level to a finer one. Thus, in examples (18)-(20), TPP and EC are the landmark-modes.

In step three, we have to decide which modes represent punctual subevents of the whole motion event. In case of continuous motion, landmark modes hold at isolated instants, thus, in the examples (18)-(20) EC and TPP turn out to be associated with instantaneous subevents. Two clarifications are required. First, in the reading of example (18) in which EC is assumed to be the initial mode, we disregard the time period prior to the beginning of the motion when saying that EC must hold at an instant. On the other hand, in the case of examples (19) and (20), this conceptual step is unnecessary, as in those cases landmark-modes are "really" punctual. Second, as Gergely Pethő pointed out in a personal comment, in the reading of sentence (18) starting from the TPP mode, Ferenc is allowed to stop for a while at the inner or the outer side of the door, and thus, TPP and EC modes can be durative. This possibility is a challenge for the present analysis. Thus, I suggest that it is possible to map real motion situations onto continuous RCC-sequences at the level of conceptual representations in such a way that intermediate stops are abstracted away.

Finally, in step four, I make use of Kiefer's above-mentioned claim according to which a sentence is perfective just in case its event structure contains a punctual subevent. Therefore I claim that in the examples (18)-(20) some non-final subevent performs the perfectivization. Note that in all the examples this non-terminative subevent (TPP or EC) is semantically linked to the implicit source-argument, as these subevents are associated to RCC-relations, which describe the location of the moving entity with respect to the source argument's referent. (For example, in sentence (18) TPP and EC relations hold between the body of Ferenc and the referent of his home.) Thus, it is possible to establish new definitions of source particles and goal particles as well (cf. section 2.2): some given instances of particles are to be classified as source particles (or goal particles) if and only if the punctual subevents perfectivizing the whole motion events are attached to RCC modes defining the location of the moving entity with respect to the source argument's referent (or with respect to the goal argument's referent, respectively).

Last but not least, we can try to answer the following question: in the examples (18) to (20), is EC or TPP mode the unique perfectivizing subevent? These sentences describe departure events instead of arrival events, and thus, considering the direction of movement, EC mode performs the perfectivization, according to my intuitions. In the case of sentences (18) and (20), EC mode describes the moment when the moving entity got his body totally outside of the referent region (Ferenc from his home, the plane from the Hungarian airspace).

Sentence (19) is different, but in that case there is only one punctual subevent to be found, according to the present analysis.

6. Conclusion and Prospects

At the beginning of this paper, I presented some data related to the Hungarian verbal particle *el* which demonstrated that this particle is able to perfectivize motion events in two ways. On the one hand, it can express the arrival at a goal, and, on the other hand, it can express the departure from a specific source without implying the arrival at a specific place. The important thing to note was that either of these uses is of perfective aspect. In section 2, I presented some evidence to my claim that it is possible to differentiate between two kinds of use of particles with respect to their perfectivizing capacity in sentences describing motion events in Hungarian. While so-called 'goal particle uses' can perfectivize only with the help of the goal argument, the so-called 'source particle uses' are able to perfectivize motion events with the help of the source argument. Some particles – like the Hungarian particle *be* 'into'- are assumed to bear goal particle uses constantly, while others – like the Hungarian particle *el* 'away/off' – are assumed to have source particle uses as well as goal particle uses. In section 3, I surveyed the traditional terminative approach to perfectivity found in the literature in connection with motion events, according to which perfective motion events always express the reaching of a goal (Tenny 1994 and É. Kiss 2005). In section 4 and 5, I introduced an alternative approach (the so-called punctual subevent approach), which was mainly based on the mereo-topological analysis and the Dominance Theory of Galton (2000).

The punctual subevent approach has several advantages over the traditional terminative approach. First of all, it handles more adequately the linguistic data related to source particle uses (cf. Hungarian *el*).

Second, this approach can maintain the traditional analysis of goal particles according to which they perform the perfectivization with the help of some motion phase determined by the goal argument. We can check that in the case of sentences containing goal particles like Hung. *be* 'into' there are subevents related to the goal argument, which are potentially punctual and, thus, able to perfectivize the event. (Albeit these subevents need not be final in an absolute sense, the only requirement for them is to be semantically related to the goal argument.[7]) So it is possible to provide a unified analysis of the classes of source and goal particles (prepositions etc.), and at the same time to maintain a distinction between them.

Third, this analysis can, in principle, be extended to the whole range of so-called topological prepositions and particles, expressing spatial changes in terms of some topological relation (like topological inclusion in the case of *into* and *out of*, cf. Talmy 1975).

And last but not least, I mention another possible extension of this approach. Let us consider the following examples:

(21) *A tapéta* *el*$_{PRT}$*.vált* *a fal.tól.*
The wallpaper PRT.got-separated the wall.from
'The wallpaper got separated from the wall.'

(22) *A [cipő talpa]* *el*$_{PRT}$*.vált.*
The [sole] PRT.got-separated
'The sole got separated (from the shoe).'

In these examples, it is not necessary for the wallpaper and the sole to become totally separated from the wall and the shoe, respectively. If we now disregard the traditional analysis of these sentences according to which perfectivity does not come from the spatial change but from the fact that the wallpaper and the sole became unusable, then we can find a spatial explanation, as well.

Cohn & Varzi (2003) differentiate several degrees of strength of connection (the common boundary is a single point or an extended boundary portion or a maximal boundary etc.). If we integrate these refinements into the RCC8 system, then it will be able to explain the perfectivity of examples (21) and (22). In other words, although we

---

7 For example, the following sentence describes an instance of the RCC-transition type [DC→EC→PO→TPP→NTPP]: *Egy madár be*$_{PRT}$*.repült a szobá.ba* A bird PRT.flew the room.into ('A bird flew in the room'). The punctual subevent perfectivizing the whole event is that determined by the TPP relation, but the absolutely final subevent may be that one characterized by NTPP.

remain inside EC mode during the whole events described in these examples (i.e. we do not reach neither PO nor DC), by dividing EC mode up into finer sub-modes we can explain why a kind of external connection (cf. maximal boundary) can be regarded as a landmark-mode with respect to another kind of external connection (extended boundary portion).

7. References

Cohn, A.G. & Varzi, A.C. (2003): Mereotopological connection. *Journal of Philosophical Logic* 32(4), 357-90.

É. Kiss, K. (2005): First steps towards a theory of the verbal particle. In: Piñon, Ch. & Siptár, P. (eds.): *Papers from the Düsseldorf Conference. Approaches to Hungarian 9.* Budapest: Akadémiai Kiadó, 59-88.

Euzenat, J. (1995): An algebraic approach to granularity in qualitative time and space representation. In: *Proceedings of the Fourteenth International Joint Conference on Artificial Intelligence.* Montreal (CA), 894-900.

Galton, A. (2000): *Qualitative spatial change.* Oxford & New York: Oxford University Press.

Jackendoff, R. (1996): The proper treatment of measuring out, telicity, and perhaps even quantification in English. *Natural Language and Linguistic Theory* 14, 305-54.

Kiefer Ferenc (2000): *Jelentéselmélet* [Semantic Theory]. Budapest: Corvina.

Krifka, M. (1998): The origins of telicity. In: Rothstein, S. (ed.): *Events and grammar.* Dordrecht: Kluwer, 197-235.

Krifka, M. (2001): The mereological approach to aspectual composition. *Conference Perspectives on Aspect.* University of Utrecht: OTS, December 12-14, 2001. Handout.

Levin, B. & Rappaport Hovav, M. (2005): *Argument realization.* Cambridge University Press.

Randell, D.A., Cui, Z. & Cohn, A.G. (1992): A spatial logic based on regions and connection. In: Nebel, B., Swarthout, W. & Rich, C. (eds.): *Proceedings of the third International Conference on Knowledge Representation and Reasoning.* San Mateo, Morgan Kaufmann, 165-176.

Talmy, L. (1975): Semantics and syntax of motion. In: Kimball, J.P. (ed.): *Syntax and semantics*, vol. 4. New York Academic Press, 181-238.

Tschander, L.B. (2003): Concepts of motion and their linguistic encoding. In: Härtl, H. & Tappe, H. (eds.): *Mediating between concepts and grammar.* Berlin: Mouton de Gruyter, 405-33.

Tenny, C. (1994): *Aspectual roles and the syntax-semantics interface.* (Studies in Linguistics and Philosophy, Vol. 52). Dordrecht & Boston & London: Kluwer Academic Publishers.

Zwarts, J. (2005): *Prepositional aspect and the algebra of paths.* Workshop on Event Structures in Linguistic Form and Interpretation, Leipzig.

METALINGUISTICA

Editor/Herausgeber: András Kertész

Bd./Vol. 1 András Kertész (Hrsg.): Sprache als Kognition - Sprache als Interaktion. Studien zum Grammatik-Pragmatik-Verhältnis. 1995.

Bd./Vol. 2 Tibor Laczkó: The Syntax of Hungarian Noun Phrases. A Lexical-Functional Approach. 1995.

Bd./Vol. 3 Péter Pelyvás: Subjectivity in English. Generative Grammar Versus the Cognitive Theory of Epistemic Grounding. 1996.

Bd./Vol. 4 András Kertész (Hrsg.): Metalinguistik im Wandel. Die 'kognitive Wende' in Wissenschaftstheorie und Linguistik. 1997.

Bd./Vol. 5 Gábor Alberti: Argument Selection. 1997.

Bd./Vol. 6 Zsuzsanna Iványi: Wortsuchprozesse. Eine gesprächsanalytische Untersuchung und ihre wissenschaftsmethodologischen Konsequenzen. 1998.

Bd./Vol. 7 Piroska Kocsány / Anna Molnár (Hrsg.): Wort und (Kon)text. 2001.

Bd./Vol. 8 Éva Sáfár: Persuasive Texte. Eine vergleichende Untersuchung sprachlicher Argumentationsstrategien. 2001.

Bd./Vol. 9 András Kertész (ed.): Approaches to the Pragmatics of Scientific Discourse. 2001.

Bd./Vol. 10 Zsuzsanna Iványi / András Kertész (Hrsg.): Gesprächsforschung. Tendenzen und Perspektiven. 2001.

Bd./Vol. 11 Peter Plöger: Wissenschaft durch Wechselwirkung. Bausteine zu einem diskursiven Modell der Wissenschaften. 2002.

Bd./Vol. 12 Anna Molnár: Die Grammatikalisierung deutscher Modalpartikeln. Fallstudien. 2002.

Bd./Vol. 13 László Hunyadi. Hungarian Sentence Prosody and Universal Grammar. On the Phonology – Syntax Interface. 2002.

Bd./vol. 14 Marcello La Matina: Texts, Pictures and Scores. Some Aspects of a Philosophy of Languages. 2002.

Bd./Vol. 15 Krisztina Károly: Lexical Repetition in Text. A Study of the Text-Organizing Function of Lexical Repetition in Foreign Language Argumentative Discourse. 2002.

Bd./Vol. 16 László Tarnay / Tamás Pólya: Specificity Recognition and Social Cognition. 2004.

Bd./Vol. 17 Gábor Tolcsvai Nagy: A Cognitive Theory of Style. 2005.

Bd./Vol. 18 Lajos Marosán: The Meaning of Word Classes. 2006.

Bd./Vol. 19 Marina Rakova / Gergely Pethő / Csilla Rákosi (eds.): The Cognitive Basis of Polysemy. New Sources of Evidence for Theories of Word Meaning. 2007.

www.peterlang.de

Peter Lang · Internationaler Verlag der Wissenschaften

Lajos Marosán

The Meaning of Word Classes

Frankfurt am Main, Berlin, Bern, Bruxelles, New York, Oxford, Wien, 2006.
X, 207 pp.
MetaLinguistica. Edited by András Kertész. Vol. 18
ISBN 978-3-631-54836-3 · pb. € 39.–*

Linguists who believe that word classes bear meaning are numerous; the author of this book, however, argues that this belief is untenable. This book proposes a new account of the claim that parts of speech have meaning – a view which has been present in grammars and some philosophical treatises ever since language was studied. The author presents questions of grammatical analysis, critically discussing the relevant views held by typologists and generativists, traditional grammarians and prototype theoreticians.

Contents: Current trends and word classes · Derivation and word classes · Prototypicality and word classes · The ontological hypothesis and word classes · Meaning and word classes

Frankfurt am Main · Berlin · Bern · Bruxelles · New York · Oxford · Wien
Distribution: Verlag Peter Lang AG
Moosstr. 1, CH-2542 Pieterlen
Telefax 00 41 (0) 32 / 376 17 27

*The €-price includes German tax rate
Prices are subject to change without notice

Homepage http://www.peterlang.de

www.ingramcontent.com/pod-product-compliance
Ingram Content Group UK Ltd.
Pitfield, Milton Keynes, MK11 3LW, UK
UKHW021238300926
15471UKWH00013B/212

9 783631 540947